Good
Clinical Practice

Pharmaceutical, Biologics, and
Medical Device
Regulations and Guidance Documents

Concise Reference

Volume 1: Regulations

D1560229

Good Clinical Practice

Pharmaceutical, Biologics, and Medical Device Regulations and Guidance Documents

Concise Reference

Volume 1: Regulations

International Conference on Harmonisation (ICH) Quality Guidelines:
Pharmaceutical, Biologics, and Medical Device Regulations and Guidance
Documents Concise Reference; Volume 1, Regulations

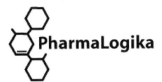

PharmaLogika, Inc.
PO Box 461
Willow Springs, NC 27592

www.pharmalogika.com

Other documents that complement these regulations and guidelines are available
from the relative branches of government and the documents contained herein
may be updated from time to time. It is the responsibility of the user to ensure
that the information is still valid and accurate.

Author / Editor: Mindy J. Allport-Settle

Published by PharmaLogika, Inc.

Printed in the United States of America. First Printing.

ISBN 0-9821476-7-8
ISBN-13 978-0-9821476-7-2

Contents

Part I

Federal Regulations Relating to Good Clinical Practice and Clinical Trials

Preface

About this Book

This book (***Volume 1 of a two volume set***) is designed to be a unified reference source for the U.S. Food and Drug Adminstration's Good Clinical Practice regulations for pharmaceutical, biologics and medical device products. Volume 2 of this set is a concise reference source for the associated guidance documents.

The included *Overview and Orientation* (Chapter 2 of this book) is designed to provide a foundation for understanding the background of the FDA, its guidelines, its relationship with other countries and its relationship with manufacturers and distributors.

This book is designed to be used both as a reference for experienced industry representatives and as a training resource for those new to the industry.

Included Documents and Features

Good Clinical Practice Regulations:

- *FDA Overview and Orientation*
- *Introduction to GCP*
- *Part I: Federal Regulations Relating to Good Clinical Practice and Clinical Trials*
  - *Parts 50 and 56*
  - *Part 54*
  - *Part 210*
  - *Part 320*
  - *Part 812*
  - *Part 814*

Reference Tools

- *Part II: Combined Glossary and Index for all Regulations*

About the Reference Tools

FDA Overview and Orientation and the Introduction to GCP

The FDA overview provides the reader with a brief history of the Food and Drug Administration (FDA) and explains not only what good clinical practice is, but why it exists and how it came to be. The introduction to GCP provides a guide to the FDA's approach to clinical trial management.

Combined Glossary

The Combined Glossary includes all of the glossaries from each regulation and guidance listed alphabetically rather than by document.

When a word or term appears multiple times in the regulation and guidance documents, the word will appear multiple times in the Combined Glossary if there is a variation in the definition. Each duplicate entry is indented to highlight that it is a duplicate and the earliest reference to the entry is listed first. The source for each entry is bracketed (i.e., [21 CFR § 50]) for ease of reference. While the definitions are similar from one regulatory or guidance document to the next, they are not always identical.

Combined Index for all Regulations

The index is composed of a list of both words and terms specific to the Good Clinical Practice regulations.

Pharmaceutical, biotechnology, and medical device companies use terminology that combines scientific and technical jargon with legal phrases and concepts.

The index provides keywords and terminology as a tool to easily locate specific references across all documents rather than having to rely on memory or paging through each document individually.

FDA Overview and Orientation

The Food and Drug Administration (FDA)

The United States Food and Drug Administration (FDA) is responsible for protecting and promoting the nation's public health.

The programs for safety regulation vary widely by the type of product, its potential risks, and the regulatory powers granted to the agency. For example, the FDA regulates almost every facet of prescription drugs, including testing, manufacturing, labeling, advertising, marketing, efficacy and safety. FDA regulation of cosmetics, however, is focused primarily on labeling and safety. The FDA regulates most products with a set of published standards enforced by a combination of facility inspections, voluntary company reporting standards, and public and consumer watchdog activity.

The FDA frequently works in conjunction with other Federal agencies including the Department of Agriculture, Drug Enforcement Administration, Customs and Border Protection, and Consumer Product Safety Commission.

Historical Origins of Federal Food and Drug Regulation

Prior to the 20th century, there were few federal laws regulating the contents and sale of domestically produced food and pharmaceuticals before the 20th century (with one exception being the short-lived Vaccine Act of 1813). Some state laws provided varying degrees of protection against unethical sales practices, such as misrepresenting the ingredients of food products or therapeutic substances.

The history of the FDA can be traced to the latter part of the 19th century and the U.S. Department of Agriculture's Division of Chemistry (later Bureau of Chemistry). Under Harvey Washington Wiley, appointed chief chemist in 1883, the Division began conducting research into the adulteration and misbranding of food and drugs on the American market. Although they had no regulatory powers, the Division published its findings from 1887 to 1902 in a ten-part series entitled Foods and Food Adulterants. Wiley used these findings, and alliances with diverse organizations (such as state regulators, the

General Federation of Women's Clubs, and national associations of physicians and pharmacists) to lobby for a new federal law to set uniform standards for food and drugs to enter into interstate commerce.

Wiley's advocacy came at a time when the public had become alert to hazards in the marketplace by journalists and became part of a general trend for increased federal regulation in matters pertinent to public safety during the Progressive Era.[1] The 1902 Biologics Control Act was put in place after diphtheria antitoxin was collected from a horse named Jim who also had tetanus, resulting in several deaths.

The 1906 Food and Drug Act and creation of the FDA

In June 1906, President Theodore Roosevelt signed into law the Food and Drug Act, also known as the "Wiley Act" after its chief advocate.[2] The Act prohibited, under penalty of seizure of goods, the interstate transport of food which had been "adulterated," with that term referring to the addition of fillers of reduced "quality or strength," coloring to conceal "damage or inferiority," formulation with additives "injurious to health," or the use of "filthy, decomposed, or putrid" substances. The act applied similar penalties to the interstate marketing of "adulterated" drugs, in which the "standard of strength, quality, or purity" of the active ingredient was not either stated clearly on the label or listed in the United States Pharmacopoeia or the National Formulary. The act also banned "misbranding" of food and drugs.[3] The responsibility for examining food and drugs for such "adulteration" or "misbranding" was given to Wiley's USDA Bureau of Chemistry.[4] Strength, quality, identity, potency, and purity (SQuIPP) are currently the key product safety standards, with only two measures added since 1906 Act.

Wiley used these new regulatory powers to pursue an aggressive campaign against the manufacturers of foods with chemical additives, but the Chemistry Bureau's authority was soon checked by judicial decisions, as well as by the creation of the Board of Food and Drug Inspection and the Referee Board of Consulting Scientific Experts as separate organizations within the USDA in 1907 and 1908 respectively. A 1911 Supreme Court decision ruled that the 1906 act

---

[1] A History of the FDA at www.FDA.gov.
[2] A History of the FDA at www.FDA.gov.
[3] Text in quotation marks is the original text of the 1906 Food and Drugs Act and Amendments.
[4] A History of the FDA at www.FDA.gov.

---

did not apply to false claims of therapeutic efficacy,[5] in response to which a 1912 amendment added "false and fraudulent" claims of "curative or therapeutic effect" to the Act's definition of "misbranded." However, these powers continued to be narrowly defined by the courts, which set high standards for proof of fraudulent intent.[6] In 1927, the Bureau of Chemistry's regulatory powers were reorganized under a new USDA body, the Food, Drug, and Insecticide organization. This name was shortened to the Food and Drug Administration (FDA) three years later.[7]

The 1938 Food, Drug, and Cosmetic Act

By the 1930s, muckraking journalists, consumer protection organizations, and federal regulators began mounting a campaign for stronger regulatory authority by publicizing a list of injurious products which had been ruled permissible under the 1906 law, including radioactive beverages, cosmetics which caused blindness, and worthless "cures" for diabetes and tuberculosis. The resulting proposed law was unable to get through the Congress of the United States for five years, but was rapidly enacted into law following the public outcry over the 1937 Elixir Sulfanilamide tragedy, in which over 100 people died after using a drug formulated with a toxic, untested solvent. The only way that the FDA could even seize the product was due to a misbranding problem: an "Elixir" was defined as a medication dissolved in ethanol, not the diethylene glycol used in the Elixir Sulfanilamide.

President Franklin Delano Roosevelt signed the new Food, Drug, and Cosmetic Act (FD&C Act) into law on June 24, 1938. The new law significantly increased federal regulatory authority over drugs by mandating a pre-market review of the safety of all new drugs, as well as banning false therapeutic claims in drug labeling without requiring that the FDA prove fraudulent intent. The law also authorized factory inspections and expanded enforcement powers, set new regulatory standards for foods, and brought cosmetics and therapeutic devices under federal regulatory authority. This law, though extensively amended in subsequent years, remains the central foundation of FDA regulatory authority to the present day.[8]

---

[5] United States v. Johnson (31 S. Ct. 627 May 29, 1911, decided).
[6] A History of the FDA at www.FDA.gov.
[7] Milestones in U.S. Food and Drug Law History at www.FDA.gov.
[8] A History of the FDA at www.FDA.gov.

Early FD&C Act amendments: 1938-1958

Soon after passage of the 1938 Act, the FDA began to designate certain drugs as safe for use only under the supervision of a medical professional, and the category of 'prescription-only' drugs was securely codified into law by the 1951 Durham-Humphrey Amendment.[9] While pre-market testing of drug efficacy was not authorized under the 1938 FD&C Act, subsequent amendments such as the Insulin Amendment and Penicillin Amendment did mandate potency testing for formulations of specific lifesaving pharmaceuticals.[10] The FDA began enforcing its new powers against drug manufacturers who could not substantiate the efficacy claims made for their drugs, and the United States Court of Appeals for the Ninth Circuit ruling in Alberty Food Products Co. v. United States (1950) found that drug manufacturers could not evade the "false therapeutic claims" provision of the 1938 act by simply omitting the intended use of a drug from the drug's label. These developments confirmed extensive powers for the FDA to enforce post-marketing recalls of ineffective drugs.[11] Much of the FDA's regulatory attentions in this era were directed towards abuse of amphetamines and barbiturates, but the agency also reviewed some 13,000 new drug applications between 1938 and 1962. While the science of toxicology was in its infancy at the start of this era, rapid advances in experimental assays for food additive and drug safety testing were made during this period by FDA regulators and others.[12]

Good Manufacturing Practices vs. Current Good Manufacturing Practices

The terms "Good Manufacturing Practices (GMPs)" and "Current Good Manufacturing Practices (CGMPs or cGMPs[13])" are often used interchangeably both in industry and by FDA inspectors.

"Good Manufacturing Practices" generally refers to the legal mandates detailed in Title 21 of the Code of Federal Regulations (21CFR). "Current Good Manufacturing Practices" refers not only to the legal

---

[9] A History of the FDA at www.FDA.gov.
[10] Milestones in U.S. Food and Drug Law History at www.FDA.gov
[11] A History of the FDA at www.FDA.gov.
[12] A History of the FDA at www.FDA.gov.
[13] The lower case "c" was coined in industry to differentiate between the law, emphasized with capital letters, and the current accepted industry practice not mandated by law.

---

requirements, but to the guidance provided by the FDA and the standards practiced in industry that are not memorialized as law.

Organizational Structure

The FDA is an agency within the United States Department of Health and Human Services responsible for protecting and promoting the nation's public health. It is organized into the following major subdivisions, each focused on a major area of regulatory responsibility:

- The Office of the Commissioner (OC)
- The Center for Drug Evaluation and Research (CDER)
- The Center for Biologics Evaluation and Research (CBER)
- The Center for Food Safety and Applied Nutrition (CFSAN)
- The Center for Devices and Radiological Health (CDRH)
- The Center for Veterinary Medicine (CVM)
- The National Center for Toxicological Research (NCTR)
- The Office of Regulatory Affairs (ORA)
- The Office of Criminal Investigations (OCI)

How does the FDA communicate with Industry?

Code of Federal Regulations[14]

The Code of Federal Regulations (CFR) is the codification of the general and permanent rules and regulations (sometimes called administrative law) published in the Federal Register by the executive departments and agencies of the Federal Government of the United States. The CFR is published by the Office of the Federal Register, an agency of the National Archives and Records Administration (NARA).

The CFR is divided into 50 titles that represent broad areas subject to Federal regulation. Title 21 is the portion of the Code of Federal Regulations that governs food and drugs within the United States for the Food and Drug Administration (FDA), the Drug Enforcement Administration (DEA), and the Office of National Drug Control Policy (ONDCP).

---

[14] Available CFR Titles on GPO Access at
http://www.access.gpo.gov/nara/cfr/cfr-table-search.html#page1

It is divided into three chapters:

- Chapter I — Food and Drug Administration
- Chapter II — Drug Enforcement Administration
- Chapter III — Office of National Drug Control Policy

Guidance Documents

Guidance documents represent the Agency's current thinking on a particular subject. They do not create or confer any rights for or on any person and do not operate to bind FDA or the public. An alternative approach may be used if such approach satisfies the requirements of the applicable statute, regulations, or both. For information on a specific guidance document, please contact the originating office. Another method of obtaining guidance documents is through the Division of Drug Information.

Federal Register

The Federal Register (since March 14, 1936), abbreviated FR, or sometimes Fed. Reg.) is the official journal of the federal government of the United States that contains most routine publications and public notices of government agencies. It is a daily (except holidays) publication.

The Federal Register is compiled by the Office of the Federal Register (within the National Archives and Records Administration) and is printed by the Government Printing Office.

There are no copyright restrictions on the Federal Register as it is a work of the U.S. government. It is in the public domain.[15]

Citations from the Federal Register are [volume] FR [page number] ([date]), e.g., 65 FR 741 (2000-10-01).

Direct Communication and Letters

The FDA interacts with consumers, health professionals, and industry representatives through letters, meetings (requested by either the FDA or the industry representatives), and telephone calls.

While not all questions can be answered over the phone, the FDA prefers telephone interactions over physical meetings (when a teleconference can reasonably replace a face-to-face meeting).

---

[15] The Federal Register at the GPO, online in both text and PDF, from 1994 on.

www.FDA.gov

The FDA maintains a website at www.fda.gov that is focused on three key audiences:

- consumers

- health professionals

- industry representatives

Through collaboration with users in testing site-wide designs, FDA.gov provides online access to its guidance documents, communication with industry, consumers, and health professionals. Information is categorized by topic, with related subjects consolidated in sections on the site.

Additionally, FDA.gov provides a search engine for Title 21 of the CFR that makes finding keyword references throughout the title more accessible.

Conferences

The FDA routinely sends speakers to industry conferences where they are available to answer questions on their particular area of expertise.

False Statement to a Federal Agency

The U.S. Code of Federal Regulations (CFR) makes it a federal crime for anyone willfully and knowingly to make a false or fraudulent statement to a department or agency of the United States. The false statement must be related to a material matter, and the defendant must have acted willfully and with knowledge of the falsity. It is not necessary to show that the government agency was in fact deceived or misled. The issue of materiality is one of law for the courts. The maximum penalty is five years' imprisonment and a $10,000 fine.

A person may be guilty of a violation without proof that he or she had knowledge that the matter was within the jurisdiction of a federal agency. A businessperson may violate this law by making a false statement to another firm or person with knowledge that the information will be submitted to a government agency. Businesses must take care to avoid exaggerations in the context of any matter that may come within the jurisdiction of a federal agency.

CFR Title 21 - Food and Drugs: Parts 1 to 1499[16]

General

(1) General enforcement regulations

(2) General administrative rulings and decisions

(3) Product jurisdiction

(5) Organization

(7) Enforcement policy

(10) Administrative practices and procedures

(11) Electronic records; electronic signatures

(12) Formal evidentiary public hearing

(13) Public hearing before a public board of inquiry

(14) Public hearing before a public advisory committee

(15) Public hearing before the commissioner

(16) Regulatory hearing before the food and drug administration

(17) Civil money penalties hearings

(19) Standards of conduct and conflicts of interest

(20) Public information

(21) Protection of privacy

(25) Environmental impact considerations

(26) Mutual recognition of pharmaceutical good manufacturing practice

(50) Protection of human subjects

(54) Financial disclosure by clinical investigators

(56) Institutional review boards

(58) Good laboratory practice for nonclinical laboratory studies

(60) Patent term restoration

---

[16] All of the 21CFR regulations can be searched online for no charge at http://www.accessdata.fda.gov/scripts/cdrh/cfdocs/cfcfr/cfrsearch.cfm

---

(70) Color additives

(71) Color additive petitions

(73) Listing of color additives exempt from certification

(74) Listing of color additives subject to certification

(80) Color additive certification

(81) General specifications and general restrictions for provisional color additives for use in foods, drugs, and cosmetics

(82) Listing of certified provisionally listed colors and specifications

(83-98) [reserved]

(99) Dissemination of information on unapproved/new uses for marketed drugs, biologics, and devices

Foods

(100) General

(101) Food labeling

(102) Common or usual name for nonstandardized foods

(104) Nutritional quality guidelines for foods

(105) Foods for special dietary use

(106) Infant formula quality control procedures

(107) Infant formula

(108) Emergency permit control

(109) Unavoidable contaminants in food for human consumption and food-packaging material

(110) Current good manufacturing practice in manufacturing, packing, or holding human food

(111) Current good manufacturing practice in manufacturing, packaging, labeling, or holding operations for dietary supplements

(113) Thermally processed low-acid foods packaged in hermetically sealed containers

(114) Acidified foods

(115) Shell eggs

(119) Dietary supplements that present a significant or unreasonable risk

(120) Hazard analysis and critical control point (HACCP) systems

(123) Fish and fishery products

(129) Processing and bottling of bottled drinking water

(130) Food standards: general

(131) Milk and cream

(133) Cheeses and related cheese products

(135) Frozen desserts

(136) Bakery products

(137) Cereal flours and related products

(139) Macaroni and noodle products

(145) Canned fruits

(146) Canned fruit juices

(150) Fruit butters, jellies, preserves, and related products

(152) Fruit pies

(155) Canned vegetables

(156) Vegetable juices

(158) Frozen vegetables

(160) Eggs and egg products

(161) Fish and shellfish

(163) Cacao products

(164) Tree nut and peanut products

(165) Beverages

(166) Margarine

(168) Sweeteners and table syrups

(169) Food dressings and flavorings

(170) Food additives

(171) Food additive petitions

(172) Food additives permitted for direct addition to food for human consumption

(173) Secondary direct food additives permitted in food for human consumption

(174) Indirect food additives: general

(175) Indirect food additives: adhesives and components of coatings

(176) Indirect food additives: paper and paperboard components

(177) Indirect food additives: polymers

(178) Indirect food additives: adjuvants, production aids, and sanitizers

(179) Irradiation in the production, processing and handling of food

(180) Food additives permitted in food or in contact with food on an interim basis pending additional study

(181) Prior-sanctioned food ingredients

(182) Substances generally recognized as safe

(184) Direct food substances affirmed as generally recognized as safe

(186) Indirect food substances affirmed as generally recognized as safe

(189) Substances prohibited from use in human food

(190) Dietary supplements

(191-199) [reserved]

Drugs

(200) General

(201) Labeling

(202) Prescription drug advertising

(203) Prescription drug marketing

(205) Guidelines for state licensing of wholesale prescription drug distributors

(206) Imprinting of solid oral dosage form drug products for human use

(207) Registration of producers of drugs and listing of drugs in commercial distribution

(208) Medication guides for prescription drug products

(209) Requirement for authorized dispensers and pharmacies to distribute a side effects statement

(210) Current good manufacturing practice in manufacturing, processing, packing, or holding of drugs; general

(211) Current good manufacturing practice for finished pharmaceuticals

(216) Pharmacy compounding

(225) Current good manufacturing practice for medicated feeds

(226) Current good manufacturing practice for type A medicated articles

(250) Special requirements for specific human drugs

(290) Controlled drugs

(299) Drugs; official names and established names

New Drugs and Over-the-Counter Drug Products

(300) General

(310) New drugs

(312) Investigational new drug application

(314) Applications for FDA approval to market a new drug

(315) Diagnostic radiopharmaceuticals

(316) Orphan drugs

(320) Bioavailability and bioequivalence requirements

(328) Over-the-counter drug products intended for oral ingestion that contain alcohol

(330) Over-the-counter (OTC) human drugs which are generally recognized as safe and effective and not misbranded

(331) Antacid products for over-the-counter (OTC) human use

(332) Antiflatulent products for over-the-counter human use

(333) Topical antimicrobial drug products for over-the-counter recognized as safe and effective and not misbranded

(335) Antidiarrheal drug products for over-the-counter human use

(336) Antiemetic drug products for over-the-counter human use

(338) Nighttime sleep-aid drug products for over-the-counter human use

(340) Stimulant drug products for over-the-counter human use

(341) Cold, cough, allergy, bronchodilator, and antiasthmatic drug products for over-the-counter human use

(343) Internal analgesic, antipyretic, and antirheumatic drug products for over-the-counter human use

(344) Topical OTIC drug products for over-the-counter human use

(346) Anorectal drug products for over-the-counter human use

(347) Skin protectant drug products for over-the-counter human use

(348) External analgesic drug products for over-the-counter human use

(349) Ophthalmic drug products for over-the-counter human use

(350) Antiperspirant drug products for over-the-counter human use

(352) Sunscreen drug products for over-the-counter human use [stayed indefinitely]

(355) Anticaries drug products for over-the-counter human use

(357) Miscellaneous internal drug products for over-the-counter human use

(358) Miscellaneous external drug products for over-the-counter human use

(361) Prescription drugs for human use generally recognized as safe and effective and not misbranded: drugs used in research

(369) Interpretative statements re warnings on drugs and devices for over-the-counter sale

(370-499) [reserved]

Veterinary Products

(500) General

(501) Animal food labeling

(502) Common or usual names for nonstandardized animal foods

(509) Unavoidable contaminants in animal food and food-packaging material

(510) New animal drugs

(511) New animal drugs for investigational use

(514) New animal drug applications

(515) Medicated feed mill license

(516) New animal drugs for minor use and minor species

(520) Oral dosage form new animal drugs

(522) Implantation or injectable dosage form new animal drugs

(524) Ophthalmic and topical dosage form new animal drugs

(526) Intramammary dosage forms

(529) Certain other dosage form new animal drugs

(530) Extralabel drug use in animals

(556) Tolerances for residues of new animal drugs in food

(558) New animal drugs for use in animal feeds

(564) [reserved]

(570) Food additives

(571) Food additive petitions

(573) Food additives permitted in feed and drinking water of animals

(579) Irradiation in the production, processing, and handling of animal feed and pet food

(582) Substances generally recognized as safe

(584) Food substances affirmed as generally recognized as safe in feed and drinking water of animals

(589) Substances prohibited from use in animal food or feed

(590-599) [reserved]

Biologics

(600) Biological products: general

(601) Licensing

(606) Current good manufacturing practice for blood and blood components

(607) Establishment registration and product listing for manufacturers of human blood and blood products

(610) General biological products standards

(630) General requirements for blood, blood components, and blood components, and blood derivatives

(640) Additional standards for human blood and blood products

(660) Additional standards for diagnostic substances for laboratory tests

(680) Additional standards for miscellaneous products

Cosmetics

(700) General

(701) Cosmetic labeling

(710) Voluntary registration of cosmetic product establishments

(720) Voluntary filing of cosmetic product ingredient composition statements

(740) Cosmetic product warning statements

(741-799) [reserved]

Medical Devices

(800) General

(801) Labeling

(803) Medical device reporting

(806) Medical devices; reports of corrections and removals

(807) Establishment registration and device listing for manufacturers and initial importers of devices

(808) Exemptions from federal preemption of state and local medical device requirements

(809) In vitro diagnostic products for human use

(810) Medical device recall authority

(812) Investigational device exemptions

(813) [reserved]

(814) Premarket approval of medical devices

(820) Quality system regulation

(821) Medical device tracking requirements

(822) Postmarket surveillance

(860) Medical device classification procedures

(861) Procedures for performance standards development

(862) Clinical chemistry and clinical toxicology devices

(864) Hematology and pathology devices

(866) Immunology and microbiology devices

(868) Anesthesiology devices

(870) Cardiovascular devices

(872) Dental devices

(874) Ear, nose, and throat devices

(876) Gastroenterology-urology devices

(878) General and plastic surgery devices

(880) General hospital and personal use devices

(882) Neurological devices

(884) Obstetrical and gynecological devices

(886) Ophthalmic devices

(888) Orthopedic devices

(890) Physical medicine devices

(892) Radiology devices

(895) Banned devices

(898) Performance standard for electrode lead wires and patient cables

Mammography

(900) Mammography

Radiological Health

(1000) General

(1002) Records and reports

(1003) Notification of defects or failure to comply

(1004) Repurchase, repairs, or replacement of electronic products

(1005) Importation of electronic products

(1010) Performance standards for electronic products: general

(1020) Performance standards for ionizing radiation emitting products

(1030) Performance standards for microwave and radio frequency emitting products

(1040) Performance standards for light-emitting products

(1050) Performance standards for sonic, infrasonic, and ultrasonic radiation-emitting products

Regulations under Certain Other Acts

(1210) Regulations under the federal import milk act

(1230) Regulations under the federal caustic poison act

(1240) Control of communicable diseases

(1250) Interstate conveyance sanitation

(1251-1269) [reserved]

(1270) Human tissue intended for transplantation

(1271) Human cells, tissues, and cellular and tissue-based products

(1272-1299) [reserved]

Controlled Substances

(1300) Definitions

(1301) Registration of manufacturers, distributors, and dispensers of controlled substances

(1302) Labeling and packaging requirements for controlled substances

(1303) Quotas

(1304) Records and reports of registrants

(1305) Orders for schedule I and II controlled substances

(1306) Prescriptions

(1307) Miscellaneous

(1308) Schedules of controlled substances

(1309) Registration of manufacturers, distributors, importers and exporters of List I chemicals

(1310) Records and reports of listed chemicals and certain machines

(1311) Digital certificates

(1312) Importation and exportation of controlled substances

(1313) Importation and exportation of list I and list II chemicals

(1314) Retail sale of scheduled listed chemical products

(1315) Importation and production quotas for ephedrine, pseudoephedrine, and phenylpropanolamine

(1316) Administrative functions, practices, and procedures

Office of National Drug Control Policy

(1400) [reserved]

(1401) Public availability of information

(1402) Mandatory declassification review

(1403) Uniform administrative requirements for grants and cooperative agreements to state and local governments

(1404) Governmentwide debarment and suspension (nonprocurement)

(1405) Governmentwide requirements for drug-free workplace (financial assistance)

(1406-1499) [reserved]

Introduction to GCP

Good Clinical Practice

FDA regulates scientific studies that are designed to develop evidence to support the safety and effectiveness of investigational drugs (human and animal), biological products, and medical devices. [17] Physicians and other qualified experts ("clinical investigators") who conduct these studies are required to comply with applicable statutes and regulations. These laws and regulations are intended to ensure the integrity of clinical data on which product approvals are based and to help protect the rights, safety, and welfare of human subjects.

The following resources are provided to help investigators, sponsors, and contract research organizations who conduct clinical studies on investigational new drugs comply with U.S. law and regulations covering good clinical practice (GCP).

General Information

- General Information for Clinical Investigators

- From test-tube to patient: New drug development in the United States

- Information and Activities Targeted Toward Specific Audiences and Populations

Institutional Review Boards (IRBs)

- Institutional Review Boards (IRBs) and Protection of Human Subjects in Clinical Trials

- Guidance for Institutional Review Boards and Clinical Investigators

- FDA Compliance Program 7348.809 - BIMO for Institutional Review Boards

---

[17] Available on the FDA website at
http://www.fda.gov/AboutFDA/CentersOffices/CDER/ucm090259.htm

---

FDA Regulations

- Institutional Review Boards (21 CFR Part 56)
- Human Subject Protection (Informed Consent) (21 CFR Part 50)
- Additional Safeguards for Children involved in Clinical Investigations of FDA-Regulated Products (Interim Rule) (21 CFR Part 50, subpart D)
- Investigational New Drug Application (IND Regulations) (21 CFR Part 312)

Sponsors, Monitors, and Contract Research Organizations

- Guidances and Enforcement Information
- Investigational New Drug Application (IND Regulations) (21 CFR Part 312)
- Regulations for Applications for FDA Approval to Market a New Drug (NDA Regulations) (21 CFR Part 314)

Office of Good Clinical Practice

The Office of Good Clinical Practice[18] is the focal point within FDA for Good Clinical Practice (GCP) and Human Subject Protection (HSP) issues arising in human research trials regulated by FDA. The Office of Good Clinical Practice:

- Advises and assists the Commissioner and other key officials on GCP and HSP issues arising in clinical trials that have an impact on policy, direction, and long-range goals.

- Leads, supports, and administers FDA's Human Subject Protection/Bioresearch Monitoring Council that manages and sets agency policy on bioresearch monitoring (BIMO), GCP, and HSP affecting both clinical and non-clinical trials regulated by FDA. The office also coordinates and provides oversight of working groups established by this Council.

- Coordinates FDA's Bioresearch Monitoring program with respect to clinical trials, working together with all FDA Centers as well as FDA's Office of Regulatory Affairs (ORA)

---

[18] Available on the FDA website at
http://www.fda.gov/AboutFDA/CentersOffices/OC/OfficeofScienceandHealth Coordination/GoodClinicalPracticesProgram/default.htm

- Plans and conducts training and outreach programs, both internally and externally.

- Serves as a liaison with other Federal agencies (e.g., the HHS Office for Human Research Protection (OHRP) and the Veterans Administration), outside organizations, regulated industry, and public interest groups on BIMO, GCP, and HSP policies and regulatory matters.

- Contributes to international Good Clinical Practice harmonization activities.

Running Clinical Trials

Adherence to the principles of good clinical practices (GCPs), including adequate human subject protection (HSP) is universally recognized as a critical requirement to the conduct of research involving human subjects. [19] Many countries have adopted GCP principles as laws and/or regulations. The Food and Drug Administration's (FDA's) regulations for the conduct of clinical trials, which have been in effect since the 1970s, address both GCP and HSP. These FDA regulations and guidance documents are accessible from this site. International GCP guidance documents on which FDA has collaborated and that have been adopted as official FDA guidance are also be found here. Finally, this site includes links to other sites relevant to the conduct of clinical trials, both nationally and internationally.

Bioresearch Monitoring

FDA's bioresearch monitoring (BIMO) program conducts on-site inspections of both clinical and nonclinical studies performed to support research and marketing applications/submissions to the agency. Links to the compliance programs for each inspection type and contact information for each Center's BIMO program are also accessible from this site.

Bioresearch Monitoring Program (BIMO)

FDA uses Compliance Program Guidance Manuals (CPGM) to direct its field personnel on the conduct of inspectional and investigational

---

[19] Available on the FDA website at
http://www.fda.gov/ScienceResearch/SpecialTopics/RunningClinicalTrials/default.htm

activities. [20] The CPGM's described below form the basis of FDA's Bioresearch Monitoring Program. The purpose of each program is to ensure the protection of research subjects and the integrity of data submitted to the agency in support of a marketing application.

- CPGM for Clinical Investigators
- CPGM for Sponsors, Monitors, and Contract Research Organizations
- CPGM for Good Laboratory Practice (Non-Clinical Laboratories)
- CPGM for In-Vivo Bioequivalence Compliance Program 7348.001
- CPGM for Institutional Review Boards

Regulations

FDA Regulations Relating to Good Clinical Practice and Clinical Trials

FDA regulations governing the conduct of clinical trials describe good clinical practices (GCPs) for studies with both human and non-human animal subjects. [21]

- Electronic Records; Electronic Signatures (21 CFR Part 11)
- Protection of Human Subjects (Informed Consent) (21 CFR Part 50)
- Financial Disclosure by Clinical Investigators (21 CFR Part 54)
- Institutional Review Boards (21 CFR Part 56)
- FDA IRB Registration Rule (21 CFR 56.106)
- FDA IRB Registration Rule (21 CFR 56.106)
- Good Laboratory Practice for Nonclinical Laboratory Studies (21 CFR Part 58)
- Investigational New Drug Application (21 CFR Part 312)
- Foreign Clinical Trials not conducted under an IND (21 CFR 312.120)

---

[20] Available on the FDA website at http://www.fda.gov/ScienceResearch/ SpecialTopics/RunningClinicalTrials/ucm160670.htm
[21] Available on the FDA website at http://www.fda.gov/ScienceResearch/ SpecialTopics/RunningClinicalTrials/ucm155713.htm#FDARegulations

- Expanded Access to Investigational Drugs for Treatment Use

- Charging for Investigational Drugs

- Form 1571 (Investigational New Drug Application)

- Form 1572 (Statement of Investigator)

- Applications for FDA Approval to Market a New Drug (21 CFR Part 314)

- Bioavailability and Bioequivalence Requirements (21 CFR Part 320)

- New Animal Drugs for Investigational Use (21 CFR Part 511)

- New Animal Drug Applications (21 CFR Part 514)

- Applications for FDA Approval of a Biologic License (21 CFR Part 601)

- Investigational Device Exemptions (21 CFR Part 812)

- Premarket Approval of Medical Devices (21 CFR Part 814)

Preambles to GCP Regulations

Each time Congress enacts a law affecting products regulated by the Food and Drug Administration, the FDA develops rules to implement the law. The FDA takes various steps to develop these rules, including publishing a variety of documents in the Federal Register announcing the FDA's interest in formulating, amending or repealing a rule, and offering the public the opportunity to comment on the agency's proposal. The Federal Register notice explains the legal issues and basis for the proposal, and provides information about how interested persons can submit written data, views, or arguments on the proposal. Any comments that are submitted are addressed in subsequent publications that are part of the agency's decision-making process.

The "preamble" to each of these publications includes all of the printed information immediately preceding the codified regulation. The preamble provides information about the regulation such as why the regulation is being proposed, the FDA's interpretation of the meaning and impact of the proposed regulation, and in those cases where the agency has solicited public comment, the agency's review and commentary on those comments. The preamble can also include an environmental impact assessment, an analysis of the cost impact, comments related to the Paperwork Reduction Act, and the effective date of the implementation or revocation (as the case may be) of the regulation.

The documents listed below include the various publications that contributed to the development of final rules related to FDA's regulations on good clinical practice and clinical trials.[22]

Parts 50 and 56

- Protection of Human Subjects; Informed Consent (January 27, 1981)

- Protection of Human Research Subjects; Standards for Institutional Review Boards for Clinical Investigations (January 27, 1981)

- Protection of Human Research Subjects; Clinical Investigations Which May Be Reviewed Through Expedited Review Procedure Set Forth in FDA Regulations (January 27, 1981)

- Protection of Human Subjects; Informed Consent; Standards for Institutional Review Boards for Clinical Investigations (November 1988)

- Federal Policy for the Protection of Human Subjects (June 18, 1991)

- FDA Policy for the Protection of Human Subjects (June 18, 1991)

- Protection of Human Subjects; Informed Consent; Proposed Rule (September 21, 1995)

- Protection of Human Subjects; Informed Consent, Part II (October 2, 1996)

- Protection of Human Subjects; Informed Consent and Waiver of Informed Consent Requirements in Certain Emergency Research; Final Rules (October 2, 1996)

- Protection of Human Subjects; Informed Consent (December 22, 1995)

- Protection of Human Subjects; Informed Consent Verification; Final Rule (November 5, 1996)

- Categories of Research That May Be Reviewed by the Institutional Review Board (IRB) Through an Expedited Review Procedure (November 9, 1998)

---

[22] Available on the FDA website at http://www.fda.gov/ScienceResearch/SpecialTopics/RunningClinicalTrials/ucm155713.htm#FDARegulations

- Protection of Human Subjects; Informed Consent, Exception from general requirements (October 5, 1999)

- Additional protections for children (66 FR 20589-600, April 24, 2001)

- Exception from General Requirements for Informed Consent (71 FR 32827, June 7, 2006) [PDF]

Part 54

- Financial Disclosures by Clinical Investigators (63 FR 5233, February 2, 1998)

- Financial Disclosures by a Clinical Investigator(63 FR 72171-81, December 31, 1998)

Part 210

- Current Good Manufacturing Practice Regulations and Investigational New Drugs (January 17, 2006)

Parts 312 and 314

- Proposed New Drug, Antibiotic, and Biologic Drug Product Regulations (June 9, 1983)

- New Drug and Antibiotic Regulations (February 22, 1985) New Drug, Antibiotic, and Biologic Drug Product Regulations (March 19, 1987)

- Investigational New Drug Applications and New Drug Applications (September 8, 1995)

- Investigational New Drug Applications and New Drug Applications (February 11, 1998)

- Disqualification of a Clinical Investigator (February 16, 1996)

- Disqualification of a Clinical Investigator (September 5, 1997)

- Expedited Safety Reporting Requirements for Human Drug and Biological Products (October 7, 1997)

- Clinical Hold for products intended for life threatening conditions (65 FR 34963-71, June 1, 2000)

Part 320

- Retention of BE and BA testing samples (April 28, 1993)

Part 812

- Quality System Regulations (October 7, 1996)

- Treatment Use of Investigational Devices (September 18, 1997)

- Withdrawal of Intraocular Lenses Regulation (Part 813) (January 29, 1997)

- Disqualification of Clinical Investigators (March 14, 1997)

- Modifications to the List of Recognized Standards (July 12, 1999)

- Modifications to the Medical Device and/or Study Protocol (November 23, 1998)

Part 814

- Medical Devices; Humanitarian Use Devices Part V (June 26, 1996)

- 30-Day Notices and 135-Day PMA Supplement Review (October 8, 1998)

- Humanitarian Use of Devices (November 3, 1998)

Miscellaneous

- Part 11 Electronic Records; Electronic Signatures (March 20, 1997)

- Use of Bioresearch Monitoring Information System (BMIS) (63 FR 55873-6, October 19, 1998)

- Presiding officer (66 FR 45317-8, August 28, 2001)

Part I

Federal Regulations Relating to Good Clinical Practice and Clinical Trials

Part 11: Electronic Records; Electronic Signatures

[Code of Federal Regulations]

[Title 21, Volume 1]

[Revised as of April 1, 2008]

[CITE: 21CFR11]

Title 21--Food and Drugs
Chapter I--Food and Drug Administration
Department Of Health And Human Services

Subchapter A--General

Part 11 Electronic Records; Electronic Signatures[1]

Subpart A--General Provisions

Sec. 11.1 Scope.

(a) The regulations in this part set forth the criteria under which the agency considers electronic records, electronic signatures, and handwritten signatures executed to electronic records to be trustworthy, reliable, and generally equivalent to paper records and handwritten signatures executed on paper.

(b) This part applies to records in electronic form that are created, modified, maintained, archived, retrieved, or transmitted, under any records requirements set forth in agency regulations. This part also applies to electronic records submitted to the agency under requirements of the Federal Food, Drug, and Cosmetic Act and

---

[1] 21CFR§11 is available through the FDA website on the internet at: http://www.accessdata.fda.gov/scripts/cdrh/cfdocs/cfcfr/CFRSearch.cfm?CFRPart=11&showFR=1

the Public Health Service Act, even if such records are not specifically identified in agency regulations. However, this part does not apply to paper records that are, or have been, transmitted by electronic means.

(c) Where electronic signatures and their associated electronic records meet the requirements of this part, the agency will consider the electronic signatures to be equivalent to full handwritten signatures, initials, and other general signings as required by agency regulations, unless specifically excepted by regulation(s) effective on or after August 20, 1997.

(d) Electronic records that meet the requirements of this part may be used in lieu of paper records, in accordance with 11.2, unless paper records are specifically required.

(e) Computer systems (including hardware and software), controls, and attendant documentation maintained under this part shall be readily available for, and subject to, FDA inspection.

(f) This part does not apply to records required to be established or maintained by 1.326 through 1.368 of this chapter. Records that satisfy the requirements of part 1, subpart J of this chapter, but that also are required under other applicable statutory provisions or regulations, remain subject to this part.

[62 FR 13464, Mar. 20, 1997, as amended at 69 FR 71655, Dec. 9, 2004]

Sec. 11.2 Implementation.

(a) For records required to be maintained but not submitted to the agency, persons may use electronic records in lieu of paper records or electronic signatures in lieu of traditional signatures, in whole or in part, provided that the requirements of this part are met.

(b) For records submitted to the agency, persons may use electronic records in lieu of paper records or electronic signatures in lieu of traditional signatures, in whole or in part, provided that:

  (1) The requirements of this part are met; and

  (2) The document or parts of a document to be submitted have been identified in public docket No. 92S-0251 as being the type of submission the agency accepts in electronic form.

This docket will identify specifically what types of documents or parts of documents are acceptable for submission in electronic form without paper records and the agency receiving unit(s) (e.g., specific center, office, division, branch) to which such submissions may be made. Documents to agency receiving unit(s) not specified in the public docket will not be considered as official if they are submitted in electronic form; paper forms of such documents will be considered as official and must accompany any electronic records. Persons are expected to consult with the intended agency receiving unit for details on how (e.g., method of transmission, media, file formats, and technical protocols) and whether to proceed with the electronic submission.

Sec. 11.3 Definitions.

(a) The definitions and interpretations of terms contained in section 201 of the act apply to those terms when used in this part.

(b) The following definitions of terms also apply to this part:

(1) *Act* means the Federal Food, Drug, and Cosmetic Act (secs. 201-903 (21 U.S.C. 321-393)).

(2) **Agency** means the Food and Drug Administration.

(3) **Biometrics** means a method of verifying an individual's identity based on measurement of the individual's physical feature(s) or repeatable action(s) where those features and/or actions are both unique to that individual and measurable.

(4) **Closed system** means an environment in which system access is controlled by persons who are responsible for the content of electronic records that are on the system.

(5) **Digital signature** means an electronic signature based upon cryptographic methods of originator authentication, computed by using a set of rules and a set of parameters such that the identity of the signer and the integrity of the data can be verified.

(6) **Electronic record** means any combination of text, graphics, data, audio, pictorial, or other information representation in digital form that is created, modified, maintained, archived, retrieved, or distributed by a computer system.

(7) **Electronic signature** means a computer data compilation of any symbol or series of symbols executed, adopted, or authorized by an individual to be the legally binding equivalent of the individual's handwritten signature.

(8) **Handwritten signature** means the scripted name or legal mark of an individual handwritten by that individual and executed or adopted with the present intention to authenticate a writing in a permanent form. The act of signing with a writing or marking instrument such as a pen or stylus is preserved. The scripted name or legal mark, while conventionally applied to paper, may also be applied to other devices that capture the name or mark.

(9) **Open system** means an environment in which system access is not controlled by persons who are responsible for the content of electronic records that are on the system.

Subpart B--Electronic Records

Sec. 11.10 Controls for closed systems.

Persons who use closed systems to create, modify, maintain, or transmit electronic records shall employ procedures and controls designed to ensure the authenticity, integrity, and, when appropriate, the confidentiality of electronic records, and to ensure that the signer cannot readily repudiate the signed record as not genuine. Such procedures and controls shall include the following:

(a) Validation of systems to ensure accuracy, reliability, consistent intended performance, and the ability to discern invalid or altered records.

(b) The ability to generate accurate and complete copies of records in both human readable and electronic form suitable for inspection, review, and copying by the agency. Persons should contact the agency if there are any questions regarding the ability of the agency to perform such review and copying of the electronic records.

(c) Protection of records to enable their accurate and ready retrieval throughout the records retention period.

(d) Limiting system access to authorized individuals.

(e) Use of secure, computer-generated, time-stamped audit trails to independently record the date and time of operator entries and actions that create, modify, or delete electronic records. Record changes shall not obscure previously recorded information. Such audit trail documentation shall be retained for a period at least as long as that required for the subject electronic records and shall be available for agency review and copying.

(f) Use of operational system checks to enforce permitted sequencing of steps and events, as appropriate.

(g) Use of authority checks to ensure that only authorized individuals can use the system, electronically sign a record, access the operation or computer system input or output device, alter a record, or perform the operation at hand.

(h) Use of device (e.g., terminal) checks to determine, as appropriate, the validity of the source of data input or operational instruction.

(i) Determination that persons who develop, maintain, or use electronic record/electronic signature systems have the education, training, and experience to perform their assigned tasks.

(j) The establishment of, and adherence to, written policies that hold individuals accountable and responsible for actions initiated under their electronic signatures, in order to deter record and signature falsification.

(k) Use of appropriate controls over systems documentation including:

   (1) Adequate controls over the distribution of, access to, and use of documentation for system operation and maintenance.

   (2) Revision and change control procedures to maintain an audit trail that documents time-sequenced development and modification of systems documentation.

Sec. 11.30 Controls for open systems.

Persons who use open systems to create, modify, maintain, or transmit electronic records shall employ procedures and controls designed to ensure the authenticity, integrity, and, as appropriate, the confidentiality of electronic records from the point of their creation to the point of their receipt. Such procedures and controls shall include those identified in 11.10, as appropriate, and additional measures such as document encryption and use of appropriate digital signature standards to ensure, as necessary under the circumstances, record authenticity, integrity, and confidentiality.

Sec. 11.50 Signature manifestations.

(a) Signed electronic records shall contain information associated with the signing that clearly indicates all of the following:

    (1) The printed name of the signer;

    (2) The date and time when the signature was executed; and

    (3) The meaning (such as review, approval, responsibility, or authorship) associated with the signature.

(b) The items identified in paragraphs (a)(1), (a)(2), and (a)(3) of this section shall be subject to the same controls as for electronic records and shall be included as part of any human readable form of the electronic record (such as electronic display or printout).

Sec. 11.70 Signature/record linking.

Electronic signatures and handwritten signatures executed to electronic records shall be linked to their respective electronic records to ensure that the signatures cannot be excised, copied, or otherwise transferred to falsify an electronic record by ordinary means.

Subpart C--Electronic Signatures

Sec. 11.100 General requirements.

(a) Each electronic signature shall be unique to one individual and shall not be reused by, or reassigned to, anyone else.

(b) Before an organization establishes, assigns, certifies, or otherwise sanctions an individual's electronic signature, or any element of such electronic signature, the organization shall verify the identity of the individual.

(c) Persons using electronic signatures shall, prior to or at the time of such use, certify to the agency that the electronic signatures in their system, used on or after August 20, 1997, are intended to be the legally binding equivalent of traditional handwritten signatures.

(1) The certification shall be submitted in paper form and signed with a traditional handwritten signature, to the Office of Regional Operations (HFC-100), 5600 Fishers Lane, Rockville, MD 20857.

(2) Persons using electronic signatures shall, upon agency request, provide additional certification or testimony that a specific electronic signature is the legally binding equivalent of the signer's handwritten signature.

Sec. 11.200 Electronic signature components and controls.

(a) Electronic signatures that are not based upon biometrics shall:

(1) Employ at least two distinct identification components such as an identification code and password.

(i) When an individual executes a series of signings during a single, continuous period of controlled system access, the first signing shall be executed using all electronic signature components; subsequent signings shall be executed using at least one electronic signature component that is only executable by, and designed to be used only by, the individual.

(ii) When an individual executes one or more signings not performed during a single, continuous period of controlled system access, each signing shall be executed using all of the electronic signature components.

(2) Be used only by their genuine owners; and

(3) Be administered and executed to ensure that attempted use of an individual's electronic signature by anyone other than its genuine owner requires collaboration of two or more individuals.

(b) Electronic signatures based upon biometrics shall be designed to ensure that they cannot be used by anyone other than their genuine owners.

Sec. 11.300 Controls for identification codes/passwords.

Persons who use electronic signatures based upon use of identification codes in combination with passwords shall employ controls to ensure their security and integrity. Such controls shall include:

(a) Maintaining the uniqueness of each combined identification code and password, such that no two individuals have the same combination of identification code and password.

(b) Ensuring that identification code and password issuances are periodically checked, recalled, or revised (e.g., to cover such events as password aging).

(c) Following loss management procedures to electronically deauthorize lost, stolen, missing, or otherwise potentially compromised tokens, cards, and other devices that bear or generate identification code or password information, and to issue temporary or permanent replacements using suitable, rigorous controls.

(d) Use of transaction safeguards to prevent unauthorized use of passwords and/or identification codes, and to detect and report in an immediate and urgent manner any attempts at their unauthorized use to the system security unit, and, as appropriate, to organizational management.

(e) Initial and periodic testing of devices, such as tokens or cards, that bear or generate identification code or password information to ensure that they function properly and have not been altered in an unauthorized manner.

Authority: 21 U.S.C. 321-393; 42 U.S.C. 262.

Source: 62 FR 13464, Mar. 20, 1997, unless otherwise noted.

Part 50:
Protection of Human Subjects

[Code of Federal Regulations]

[Title 21, Volume 1]

[Revised as of April 1, 2009]

[CITE: 21CFR50][1]

Title 21--Food and Drugs

Chapter I--Food and Drug Administration

Department of Health and Human Services

Subchapter A--General

Part 50 Protection of Human Subjects

Subpart A--General Provisions

Sec. 50.1 Scope.

(a) This part applies to all clinical investigations regulated by the Food and Drug Administration under sections 505(i) and 520(g) of the Federal Food, Drug, and Cosmetic Act, as well as clinical investigations that support applications for research or marketing permits for products regulated by the Food and Drug Administration, including foods, including dietary supplements, that bear a nutrient content claim or a health claim, infant formulas, food and color additives, drugs for human use, medical devices for human use, biological products for human use, and electronic products. Additional specific obligations and commitments of, and standards of conduct for, persons who sponsor or monitor clinical investigations involving particular test articles may also be found in other parts (e.g., parts 312 and 812).

---

[1] Available on the FDA website at http://www.accessdata.fda.gov/scripts/cdrh/cfdocs/cfcfr/CFRSearch.cfm?CFRPart=50&showFR=1

Compliance with these parts is intended to protect the rights and safety of subjects involved in investigations filed with the Food and Drug Administration pursuant to sections 403, 406, 409, 412, 413, 502, 503, 505, 510, 513-516, 518-520, 721, and 801 of the Federal Food, Drug, and Cosmetic Act and sections 351 and 354-360F of the Public Health Service Act.

(b) References in this part to regulatory sections of the Code of Federal Regulations are to chapter I of title 21, unless otherwise noted.

[45 FR 36390, May 30, 1980; 46 FR 8979, Jan. 27, 1981, as amended at 63 FR 26697, May 13, 1998; 64 FR 399, Jan. 5, 1999; 66 FR 20597, Apr. 24, 2001]

Sec. 50.3 Definitions.

As used in this part:

(a) *Act* means the Federal Food, Drug, and Cosmetic Act, as amended (secs. 201-902, 52 Stat. 1040et seq. as amended (21 U.S.C. 321-392)).

(b) *Application for research or marketing permit* includes:

(1) A color additive petition, described in part 71.

(2) A food additive petition, described in parts 171 and 571.

(3) Data and information about a substance submitted as part of the procedures for establishing that the substance is generally recognized as safe for use that results or may reasonably be expected to result, directly or indirectly, in its becoming a component or otherwise affecting the characteristics of any food, described in 170.30 and 570.30.

(4) Data and information about a food additive submitted as part of the procedures for food additives permitted to be used on an interim basis pending additional study, described in 180.1.

(5) Data and information about a substance submitted as part of the procedures for establishing a tolerance for unavoidable contaminants in food and food-packaging materials, described in section 406 of the act.

(6) An investigational new drug application, described in part 312 of this chapter.

(7) A new drug application, described in part 314.

(8) Data and information about the bioavailability or bioequivalence of drugs for human use submitted as part of the procedures for issuing, amending, or repealing a bioequivalence requirement, described in part 320.

(9) Data and information about an over-the-counter drug for human use submitted as part of the procedures for classifying these drugs as generally recognized as safe and effective and not misbranded, described in part 330.

(10) Data and information about a prescription drug for human use submitted as part of the procedures for classifying these drugs as generally recognized as safe and effective and not misbranded, described in this chapter.

(11) [Reserved]

(12) An application for a biologics license, described in part 601 of this chapter.

(13) Data and information about a biological product submitted as part of the procedures for determining that licensed biological products are safe and effective and not misbranded, described in part 601.

(14) Data and information about an in vitro diagnostic product submitted as part of the procedures for establishing, amending, or repealing a standard for these products, described in part 809.

(15) An Application for an Investigational Device Exemption, described in part 812.

(16) Data and information about a medical device submitted as part of the procedures for classifying these devices, described in section 513.

(17) Data and information about a medical device submitted as part of the procedures for establishing, amending, or repealing a standard for these devices, described in section 514.

(18) An application for premarket approval of a medical device, described in section 515.

(19) A product development protocol for a medical device, described in section 515.

Part 50

(20) Data and information about an electronic product submitted as part of the procedures for establishing, amending, or repealing a standard for these products, described in section 358 of the Public Health Service Act.

(21) Data and information about an electronic product submitted as part of the procedures for obtaining a variance from any electronic product performance standard, as described in 1010.4.

(22) Data and information about an electronic product submitted as part of the procedures for granting, amending, or extending an exemption from a radiation safety performance standard, as described in 1010.5.

(23) Data and information about a clinical study of an infant formula when submitted as part of an infant formula notification under section 412(c) of the Federal Food, Drug, and Cosmetic Act.

(24) Data and information submitted in a petition for a nutrient content claim, described in 101.69 of this chapter, or for a health claim, described in 101.70 of this chapter.

(25) Data and information from investigations involving children submitted in a new dietary ingredient notification, described in 190.6 of this chapter.

(c) *Clinical investigation* means any experiment that involves a test article and one or more human subjects and that either is subject to requirements for prior submission to the Food and Drug Administration under section 505(i) or 520(g) of the act, or is not subject to requirements for prior submission to the Food and Drug Administration under these sections of the act, but the results of which are intended to be submitted later to, or held for inspection by, the Food and Drug Administration as part of an application for a research or marketing permit. The term does not include experiments that are subject to the provisions of part 58 of this chapter, regarding nonclinical laboratory studies.

(d) *Investigator* means an individual who actually conducts a clinical investigation, i.e., under whose immediate direction the test article is administered or dispensed to, or used involving, a subject, or, in the event of an investigation conducted by a team of individuals, is the responsible leader of that team.

(e) *Sponsor* means a person who initiates a clinical investigation, but who does not actually conduct the investigation, i.e., the test article is administered or dispensed to or used involving, a subject under the immediate direction of another individual. A person other than an individual (e.g., corporation or agency) that uses one or more of its own employees to conduct a clinical investigation it has initiated is considered to be a sponsor (not a sponsor-investigator), and the employees are considered to be investigators.

(f) *Sponsor-investigator* means an individual who both initiates and actually conducts, alone or with others, a clinical investigation, i.e., under whose immediate direction the test article is administered or dispensed to, or used involving, a subject. The term does not include any person other than an individual, e.g., corporation or agency.

(g) *Human subject* means an individual who is or becomes a participant in research, either as a recipient of the test article or as a control. A subject may be either a healthy human or a patient.

(h) *Institution* means any public or private entity or agency (including Federal, State, and other agencies). The wordfacility as used in section 520(g) of the act is deemed to be synonymous with the terminstitution for purposes of this part.

(i) *Institutional review board (IRB)* means any board, committee, or other group formally designated by an institution to review biomedical research involving humans as subjects, to approve the initiation of and conduct periodic review of such research. The term has the same meaning as the phraseinstitutional review committee as used in section 520(g) of the act.

(j) *Test article* means any drug (including a biological product for human use), medical device for human use, human food additive, color additive, electronic product, or any other article subject to regulation under the act or under sections 351 and 354-360F of the Public Health Service Act (42 U.S.C. 262 and 263b-263n).

(k) *Minimal risk* means that the probability and magnitude of harm or discomfort anticipated in the research are not greater in and of themselves than those ordinarily encountered in daily life or during the performance of routine physical or psychological examinations or tests.

(l) *Legally authorized representative* means an individual or judicial or other body authorized under applicable law to consent on behalf of a prospective subject to the subject's particpation in the procedure(s) involved in the research.

(m) *Family member* means any one of the following legally competent persons: Spouse; parents; children (including adopted children); brothers, sisters, and spouses of brothers and sisters; and any individual related by blood or affinity whose close association with the subject is the equivalent of a family relationship.

(n) *Assent* means a child's affirmative agreement to participate in a clinical investigation. Mere failure to object may not, absent affirmative agreement, be construed as assent.

(o) *Children* means persons who have not attained the legal age for consent to treatments or procedures involved in clinical investigations, under the applicable law of the jurisdiction in which the clinical investigation will be conducted.

(p) *Parent* means a child's biological or adoptive parent.

(q) *Ward* means a child who is placed in the legal custody of the State or other agency, institution, or entity, consistent with applicable Federal, State, or local law.

(r) *Permission* means the agreement of parent(s) or guardian to the participation of their child or ward in a clinical investigation. Permission must be obtained in compliance with subpart B of this part and must include the elements of informed consent described in 50.25.

(s) *Guardian* means an individual who is authorized under applicable State or local law to consent on behalf of a child to general medical care when general medical care includes participation in research. For purposes of subpart D of this part, a guardian also means an individual who is authorized to consent on behalf of a child to participate in research.

[45 FR 36390, May 30, 1980, as amended at 46 FR 8950, Jan. 27, 1981; 54 FR 9038, Mar. 3, 1989; 56 FR 28028, June 18, 1991; 61 FR 51528, Oct. 2, 1996; 62 FR 39440, July 23, 1997; 64 FR 399, Jan. 5, 1999; 64 FR 56448, Oct. 20, 1999; 66 FR 20597, Apr. 24, 2001]

Subpart B--Informed Consent of Human Subjects

Sec. 50.20 General requirements for informed consent.

Except as provided in 50.23 and 50.24, no investigator may involve a human being as a subject in research covered by these regulations unless the investigator has obtained the legally effective informed consent of the subject or the subject's legally authorized representative. An investigator shall seek such consent only under circumstances that provide the prospective subject or the representative sufficient opportunity to consider whether or not to participate and that minimize the possibility of coercion or undue influence. The information that is given to the subject or the representative shall be in language understandable to the subject or the representative. No informed consent, whether oral or written, may include any exculpatory language through which the subject or the representative is made to waive or appear to waive any of the subject's legal rights, or releases or appears to release the investigator, the sponsor, the institution, or its agents from liability for negligence.

[46 FR 8951, Jan. 27, 1981, as amended at 64 FR 10942, Mar. 8, 1999]

Sec. 50.23 Exception from general requirements.

(a) The obtaining of informed consent shall be deemed feasible unless, before use of the test article (except as provided in paragraph (b) of this section), both the investigator and a physician who is not otherwise participating in the clinical investigation certify in writing all of the following:

   (1) The human subject is confronted by a life-threatening situation necessitating the use of the test article.

   (2) Informed consent cannot be obtained from the subject because of an inability to communicate with, or obtain legally effective consent from, the subject.

   (3) Time is not sufficient to obtain consent from the subject's legal representative.

   (4) There is available no alternative method of approved or generally recognized therapy that provides an equal or greater likelihood of saving the life of the subject.

(b) If immediate use of the test article is, in the investigator's opinion, required to preserve the life of the subject, and time is not sufficient to obtain the independent determination required in paragraph (a) of this section in advance of using the test article, the determinations of the clinical investigator shall be made and, within 5 working days after the use of the article, be reviewed and evaluated in writing by a physician who is not participating in the clinical investigation.

(c) The documentation required in paragraph (a) or (b) of this section shall be submitted to the IRB within 5 working days after the use of the test article.

(d)(1)   Under 10 U.S.C. 1107(f) the President may waive the prior consent requirement for the administration of an investigational new drug to a member of the armed forces in connection with the member's participation in a particular military operation. The statute specifies that only the President may waive informed consent in this connection and the President may grant such a waiver only if the President determines in writing that obtaining consent: Is not feasible; is contrary to the best interests of the military member; or is not in the interests of national security. The statute further provides that in making a determination to waive prior informed consent on the ground that it is not feasible or the ground that it is contrary to the best interests of the military members involved, the President shall apply the standards and criteria that are set forth in the relevant FDA regulations for a waiver of the prior informed consent requirements of section 505(i)(4) of the Federal Food, Drug, and Cosmetic Act (21 U.S.C. 355(i)(4)). Before such a determination may be made that obtaining informed consent from military personnel prior to the use of an investigational drug (including an antibiotic or biological product) in a specific protocol under an investigational new drug application (IND) sponsored by the Department of Defense (DOD) and limited to specific military personnel involved in a particular military operation is not feasible or is contrary to the best interests of the military members involved the Secretary of Defense must first request such a determination from the President, and certify and document to the President that the following standards and criteria contained in paragraphs (d)(1) through (d)(4) of this section have been met.

(i)   The extent and strength of evidence of the safety and effectiveness of the investigational new drug in relation to the medical risk that could be encountered during the military operation supports the drug's administration under an IND.

(ii) The military operation presents a substantial risk that military personnel may be subject to a chemical, biological, nuclear, or other exposure likely to produce death or serious or life-threatening injury or illness.

(iii) There is no available satisfactory alternative therapeutic or preventive treatment in relation to the intended use of the investigational new drug.

(iv) Conditioning use of the investigational new drug on the voluntary participation of each member could significantly risk the safety and health of any individual member who would decline its use, the safety of other military personnel, and the accomplishment of the military mission.

(v) A duly constituted institutional review board (IRB) established and operated in accordance with the requirements of paragraphs (d)(2) and (d)(3) of this section, responsible for review of the study, has reviewed and approved the investigational new drug protocol and the administration of the investigational new drug without informed consent. DOD's request is to include the documentation required by 56.115(a)(2) of this chapter.

(vi) DOD has explained:

(A) The context in which the investigational drug will be administered, e.g., the setting or whether it will be self-administered or it will be administered by a health professional;

(B) The nature of the disease or condition for which the preventive or therapeutic treatment is intended; and

(C) To the extent there are existing data or information available, information on conditions that could alter the effects of the investigational drug.

(vii) DOD's recordkeeping system is capable of tracking and will be used to track the proposed treatment from supplier to the individual recipient.

(viii) Each member involved in the military operation will be given, prior to the administration of the investigational new drug, a specific written information sheet (including information required by 10 U.S.C. 1107(d)) concerning the investigational new drug, the risks and benefits of its use, potential side effects, and other pertinent information about the appropriate use of the product.

(ix) Medical records of members involved in the military operation will accurately document the receipt by members of the notification required by paragraph (d)(1)(viii) of this section.

(x) Medical records of members involved in the military operation will accurately document the receipt by members of any investigational new drugs in accordance with FDA regulations including part 312 of this chapter.

(xi) DOD will provide adequate followup to assess whether there are beneficial or adverse health consequences that result from the use of the investigational product.

(xii) DOD is pursuing drug development, including a time line, and marketing approval with due diligence.

(xiii) FDA has concluded that the investigational new drug protocol may proceed subject to a decision by the President on the informed consent waiver request.

(xiv) DOD will provide training to the appropriate medical personnel and potential recipients on the specific investigational new drug to be administered prior to its use.

(xv) DOD has stated and justified the time period for which the waiver is needed, not to exceed one year, unless separately renewed under these standards and criteria.

(xvi) DOD shall have a continuing obligation to report to the FDA and to the President any changed circumstances relating to these standards and criteria (including the time period referred to in paragraph (d)(1)(xv) of this section) or that otherwise might affect the determination to use an investigational new drug without informed consent.

(xvii) DOD is to provide public notice as soon as practicable and consistent with classification requirements through notice in theFederal Registerdescribing each waiver of informed consent determination, a summary of the most updated scientific information on the products used, and other pertinent information.

(xviii) Use of the investigational drug without informed consent otherwise conforms with applicable law.

(2) The duly constituted institutional review board, described in paragraph (d)(1)(v) of this section, must include at least 3 nonaffiliated members who shall not be employees or officers of the Federal Government (other than for purposes of membership on the IRB) and shall be required to obtain any necessary security clearances. This IRB shall review the proposed IND protocol at a convened meeting at which a majority of the members are present including at least one member whose primary concerns are in nonscientific areas and, if feasible, including a majority of the nonaffiliated members. The information required by 56.115(a)(2) of this chapter is to be provided to the Secretary of Defense for further review.

(3) The duly constituted institutional review board, described in paragraph (d)(1)(v) of this section, must review and approve:

  (i) The required information sheet;

  (ii) The adequacy of the plan to disseminate information, including distribution of the information sheet to potential recipients, on the investigational product (e.g., in forms other than written);

  (iii) The adequacy of the information and plans for its dissemination to health care providers, including potential side effects, contraindications, potential interactions, and other pertinent considerations; and

  (iv) An informed consent form as required by part 50 of this chapter, in those circumstances in which DOD determines that informed consent may be obtained from some or all personnel involved.

(4) DOD is to submit to FDA summaries of institutional review board meetings at which the proposed protocol has been reviewed.

(5) Nothing in these criteria or standards is intended to preempt or limit FDA's and DOD's authority or obligations under applicable statutes and regulations.

(e)(1) Obtaining informed consent for investigational in vitro diagnostic devices used to identify chemical, biological, radiological, or nuclear agents will be deemed feasible unless, before use of the test article, both the investigator (e.g., clinical laboratory director or other responsible individual) and a physician who is not otherwise participating in the clinical investigation make the determinations and later certify in writing all of the following:

(i)   The human subject is confronted by a life-threatening situation necessitating the use of the investigational in vitro diagnostic device to identify a chemical, biological, radiological, or nuclear agent that would suggest a terrorism event or other public health emergency.

(ii) Informed consent cannot be obtained from the subject because:

(A) There was no reasonable way for the person directing that the specimen be collected to know, at the time the specimen was collected, that there would be a need to use the investigational in vitro diagnostic device on that subject's specimen; and

(B) Time is not sufficient to obtain consent from the subject without risking the life of the subject.

(iii) Time is not sufficient to obtain consent from the subject's legally authorized representative.

(iv) There is no cleared or approved available alternative method of diagnosis, to identify the chemical, biological, radiological, or nuclear agent that provides an equal or greater likelihood of saving the life of the subject.

(2) If use of the investigational device is, in the opinion of the investigator (e.g., clinical laboratory director or other responsible person), required to preserve the life of the subject, and time is not sufficient to obtain the independent determination required in paragraph (e)(1) of this section in advance of using the investigational device, the determinations of the investigator shall be made and, within 5 working days after the use of the device, be reviewed and evaluated in writing by a physician who is not participating in the clinical investigation.

(3) The investigator must submit the documentation required in paragraph (e)(1) or (e)(2) of this section to the IRB within 5 working days after the use of the device.

(4) An investigator must disclose the investigational status of the in vitro diagnostic device and what is known about the performance characteristics of the device in the report to the subject's health

care provider and in any report to public health authorities. The investigator must provide the IRB with the information required in 50.25 (except for the information described in 50.25(a)(8)) and the procedures that will be used to provide this information to each subject or the subject's legally authorized representative at the time the test results are provided to the subject's health care provider and public health authorities.

(5) The IRB is responsible for ensuring the adequacy of the information required in section 50.25 (except for the information described in 50.25(a)(8)) and for ensuring that procedures are in place to provide this information to each subject or the subject's legally authorized representative.

(6) No State or political subdivision of a State may establish or continue in effect any law, rule, regulation or other requirement that informed consent be obtained before an investigational in vitro diagnostic device may be used to identify chemical, biological, radiological, or nuclear agent in suspected terrorism events and other potential public health emergencies that is different from, or in addition to, the requirements of this regulation.

[46 FR 8951, Jan. 27, 1981, as amended at 55 FR 52817, Dec. 21, 1990; 64 FR 399, Jan. 5, 1999; 64 FR 54188, Oct. 5, 1999; 71 FR 32833, June 7, 2006]

Sec. 50.24 Exception from informed consent requirements for emergency research.

(a) The IRB responsible for the review, approval, and continuing review of the clinical investigation described in this section may approve that investigation without requiring that informed consent of all research subjects be obtained if the IRB (with the concurrence of a licensed physician who is a member of or consultant to the IRB and who is not otherwise participating in the clinical investigation) finds and documents each of the following:

(1) The human subjects are in a life-threatening situation, available treatments are unproven or unsatisfactory, and the collection of valid scientific evidence, which may include evidence obtained through randomized placebo-controlled investigations, is necessary to determine the safety and effectiveness of particular interventions.

Part 50

(2) Obtaining informed consent is not feasible because:

   (i) The subjects will not be able to give their informed consent as a result of their medical condition;

   (ii) The intervention under investigation must be administered before consent from the subjects' legally authorized representatives is feasible; and

   (iii) There is no reasonable way to identify prospectively the individuals likely to become eligible for participation in the clinical investigation.

(3) Participation in the research holds out the prospect of direct benefit to the subjects because:

   (i) Subjects are facing a life-threatening situation that necessitates intervention;

   (ii) Appropriate animal and other preclinical studies have been conducted, and the information derived from those studies and related evidence support the potential for the intervention to provide a direct benefit to the individual subjects; and

   (iii) Risks associated with the investigation are reasonable in relation to what is known about the medical condition of the potential class of subjects, the risks and benefits of standard therapy, if any, and what is known about the risks and benefits of the proposed intervention or activity.

(4) The clinical investigation could not practicably be carried out without the waiver.

(5) The proposed investigational plan defines the length of the potential therapeutic window based on scientific evidence, and the investigator has committed to attempting to contact a legally authorized representative for each subject within that window of time and, if feasible, to asking the legally authorized representative contacted for consent within that window rather than proceeding without consent. The investigator will summarize efforts made to contact legally authorized representatives and make this information available to the IRB at the time of continuing review.

(6) The IRB has reviewed and approved informed consent procedures and an informed consent document consistent with 50.25. These procedures and the informed consent

document are to be used with subjects or their legally authorized representatives in situations where use of such procedures and documents is feasible. The IRB has reviewed and approved procedures and information to be used when providing an opportunity for a family member to object to a subject's participation in the clinical investigation consistent with paragraph (a)(7)(v) of this section.

(7) Additional protections of the rights and welfare of the subjects will be provided, including, at least:

(i) Consultation (including, where appropriate, consultation carried out by the IRB) with representatives of the communities in which the clinical investigation will be conducted and from which the subjects will be drawn;

(ii) Public disclosure to the communities in which the clinical investigation will be conducted and from which the subjects will be drawn, prior to initiation of the clinical investigation, of plans for the investigation and its risks and expected benefits;

(iii) Public disclosure of sufficient information following completion of the clinical investigation to apprise the community and researchers of the study, including the demographic characteristics of the research population, and its results;

(iv) Establishment of an independent data monitoring committee to exercise oversight of the clinical investigation; and

(v) If obtaining informed consent is not feasible and a legally authorized representative is not reasonably available, the investigator has committed, if feasible, to attempting to contact within the therapeutic window the subject's family member who is not a legally authorized representative, and asking whether he or she objects to the subject's participation in the clinical investigation. The investigator will summarize efforts made to contact family members and make this information available to the IRB at the time of continuing review.

(b) The IRB is responsible for ensuring that procedures are in place to inform, at the earliest feasible opportunity, each subject, or if the subject remains incapacitated, a legally authorized representative of the subject, or if such a representative is not reasonably available, a family member, of the subject's inclusion in the clinical investigation, the details of the investigation and other information contained in the informed consent document. The IRB shall also ensure that there is a procedure to inform the subject, or if the subject remains incapacitated, a legally authorized representative of the subject, or if such a representative is not reasonably available, a family member, that he or she may discontinue the subject's participation at any time without penalty or loss of benefits to which the subject is otherwise entitled. If a legally authorized representative or family member is told about the clinical investigation and the subject's condition improves, the subject is also to be informed as soon as feasible. If a subject is entered into a clinical investigation with waived consent and the subject dies before a legally authorized representative or family member can be contacted, information about the clinical investigation is to be provided to the subject's legally authorized representative or family member, if feasible.

(c) The IRB determinations required by paragraph (a) of this section and the documentation required by paragraph (e) of this section are to be retained by the IRB for at least 3 years after completion of the clinical investigation, and the records shall be accessible for inspection and copying by FDA in accordance with 56.115(b) of this chapter.

(d) Protocols involving an exception to the informed consent requirement under this section must be performed under a separate investigational new drug application (IND) or investigational device exemption (IDE) that clearly identifies such protocols as protocols that may include subjects who are unable to consent. The submission of those protocols in a separate IND/IDE is required even if an IND for the same drug product or an IDE for the same device already exists. Applications for investigations under this section may not be submitted as amendments under 312.30 or 812.35 of this chapter.

(e) If an IRB determines that it cannot approve a clinical investigation because the investigation does not meet the criteria in the exception provided under paragraph (a) of this section or because of other relevant ethical concerns, the IRB must document its findings and provide these findings promptly in writing to the clinical investigator and to the sponsor of the clinical investigation. The sponsor of the clinical investigation must promptly disclose this information to FDA and to the sponsor's clinical investigators who are participating or are asked to participate in this or a substantially equivalent clinical investigation of the sponsor, and to other IRB's that have been, or are, asked to review this or a substantially equivalent investigation by that sponsor.

[61 FR 51528, Oct. 2, 1996]

Sec. 50.25 Elements of informed consent.

(a) Basic elements of informed consent. In seeking informed consent, the following information shall be provided to each subject:

(1) A statement that the study involves research, an explanation of the purposes of the research and the expected duration of the subject's participation, a description of the procedures to be followed, and identification of any procedures which are experimental.

(2) A description of any reasonably foreseeable risks or discomforts to the subject.

(3) A description of any benefits to the subject or to others which may reasonably be expected from the research.

(4) A disclosure of appropriate alternative procedures or courses of treatment, if any, that might be advantageous to the subject.

(5) A statement describing the extent, if any, to which confidentiality of records identifying the subject will be maintained and that notes the possibility that the Food and Drug Administration may inspect the records.

(6) For research involving more than minimal risk, an explanation as to whether any compensation and an explanation as to whether any medical treatments are available if injury occurs and, if so, what they consist of, or where further information may be obtained.

(7) An explanation of whom to contact for answers to pertinent questions about the research and research subjects' rights, and whom to contact in the event of a research-related injury to the subject.

(8) A statement that participation is voluntary, that refusal to participate will involve no penalty or loss of benefits to which the subject is otherwise entitled, and that the subject may

discontinue participation at any time without penalty or loss of benefits to which the subject is otherwise entitled.

(b) Additional elements of informed consent. When appropriate, one or more of the following elements of information shall also be provided to each subject:

    (1) A statement that the particular treatment or procedure may involve risks to the subject (or to the embryo or fetus, if the subject is or may become pregnant) which are currently unforeseeable.

    (2) Anticipated circumstances under which the subject's participation may be terminated by the investigator without regard to the subject's consent.

    (3) Any additional costs to the subject that may result from participation in the research.

    (4) The consequences of a subject's decision to withdraw from the research and procedures for orderly termination of participation by the subject.

    (5) A statement that significant new findings developed during the course of the research which may relate to the subject's willingness to continue participation will be provided to the subject.

    (6) The approximate number of subjects involved in the study.

(c) The informed consent requirements in these regulations are not intended to preempt any applicable Federal, State, or local laws which require additional information to be disclosed for informed consent to be legally effective.

(d) Nothing in these regulations is intended to limit the authority of a physician to provide emergency medical care to the extent the physician is permitted to do so under applicable Federal, State, or local law.

Sec. 50.27 Documentation of informed consent.

(a) Except as provided in 56.109(c), informed consent shall be documented by the use of a written consent form approved by the IRB and signed and dated by the subject or the subject's legally authorized representative at the time of consent. A copy shall be given to the person signing the form.

(b) Except as provided in 56.109(c), the consent form may be either of the following:

(1) A written consent document that embodies the elements of informed consent required by 50.25. This form may be read to the subject or the subject's legally authorized representative, but, in any event, the investigator shall give either the subject or the representative adequate opportunity to read it before it is signed.

(2) A short form written consent document stating that the elements of informed consent required by 50.25 have been presented orally to the subject or the subject's legally authorized representative. When this method is used, there shall be a witness to the oral presentation. Also, the IRB shall approve a written summary of what is to be said to the subject or the representative. Only the short form itself is to be signed by the subject or the representative. However, the witness shall sign both the short form and a copy of the summary, and the person actually obtaining the consent shall sign a copy of the summary. A copy of the summary shall be given to the subject or the representative in addition to a copy of the short form.

[46 FR 8951, Jan. 27, 1981, as amended at 61 FR 57280, Nov. 5, 1996]

Part 50

Subpart C [Reserved]

Subpart D--Additional Safeguards for Children in Clinical Investigations

Sec. 50.50 IRB duties.

In addition to other responsibilities assigned to IRBs under this part and part 56 of this chapter, each IRB must review clinical investigations involving children as subjects covered by this subpart D and approve only those clinical investigations that satisfy the criteria described in 50.51, 50.52, or 50.53 and the conditions of all other applicable sections of this subpart D.

Sec. 50.51 Clinical investigations not involving greater than minimal risk.

Any clinical investigation within the scope described in 50.1 and 56.101 of this chapter in which no greater than minimal risk to children is presented may involve children as subjects only if the IRB finds and documents that adequate provisions are made for soliciting the assent of the children and the permission of their parents or guardians as set forth in 50.55.

Sec. 50.52 Clinical investigations involving greater than minimal risk but presenting the prospect of direct benefit to individual subjects.

Any clinical investigation within the scope described in 50.1 and 56.101 of this chapter in which more than minimal risk to children is presented by an intervention or procedure that holds out the prospect of direct benefit for the individual subject, or by a monitoring procedure that is likely to contribute to the subject's well-being, may involve children as subjects only if the IRB finds and documents that:

(a) The risk is justified by the anticipated benefit to the subjects;

(b) The relation of the anticipated benefit to the risk is at least as favorable to the subjects as that presented by available alternative approaches; and

(c) Adequate provisions are made for soliciting the assent of the children and permission of their parents or guardians as set forth in 50.55.

Sec. 50.53 Clinical investigations involving greater than minimal risk and no prospect of direct benefit to individual subjects, but likely to yield generalizable knowledge about the subjects' disorder or condition.

Any clinical investigation within the scope described in 50.1 and 56.101 of this chapter in which more than minimal risk to children is presented by an intervention or procedure that does not hold out the prospect of direct benefit for the individual subject, or by a monitoring procedure that is not likely to contribute to the well-being of the subject, may involve children as subjects only if the IRB finds and documents that:

(a) The risk represents a minor increase over minimal risk;

(b) The intervention or procedure presents experiences to subjects that are reasonably commensurate with those inherent in their actual or expected medical, dental, psychological, social, or educational situations;

(c) The intervention or procedure is likely to yield generalizable knowledge about the subjects' disorder or condition that is of vital importance for the understanding or amelioration of the subjects' disorder or condition; and

(d) Adequate provisions are made for soliciting the assent of the children and permission of their parents or guardians as set forth in 50.55.

Sec. 50.54 Clinical investigations not otherwise approvable that present an opportunity to understand, prevent, or alleviate a serious problem affecting the health or welfare of children.

If an IRB does not believe that a clinical investigation within the scope described in 50.1 and 56.101 of this chapter and involving children as subjects meets the requirements of 50.51, 50.52, or 50.53, the clinical investigation may proceed only if:

(a) The IRB finds and documents that the clinical investigation presents a reasonable opportunity to further the understanding, prevention, or alleviation of a serious problem affecting the health or welfare of children; and

(b) The Commissioner of Food and Drugs, after consultation with a panel of experts in pertinent disciplines (for example: science, medicine, education, ethics, law) and following opportunity for public review and comment, determines either:

(1) That the clinical investigation in fact satisfies the conditions of 50.51, 50.52, or 50.53, as applicable, or

(2) That the following conditions are met:

(i) The clinical investigation presents a reasonable opportunity to further the understanding, prevention, or alleviation of a serious problem affecting the health or welfare of children;

(ii) The clinical investigation will be conducted in accordance with sound ethical principles; and

(iii) Adequate provisions are made for soliciting the assent of children and the permission of their parents or guardians as set forth in 50.55.

Sec. 50.55 Requirements for permission by parents or guardians and for assent by children.

(a) In addition to the determinations required under other applicable sections of this subpart D, the IRB must determine that adequate provisions are made for soliciting the assent of the children when in the judgment of the IRB the children are capable of providing assent.

(b) In determining whether children are capable of providing assent, the IRB must take into account the ages, maturity, and psychological state of the children involved. This judgment may be made for all children to be involved in clinical investigations under a particular protocol, or for each child, as the IRB deems appropriate.

(c) The assent of the children is not a necessary condition for proceeding with the clinical investigation if the IRB determines:

(1) That the capability of some or all of the children is so limited that they cannot reasonably be consulted, or

(2) That the intervention or procedure involved in the clinical investigation holds out a prospect of direct benefit that is important to the health or well-being of the children and is available only in the context of the clinical investigation.

(d) Even where the IRB determines that the subjects are capable of assenting, the IRB may still waive the assent requirement if it finds and documents that:

(1) The clinical investigation involves no more than minimal risk to the subjects;

(2) The waiver will not adversely affect the rights and welfare of the subjects;

(3) The clinical investigation could not practicably be carried out without the waiver; and

(4) Whenever appropriate, the subjects will be provided with additional pertinent information after participation.

(e) In addition to the determinations required under other applicable sections of this subpart D, the IRB must determine that the permission of each child's parents or guardian is granted.

    (1) Where parental permission is to be obtained, the IRB may find that the permission of one parent is sufficient, if consistent with State law, for clinical investigations to be conducted under 50.51 or 50.52.

    (2) Where clinical investigations are covered by 50.53 or 50.54 and permission is to be obtained from parents, both parents must give their permission unless one parent is deceased, unknown, incompetent, or not reasonably available, or when only one parent has legal responsibility for the care and custody of the child if consistent with State law.

(f) Permission by parents or guardians must be documented in accordance with and to the extent required by 50.27.

(g) When the IRB determines that assent is required, it must also determine whether and how assent must be documented.

Sec. 50.56 Wards.

(a) Children who are wards of the State or any other agency, institution, or entity can be included in clinical investigations approved under 50.53 or 50.54 only if such clinical investigations are:

    (1) Related to their status as wards; or

    (2) Conducted in schools, camps, hospitals, institutions, or similar settings in which the majority of children involved as subjects are not wards.

(b) If the clinical investigation is approved under paragraph (a) of this section, the IRB must require appointment of an advocate for each child who is a ward.

    (1) The advocate will serve in addition to any other individual acting on behalf of the child as guardian or in loco parentis.

    (2) One individual may serve as advocate for more than one child.

    (3) The advocate must be an individual who has the background and experience to act in, and agrees to act in, the best interest

Part 50

of the child for the duration of the child's participation in the clinical investigation.

(4) The advocate must not be associated in any way (except in the role as advocate or member of the IRB) with the clinical investigation, the investigator(s), or the guardian organization.

Authority: 21 U.S.C 321, 343, 346, 346a, 348, 350a, 350b, 352, 353, 355, 360, 360c-360f, 360h-360j, 371, 379e, 381; 42 U.S.C. 216, 241, 262, 263b-263n.

Source: 45 FR 36390, May 30, 1980, unless otherwise noted.

Part 54: Financial Disclosure by Clinical Investigators

[Code of Federal Regulations]

[Title 21, Volume 1]

[Revised as of April 1, 2009]

[CITE: 21CFR54]

Title 21--Food and Drugs

Chapter I--Food and Drug Administration

Department of Health and Human Services

Subchapter A--General

Part 54 Financial Disclosure by Clinical Investigators[1]

Sec. 54.1 Purpose.

(a) The Food and Drug Administration (FDA) evaluates clinical studies submitted in marketing applications, required by law, for new human drugs and biological products and marketing applications and reclassification petitions for medical devices.

(b) The agency reviews data generated in these clinical studies to determine whether the applications are approvable under the statutory requirements. FDA may consider clinical studies inadequate and the data inadequate if, among other things, appropriate steps have not been taken in the design, conduct, reporting, and analysis of the studies to minimize bias. One potential source of bias in clinical studies is a financial interest of

---

[1] Available on the FDA website at http://www.accessdata.fda.gov/scripts/cdrh/cfdocs/cfCFR/CFRSearch.cfm?CFRPart=54&showFR=1

the clinical investigator in the outcome of the study because of the way payment is arranged (e.g., a royalty) or because the investigator has a proprietary interest in the product (e.g., a patent) or because the investigator has an equity interest in the sponsor of the covered study. This section and conforming regulations require an applicant whose submission relies in part on clinical data to disclose certain financial arrangements between sponsor(s) of the covered studies and the clinical investigators and certain interests of the clinical investigators in the product under study or in the sponsor of the covered studies. FDA will use this information, in conjunction with information about the design and purpose of the study, as well as information obtained through on-site inspections, in the agency's assessment of the reliability of the data.

Sec. 54.2 Definitions.

For the purposes of this part:

(a) *Compensation affected by the outcome of clinical studies* means compensation that could be higher for a favorable outcome than for an unfavorable outcome, such as compensation that is explicitly greater for a favorable result or compensation to the investigator in the form of an equity interest in the sponsor of a covered study or in the form of compensation tied to sales of the product, such as a royalty interest.

(b) *Significant equity interest in the sponsor of a covered study* means any ownership interest, stock options, or other financial interest whose value cannot be readily determined through reference to public prices (generally, interests in a nonpublicly traded corporation), or any equity interest in a publicly traded corporation that exceeds $50,000 during the time the clinical investigator is carrying out the study and for 1 year following completion of the study.

(c) *Proprietary interest in the tested product* means property or other financial interest in the product including, but not limited to, a patent, trademark, copyright or licensing agreement.

(d) *Clinical investigator* means only a listed or identified investigator or subinvestigator who is directly involved in the treatment or evaluation of research subjects. The term also includes the spouse and each dependent child of the investigator.

(e) ***Covered clinical study*** means any study of a drug or device in humans submitted in a marketing application or reclassification petition subject to this part that the applicant or FDA relies on to establish that the product is effective (including studies that show equivalence to an effective product) or any study in which a single investigator makes a significant contribution to the demonstration of safety. This would, in general, not include phase 1 tolerance studies or pharmacokinetic studies, most clinical pharmacology studies (unless they are critical to an efficacy determination), large open safety studies conducted at multiple sites, treatment protocols, and parallel track protocols. An applicant may consult with FDA as to which clinical studies constitute "covered clinical studies" for purposes of complying with financial disclosure requirements.

(f) ***Significant payments of other sorts*** means payments made by the sponsor of a covered study to the investigator or the institution to support activities of the investigator that have a monetary value of more than $25,000, exclusive of the costs of conducting the clinical study or other clinical studies, (e.g., a grant to fund ongoing research, compensation in the form of equipment or retainers for ongoing consultation or honoraria) during the time the clinical investigator is carrying out the study and for 1 year following the completion of the study.

(g) ***Applicant*** means the party who submits a marketing application to FDA for approval of a drug, device, or biologic product. The applicant is responsible for submitting the appropriate certification and disclosure statements required in this part.

(h) ***Sponsor of the covered clinical study*** means the party supporting a particular study at the time it was carried out.

[63 FR 5250, Feb. 2, 1998, as amended at 63 FR 72181, Dec. 31, 1998]

Sec. 54.3 Scope.

The requirements in this part apply to any applicant who submits a marketing application for a human drug, biological product, or device and who submits covered clinical studies. The applicant is responsible for making the appropriate certification or disclosure statement where the applicant either contracted with one or more clinical investigators to conduct the studies or submitted studies conducted by others not under contract to the applicant.

Part 54

Sec. 54.4 Certification and disclosure requirements.

For purposes of this part, an applicant must submit a list of all clinical investigators who conducted covered clinical studies to determine whether the applicant's product meets FDA's marketing requirements, identifying those clinical investigators who are full-time or part-time employees of the sponsor of each covered study. The applicant must also completely and accurately disclose or certify information concerning the financial interests of a clinical investigator who is not a full-time or part-time employee of the sponsor for each covered clinical study. Clinical investigators subject to investigational new drug or investigational device exemption regulations must provide the sponsor of the study with sufficient accurate information needed to allow subsequent disclosure or certification. The applicant is required to submit for each clinical investigator who participates in a covered study, either a certification that none of the financial arrangements described in 54.2 exist, or disclose the nature of those arrangements to the agency. Where the applicant acts with due diligence to obtain the information required in this section but is unable to do so, the applicant shall certify that despite the applicant's due diligence in attempting to obtain the information, the applicant was unable to obtain the information and shall include the reason.

(a) The applicant (of an application submitted under sections 505, 506, 510(k), 513, or 515 of the Federal Food, Drug, and Cosmetic Act, or section 351 of the Public Health Service Act) that relies in whole or in part on clinical studies shall submit, for each clinical investigator who participated in a covered clinical study, either a certification described in paragraph (a)(1) of this section or a disclosure statement described in paragraph (a)(3) of this section.

  (1) Certification: The applicant covered by this section shall submit for all clinical investigators (as defined in 54.2(d)), to whom the certification applies, a completed Form FDA 3454 attesting to the absence of financial interests and arrangements described in paragraph (a)(3) of this section. The form shall be dated and signed by the chief financial officer or other responsible corporate official or representative.

  (2) If the certification covers less than all covered clinical data in the application, the applicant shall include in the certification a list of the studies covered by this certification.

  (3) Disclosure Statement: For any clinical investigator defined in 54.2(d) for whom the applicant does not submit the

certification described in paragraph (a)(1) of this section, the applicant shall submit a completed Form FDA 3455 disclosing completely and accurately the following:

(i) Any financial arrangement entered into between the sponsor of the covered study and the clinical investigator involved in the conduct of a covered clinical trial, whereby the value of the compensation to the clinical investigator for conducting the study could be influenced by the outcome of the study;

(ii) Any significant payments of other sorts from the sponsor of the covered study, such as a grant to fund ongoing research, compensation in the form of equipment, retainer for ongoing consultation, or honoraria;

(iii) Any proprietary interest in the tested product held by any clinical investigator involved in a study;

(iv) Any significant equity interest in the sponsor of the covered study held by any clinical investigator involved in any clinical study; and

(v) Any steps taken to minimize the potential for bias resulting from any of the disclosed arrangements, interests, or payments.

(b) The clinical investigator shall provide to the sponsor of the covered study sufficient accurate financial information to allow the sponsor to submit complete and accurate certification or disclosure statements as required in paragraph (a) of this section. The investigator shall promptly update this information if any relevant changes occur in the course of the investigation or for 1 year following completion of the study.

(c) Refusal to file application. FDA may refuse to file any marketing application described in paragraph (a) of this section that does not contain the information required by this section or a certification by the applicant that the applicant has acted with due diligence to obtain the information but was unable to do so and stating the reason.

[63 FR 5250, Feb. 2, 1998; 63 FR 35134, June 29, 1998, as amended at 64 FR 399, Jan. 5, 1999]

Part 54

Sec. 54.5 Agency evaluation of financial interests.

(a) Evaluation of disclosure statement. FDA will evaluate the information disclosed under 54.4(a)(2) about each covered clinical study in an application to determine the impact of any disclosed financial interests on the reliability of the study. FDA may consider both the size and nature of a disclosed financial interest (including the potential increase in the value of the interest if the product is approved) and steps that have been taken to minimize the potential for bias.

(b) Effect of study design. In assessing the potential of an investigator's financial interests to bias a study, FDA will take into account the design and purpose of the study. Study designs that utilize such approaches as multiple investigators (most of whom do not have a disclosable interest), blinding, objective endpoints, or measurement of endpoints by someone other than the investigator may adequately protect against any bias created by a disclosable financial interest.

(c) Agency actions to ensure reliability of data. If FDA determines that the financial interests of any clinical investigator raise a serious question about the integrity of the data, FDA will take any action it deems necessary to ensure the reliability of the data including:

　　(1) Initiating agency audits of the data derived from the clinical investigator in question;

　　(2) Requesting that the applicant submit further analyses of data, e.g., to evaluate the effect of the clinical investigator's data on overall study outcome;

　　(3) Requesting that the applicant conduct additional independent studies to confirm the results of the questioned study; and

　　(4) Refusing to treat the covered clinical study as providing data that can be the basis for an agency action.

Sec. 54.6 Recordkeeping and record retention.

(a) Financial records of clinical investigators to be retained. An applicant who has submitted a marketing application containing covered clinical studies shall keep on file certain information pertaining to the financial interests of clinical investigators who conducted studies on which the application relies and who are not full or part-time employees of the applicant, as follows:

(1) Complete records showing any financial interest or arrangement as described in 54.4(a)(3)(i) paid to such clinical investigators by the sponsor of the covered study.

(2) Complete records showing significant payments of other sorts, as described in 54.4(a)(3)(ii), made by the sponsor of the covered clinical study to the clinical investigator.

(3) Complete records showing any financial interests held by clinical investigators as set forth in 54.4(a)(3)(iii) and (a)(3)(iv).

(b) Requirements for maintenance of clinical investigators' financial records. (1) For any application submitted for a covered product, an applicant shall retain records as described in paragraph (a) of this section for 2 years after the date of approval of the application.

(2) The person maintaining these records shall, upon request from any properly authorized officer or employee of FDA, at reasonable times, permit such officer or employee to have access to and copy and verify these records.

Part 54

Authority: 21 U.S.C. 321, 331, 351, 352, 353, 355, 360, 360c-360j, 371, 372, 373, 374, 375, 376, 379; 42 U.S.C. 262.

Source: 63 FR 5250, Feb. 2, 1998, unless otherwise noted.

Part 56:
Institutional Review Boards

[Code of Federal Regulations]

[Title 21, Volume 1]

[Revised as of April 1, 2009]

[CITE: 21CFR56]

Title 21--Food and Drugs

Chapter I--Food and Drug Administration

Department of Health and Human Services

Subchapter A--General

Part 56 Institutional Review Boards[1]

Subpart A--General Provisions

Sec. 56.101 Scope.

(a) This part contains the general standards for the composition, operation, and responsibility of an Institutional Review Board (IRB) that reviews clinical investigations regulated by the Food and Drug Administration under sections 505(i) and 520(g) of the act, as well as clinical investigations that support applications for research or marketing permits for products regulated by the Food and Drug Administration, including foods, including dietary supplements, that bear a nutrient content claim or a health claim, infant formulas, food and color additives, drugs for human use, medical devices for human use, biological products for human use, and electronic products. Compliance with this part is intended to

---

[1] Available on the FDA website at http://www.accessdata.fda.gov/scripts/cdrh/cfdocs/cfCFR/CFRSearch.cfm?CFRPart=56&showFR=1

protect the rights and welfare of human subjects involved in such investigations.

(b) References in this part to regulatory sections of the Code of Federal Regulations are to chapter I of title 21, unless otherwise noted.

[46 FR 8975, Jan. 27, 1981, as amended at 64 FR 399, Jan. 5, 1999; 66 FR 20599, Apr. 24, 2001]

Sec. 56.102 Definitions.

As used in this part:

(a) *Act* means the Federal Food, Drug, and Cosmetic Act, as amended (secs. 201-902, 52 Stat. 1040et seq., as amended (21 U.S.C. 321-392)).

(b) *Application for research or marketing permit* includes:

(1) A color additive petition, described in part 71.

(2) Data and information regarding a substance submitted as part of the procedures for establishing that a substance is generally recognized as safe for a use which results or may reasonably be expected to result, directly or indirectly, in its becoming a component or otherwise affecting the characteristics of any food, described in 170.35.

(3) A food additive petition, described in part 171.

(4) Data and information regarding a food additive submitted as part of the procedures regarding food additives permitted to be used on an interim basis pending additional study, described in 180.1.

(5) Data and information regarding a substance submitted as part of the procedures for establishing a tolerance for unavoidable contaminants in food and food-packaging materials, described in section 406 of the act.

(6) An investigational new drug application, described in part 312 of this chapter.

(7) A new drug application, described in part 314.

(8) Data and information regarding the bioavailability or bioequivalence of drugs for human use submitted as part of

the procedures for issuing, amending, or repealing a bioequivalence requirement, described in part 320.

(9) Data and information regarding an over-the-counter drug for human use submitted as part of the procedures for classifying such drugs as generally recognized as safe and effective and not misbranded, described in part 330.

(10) An application for a biologics license, described in part 601 of this chapter.

(11) Data and information regarding a biological product submitted as part of the procedures for determining that licensed biological products are safe and effective and not misbranded, as described in part 601 of this chapter.

(12) An Application for an Investigational Device Exemption, described in part 812.

(13) Data and information regarding a medical device for human use submitted as part of the procedures for classifying such devices, described in part 860.

(14) Data and information regarding a medical device for human use submitted as part of the procedures for establishing, amending, or repealing a standard for such device, described in part 861.

(15) An application for premarket approval of a medical device for human use, described in section 515 of the act.

(16) A product development protocol for a medical device for human use, described in section 515 of the act.

Part 56

(17) Data and information regarding an electronic product submitted as part of the procedures for establishing, amending, or repealing a standard for such products, described in section 358 of the Public Health Service Act.

(18) Data and information regarding an electronic product submitted as part of the procedures for obtaining a variance from any electronic product performance standard, as described in 1010.4.

(19) Data and information regarding an electronic product submitted as part of the procedures for granting, amending, or extending an exemption from a radiation safety performance standard, as described in 1010.5.

(20) Data and information regarding an electronic product submitted as part of the procedures for obtaining an exemption from notification of a radiation safety defect or failure of compliance with a radiation safety performance standard, described in subpart D of part 1003.

(21) Data and information about a clinical study of an infant formula when submitted as part of an infant formula notification under section 412(c) of the Federal Food, Drug, and Cosmetic Act.

(22) Data and information submitted in a petition for a nutrient content claim, described in 101.69 of this chapter, and for a health claim, described in 101.70 of this chapter.

(23) Data and information from investigations involving children submitted in a new dietary ingredient notification, described in 190.6 of this chapter.

(c) **Clinical investigation** means any experiment that involves a test article and one or more human subjects, and that either must meet the requirements for prior submission to the Food and Drug Administration under section 505(i) or 520(g) of the act, or need not meet the requirements for prior submission to the Food and Drug Administration under these sections of the act, but the results of which are intended to be later submitted to, or held for inspection by, the Food and Drug Administration as part of an application for a research or marketing permit. The term does not include experiments that must meet the provisions of part 58, regarding nonclinical laboratory studies. The termsresearch, clinical research, clinical study, study, andclinical investigation are deemed to be synonymous for purposes of this part.

(d) **Emergency use** means the use of a test article on a human subject in a life-threatening situation in which no standard acceptable treatment is available, and in which there is not sufficient time to obtain IRB approval.

(e) **Human subject** means an individual who is or becomes a participant in research, either as a recipient of the test article or as a control. A subject may be either a healthy individual or a patient.

(f) **Institution** means any public or private entity or agency (including Federal, State, and other agencies). The termfacility as used in section 520(g) of the act is deemed to be synonymous with the terminstitution for purposes of this part.

(g) **Institutional Review Board (IRB)** means any board, committee, or other group formally designated by an institution to review, to approve the initiation of, and to conduct periodic review of, biomedical research involving human subjects. The primary purpose of such review is to assure the protection of the rights and welfare of the human subjects. The term has the same meaning as the phrase institutional review committee as used in section 520(g) of the act.

(h) **Investigator** means an individual who actually conducts a clinical investigation (i.e., under whose immediate direction the test article is administered or dispensed to, or used involving, a subject) or, in the event of an investigation conducted by a team of individuals, is the responsible leader of that team.

(i) **Minimal risk** means that the probability and magnitude of harm or discomfort anticipated in the research are not greater in and of themselves than those ordinarily encountered in daily life or during the performance of routine physical or psychological examinations or tests.

(j) **Sponsor** means a person or other entity that initiates a clinical investigation, but that does not actually conduct the investigation, i.e., the test article is administered or dispensed to, or used involving, a subject under the immediate direction of another individual. A person other than an individual (e.g., a corporation or agency) that uses one or more of its own employees to conduct an investigation that it has initiated is considered to be a sponsor (not a sponsor-investigator), and the employees are considered to be investigators.

(k) **Sponsor-investigator** means an individual who both initiates and actually conducts, alone or with others, a clinical investigation, i.e., under whose immediate direction the test article is administered or dispensed to, or used involving, a subject. The term does not include any person other than an individual, e.g., it does not include a corporation or agency. The obligations of a sponsor-investigator under this part include both those of a sponsor and those of an investigator.

(l) **Test article** means any drug for human use, biological product for human use, medical device for human use, human food additive, color additive, electronic product, or any other article subject to

Part 56

regulation under the act or under sections 351 or 354-360F of the Public Health Service Act.

(m) **IRB approval** means the determination of the IRB that the clinical investigation has been reviewed and may be conducted at an institution within the constraints set forth by the IRB and by other institutional and Federal requirements.

[46 FR 8975, Jan. 27, 1981, as amended at 54 FR 9038, Mar. 3, 1989; 56 FR 28028, June 18, 1991; 64 FR 399, Jan. 5, 1999; 64 FR 56448, Oct. 20, 1999; 65 FR 52302, Aug. 29, 2000; 66 FR 20599, Apr. 24, 2001; 74 FR 2368, Jan. 15, 2009]

Sec. 56.103 Circumstances in which IRB review is required.

(a) Except as provided in 56.104 and 56.105, any clinical investigation which must meet the requirements for prior submission (as required in parts 312, 812, and 813) to the Food and Drug Administration shall not be initiated unless that investigation has been reviewed and approved by, and remains subject to continuing review by, an IRB meeting the requirements of this part.

(b) Except as provided in 56.104 and 56.105, the Food and Drug Administration may decide not to consider in support of an application for a research or marketing permit any data or information that has been derived from a clinical investigation that has not been approved by, and that was not subject to initial and continuing review by, an IRB meeting the requirements of this part. The determination that a clinical investigation may not be considered in support of an application for a research or marketing permit does not, however, relieve the applicant for such a permit of any obligation under any other applicable regulations to submit the results of the investigation to the Food and Drug Administration.

(c) Compliance with these regulations will in no way render inapplicable pertinent Federal, State, or local laws or regulations.

[46 FR 8975, Jan. 27, 1981; 46 FR 14340, Feb. 27, 1981]

Sec. 56.104 Exemptions from IRB requirement.

The following categories of clinical investigations are exempt from the requirements of this part for IRB review:

(a) Any investigation which commenced before July 27, 1981 and was subject to requirements for IRB review under FDA regulations before that date, provided that the investigation remains subject to review of an IRB which meets the FDA requirements in effect before July 27, 1981.

(b) Any investigation commenced before July 27, 1981 and was not otherwise subject to requirements for IRB review under Food and Drug Administration regulations before that date.

(c) Emergency use of a test article, provided that such emergency use is reported to the IRB within 5 working days. Any subsequent use of the test article at the institution is subject to IRB review.

(d) Taste and food quality evaluations and consumer acceptance studies, if wholesome foods without additives are consumed or if a food is consumed that contains a food ingredient at or below the level and for a use found to be safe, or agricultural, chemical, or environmental contaminant at or below the level found to be safe, by the Food and Drug Administration or approved by the Environmental Protection Agency or the Food Safety and Inspection Service of the U.S. Department of Agriculture.

[46 FR 8975, Jan. 27, 1981, as amended at 56 FR 28028, June 18, 1991]

Sec. 56.105 Waiver of IRB requirement.

On the application of a sponsor or sponsor-investigator, the Food and Drug Administration may waive any of the requirements contained in these regulations, including the requirements for IRB review, for specific research activities or for classes of research activities, otherwise covered by these regulations.

Subpart B--Organization and Personnel

Sec. 56.106 Registration.

(a) Who must register ? Each IRB in the United States that reviews clinical investigations regulated by FDA under sections 505(i) or 520(g) of the act and each IRB in the United States that reviews clinical investigations that are intended to support applications for research or marketing permits for FDA-regulated products must register at a site maintained by the Department of Health and Human Services (HHS). (A research permit under section 505(i) of the act is usually known as an investigational new drug application (IND), while a research permit under section 520(g) of the act is usually known as an investigational device exemption (IDE).) An individual authorized to act on the IRB's behalf must submit the registration information. All other IRBs may register voluntarily.

(b) What information must an IRB register ? Each IRB must provide the following information:

(1) The name, mailing address, and street address (if different from the mailing address) of the institution operating the IRB and the name, mailing address, phone number, facsimile number, and electronic mail address of the senior officer of that institution who is responsible for overseeing activities performed by the IRB;

(2) The IRB's name, mailing address, street address (if different from the mailing address), phone number, facsimile number, and electronic mail address; each IRB chairperson's name, phone number, and electronic mail address; and the name, mailing address, phone number, facsimile number, and electronic mail address of the contact person providing the registration information.

(3) The approximate number of active protocols involving FDA-regulated products reviewed. For purposes of this rule, an "active protocol" is any protocol for which an IRB conducted an initial review or a continuing review at a convened meeting or under an expedited review procedure during the preceding 12 months; and

(4) A description of the types of FDA-regulated products (such as biological products, color additives, food additives, human drugs, or medical devices) involved in the protocols that the IRB reviews.

(c) When must an IRB register ? Each IRB must submit an initial registration. The initial registration must occur before the IRB begins to review a clinical investigation described in paragraph (a) of this section. Each IRB must renew its registration every 3 years. IRB registration becomes effective after review and acceptance by HHS.

(d) Where can an IRB register ? Each IRB may register electronically throughhttp://ohrp.cit.nih.gov/efile. If an IRB lacks the ability to register electronically, it must send its registration information, in writing, to the Good Clinical Practice Program (HF-34), Office of Science and Health Coordination, Food and Drug Administration, 5600 Fishers Lane, Rockville, MD 20857.

(e) How does an IRB revise its registration information ? If an IRB's contact or chair person information changes, the IRB must revise its registration information by submitting any changes in that information within 90 days of the change. An IRB's decision to review new types of FDA-regulated products (such as a decision to review studies pertaining to food additives whereas the IRB previously reviewed studies pertaining to drug products), or to discontinue reviewing clinical investigations regulated by FDA is a change that must be reported within 30 days of the change. An IRB's decision to disband is a change that must be reported within 30 days of permanent cessation of the IRB's review of research. All other information changes may be reported when the IRB renews its registration. The revised information must be sent to FDA either electronically or in writing in accordance with paragraph (d) of this section.

[74 FR 2368, Jan. 15, 2009]

Sec. 56.107 IRB membership.

(a) Each IRB shall have at least five members, with varying backgrounds to promote complete and adequate review of research activities commonly conducted by the institution. The IRB shall be sufficiently qualified through the experience and expertise of its members, and the diversity of the members, including consideration of race, gender, cultural backgrounds, and sensitivity to such issues as community attitudes, to promote respect for its advice and counsel in safeguarding the rights and welfare of human subjects. In addition to possessing the professional competence necessary to review the specific research activities, the IRB shall be able to ascertain the acceptability of proposed research in terms of institutional commitments and regulations, applicable law, and standards or professional conduct and practice. The IRB shall therefore include persons knowledgeable in these areas. If an IRB regularly reviews research that involves a vulnerable category of subjects, such as children, prisoners, pregnant women, or handicapped or mentally disabled persons, consideration shall be given to the inclusion of one or

Part 56

more individuals who are knowledgeable about and experienced in working with those subjects.

b) Every nondiscriminatory effort will be made to ensure that no IRB consists entirely of men or entirely of women, including the instituton's consideration of qualified persons of both sexes, so long as no selection is made to the IRB on the basis of gender. No IRB may consist entirely of members of one profession.

(c) Each IRB shall include at least one member whose primary concerns are in the scientific area and at least one member whose primary concerns are in nonscientific areas.

(d) Each IRB shall include at least one member who is not otherwise affiliated with the institution and who is not part of the immediate family of a person who is affiliated with the institution.

(e) No IRB may have a member participate in the IRB's initial or continuing review of any project in which the member has a conflicting interest, except to provide information requested by the IRB.

(f) An IRB may, in its discretion, invite individuals with competence in special areas to assist in the review of complex issues which require expertise beyond or in addition to that available on the IRB. These individuals may not vote with the IRB.

[46 FR 8975, Jan 27, 1981, as amended at 56 FR 28028, June 18, 1991; 56 FR 29756, June 28, 1991]

Subpart C--IRB Functions and Operations

Sec. 56.108 IRB functions and operations.

In order to fulfill the requirements of these regulations, each IRB shall:

(a) Follow written procedures: (1) For conducting its initial and continuing review of research and for reporting its findings and actions to the investigator and the institution; (2) for determining which projects require review more often than annually and which projects need verification from sources other than the investigator that no material changes have occurred since previous IRB review; (3) for ensuring prompt reporting to the IRB of changes in research activity; and (4) for ensuring that changes in approved research, during the period for which IRB approval has already been given, may not be initiated without IRB review and approval except where necessary to eliminate apparent immediate hazards to the human subjects.

(b) Follow written procedures for ensuring prompt reporting to the IRB, appropriate institutional officials, and the Food and Drug Administration of: (1) Any unanticipated problems involving risks to human subjects or others; (2) any instance of serious or continuing noncompliance with these regulations or the requirements or determinations of the IRB; or (3) any suspension or termination of IRB approval.

(c) Except when an expedited review procedure is used (see 56.110), review proposed research at convened meetings at which a majority of the members of the IRB are present, including at least one member whose primary concerns are in nonscientific areas. In order for the research to be approved, it shall receive the approval of a majority of those members present at the meeting.

[46 FR 8975, Jan. 27, 1981, as amended at 56 FR 28028, June 18, 1991; 67 FR 9585, Mar. 4, 2002]

Sec. 56.109 IRB review of research.

(a) An IRB shall review and have authority to approve, require modifications in (to secure approval), or disapprove all research activities covered by these regulations.

(b) An IRB shall require that information given to subjects as part of informed consent is in accordance with 50.25. The IRB may require that information, in addition to that specifically mentioned in 50.25, be given to the subjects when in the IRB's judgment the information would meaningfully add to the protection of the rights and welfare of subjects.

(c) An IRB shall require documentation of informed consent in accordance with 50.27 of this chapter, except as follows:

  (1) The IRB may, for some or all subjects, waive the requirement that the subject, or the subject's legally authorized representative, sign a written consent form if it finds that the research presents no more than minimal risk of harm to

Part 56

subjects and involves no procedures for which written consent is normally required outside the research context; or

(2) The IRB may, for some or all subjects, find that the requirements in 50.24 of this chapter for an exception from informed consent for emergency research are met.

(d) In cases where the documentation requirement is waived under paragraph (c)(1) of this section, the IRB may require the investigator to provide subjects with a written statement regarding the research.

(e) An IRB shall notify investigators and the institution in writing of its decision to approve or disapprove the proposed research activity, or of modifications required to secure IRB approval of the research activity. If the IRB decides to disapprove a research activity, it shall include in its written notification a statement of the reasons for its decision and give the investigator an opportunity to respond in person or in writing. For investigations involving an exception to informed consent under 50.24 of this chapter, an IRB shall promptly notify in writing the investigator and the sponsor of the research when an IRB determines that it cannot approve the research because it does not meet the criteria in the exception provided under 50.24(a) of this chapter or because of other relevant ethical concerns. The written notification shall include a statement of the reasons for the IRB's determination.

(f) An IRB shall conduct continuing review of research covered by these regulations at intervals appropriate to the degree of risk, but not less than once per year, and shall have authority to observe or have a third party observe the consent process and the research.

(g) An IRB shall provide in writing to the sponsor of research involving an exception to informed consent under 50.24 of this chapter a copy of information that has been publicly disclosed under 50.24(a)(7)(ii) and (a)(7)(iii) of this chapter. The IRB shall provide this information to the sponsor promptly so that the sponsor is aware that such disclosure has occurred. Upon receipt, the sponsor shall provide copies of the information disclosed to FDA.

(h) When some or all of the subjects in a study are children, an IRB must determine that the research study is in compliance with part 50, subpart D of this chapter, at the time of its initial review of the research. When some or all of the subjects in a study that is ongoing on April 30, 2001 are children, an IRB must conduct a review of the research to determine compliance with part 50, subpart D of this chapter, either at the time of continuing review or, at the discretion of the IRB, at an earlier date.

[46 FR 8975, Jan. 27, 1981, as amended at 61 FR 51529, Oct. 2, 1996; 66 FR 20599, Apr. 24, 2001]

Sec. 56.110 Expedited review procedures for certain kinds of research involving no more than minimal risk, and for minor changes in approved research.

(a) The Food and Drug Administration has established, and published in theFederal Register,a list of categories of research that may be reviewed by the IRB through an expedited review procedure. The list will be amended, as appropriate, through periodic republication in theFederal Register.

(b) An IRB may use the expedited review procedure to review either or both of the following: (1) Some or all of the research appearing on the list and found by the reviewer(s) to involve no more than minimal risk, (2) minor changes in previously approved research during the period (of 1 year or less) for which approval is authorized. Under an expedited review procedure, the review may be carried out by the IRB chairperson or by one or more experienced reviewers designated by the IRB chairperson from among the members of the IRB. In reviewing the research, the reviewers may exercise all of the authorities of the IRB except that the reviewers may not disapprove the research. A research activity may be disapproved only after review in accordance with the nonexpedited review procedure set forth in 56.108(c).

(c) Each IRB which uses an expedited review procedure shall adopt a method for keeping all members advised of research proposals which have been approved under the procedure.

(d) The Food and Drug Administration may restrict, suspend, or terminate an institution's or IRB's use of the expedited review procedure when necessary to protect the rights or welfare of subjects.

[46 FR 8975, Jan. 27, 1981, as amended at 56 FR 28029, June 18, 1991]

Sec. 56.111 Criteria for IRB approval of research.

(a) In order to approve research covered by these regulations the IRB shall determine that all of the following requirements are satisfied:

(1) Risks to subjects are minimized: (i) By using procedures which are consistent with sound research design and which do not unnecessarily expose subjects to risk, and (ii) whenever appropriate, by using procedures already being performed on the subjects for diagnostic or treatment purposes.

(2) Risks to subjects are reasonable in relation to anticipated benefits, if any, to subjects, and the importance of the knowledge that may be expected to result. In evaluating risks and benefits, the IRB should consider only those risks and benefits that may result from the research (as distinguished from risks and benefits of therapies that subjects would receive even if not participating in the research). The IRB should not consider possible long-range effects of applying knowledge gained in the research (for example, the possible effects of the research on public policy) as among those research risks that fall within the purview of its responsibility.

(3) Selection of subjects is equitable. In making this assessment the IRB should take into account the purposes of the research and the setting in which the research will be conducted and should be particularly cognizant of the special problems of research involving vulnerable populations, such as children, prisoners, pregnant women, handicapped, or mentally disabled persons, or economically or educationally disadvantaged persons.

(4) Informed consent will be sought from each prospective subject or the subject's legally authorized representative, in accordance with and to the extent required by part 50.

(5) Informed consent will be appropriately documented, in accordance with and to the extent required by 50.27.

(6) Where appropriate, the research plan makes adequate provision for monitoring the data collected to ensure the safety of subjects.

(7) Where appropriate, there are adequate provisions to protect the privacy of subjects and to maintain the confidentiality of data.

(b) When some or all of the subjects, such as children, prisoners, pregnant women, handicapped, or mentally disabled persons, or economically or educationally disadvantaged persons, are likely to be vulnerable to coercion or undue influence additional safeguards have been included in the study to protect the rights and welfare of these subjects.

(c) In order to approve research in which some or all of the subjects are children, an IRB must determine that all research is in compliance with part 50, subpart D of this chapter.

[46 FR 8975, Jan. 27, 1981, as amended at 56 FR 28029, June 18, 1991; 66 FR 20599, Apr. 24, 2001]

Sec. 56.112 Review by institution.

Research covered by these regulations that has been approved by an IRB may be subject to further appropriate review and approval or disapproval by officials of the institution. However, those officials may not approve the research if it has not been approved by an IRB.

Sec. 56.113 Suspension or termination of IRB approval of research.

An IRB shall have authority to suspend or terminate approval of research that is not being conducted in accordance with the IRB's requirements or that has been associated with unexpected serious harm to subjects. Any suspension or termination of approval shall include a statement of the reasons for the IRB's action and shall be reported promptly to the investigator, appropriate institutional officials, and the Food and Drug Administration.

Sec. 56.114 Cooperative research.

In complying with these regulations, institutions involved in multi-institutional studies may use joint review, reliance upon the review of another qualified IRB, or similar arrangements aimed at avoidance of duplication of effort.

Part 56

Subpart D--Records and Reports

Sec. 56.115 IRB records.

(a) An institution, or where appropriate an IRB, shall prepare and maintain adequate documentation of IRB activities, including the following:

    (1) Copies of all research proposals reviewed, scientific evaluations, if any, that accompany the proposals, approved sample consent documents, progress reports submitted by investigators, and reports of injuries to subjects.

    (2) Minutes of IRB meetings which shall be in sufficient detail to show attendance at the meetings; actions taken by the IRB; the vote on these actions including the number of members voting for, against, and abstaining; the basis for requiring changes in or disapproving research; and a written summary of the discussion of controverted issues and their resolution.

    (3) Records of continuing review activities.

    (4) Copies of all correspondence between the IRB and the investigators.

    (5) A list of IRB members identified by name; earned degrees; representative capacity; indications of experience such as board certifications, licenses, etc., sufficient to describe each member's chief anticipated contributions to IRB deliberations; and any employment or other relationship between each member and the institution; for example: full-time employee, part-time employee, a member of governing panel or board, stockholder, paid or unpaid consultant.

    (6) Written procedures for the IRB as required by 56.108 (a) and (b).

    (7) Statements of significant new findings provided to subjects, as required by 50.25.

(b) The records required by this regulation shall be retained for at least 3 years after completion of the research, and the records shall be accessible for inspection and copying by authorized representatives of the Food and Drug Administration at reasonable times and in a reasonable manner.

(c) The Food and Drug Administration may refuse to consider a clinical investigation in support of an application for a research or marketing permit if the institution or the IRB that reviewed the investigation refuses to allow an inspection under this section.

[46 FR 8975, Jan. 27, 1981, as amended at 56 FR 28029, June 18, 1991; 67 FR 9585, Mar. 4, 2002]

Subpart E--Administrative Actions for Noncompliance

Sec. 56.120 Lesser administrative actions.

(a) If apparent noncompliance with these regulations in the operation of an IRB is observed by an FDA investigator during an inspection, the inspector will present an oral or written summary of observations to an appropriate representative of the IRB. The Food and Drug Administration may subsequently send a letter describing the noncompliance to the IRB and to the parent institution. The agency will require that the IRB or the parent institution respond to this letter within a time period specified by FDA and describe the corrective actions that will be taken by the IRB, the institution, or both to achieve compliance with these regulations.

(b) On the basis of the IRB's or the institution's response, FDA may schedule a reinspection to confirm the adequacy of corrective actions. In addition, until the IRB or the parent institution takes appropriate corrective action, the agency may:

   (1) Withhold approval of new studies subject to the requirements of this part that are conducted at the institution or reviewed by the IRB;

   (2) Direct that no new subjects be added to ongoing studies subject to this part;

   (3) Terminate ongoing studies subject to this part when doing so would not endanger the subjects; or

   (4) When the apparent noncompliance creates a significant threat to the rights and welfare of human subjects, notify relevant State and Federal regulatory agencies and other parties with a direct interest in the agency's action of the deficiencies in the operation of the IRB.

Part 56

(c) The parent institution is presumed to be responsible for the operation of an IRB, and the Food and Drug Administration will ordinarily direct any administrative action under this subpart against the institution. However, depending on the evidence of responsibility for deficiencies, determined during the investigation, the Food and Drug Administration may restrict its administrative actions to the IRB or to a component of the parent institution determined to be responsible for formal designation of the IRB.

Sec. 56.121 Disqualification of an IRB or an institution.

(a) Whenever the IRB or the institution has failed to take adequate steps to correct the noncompliance stated in the letter sent by the agency under 56.120(a), and the Commissioner of Food and Drugs determines that this noncompliance may justify the disqualification of the IRB or of the parent institution, the Commissioner will institute proceedings in accordance with the requirements for a regulatory hearing set forth in part 16.

(b) The Commissioner may disqualify an IRB or the parent institution if the Commissioner determines that:

(1) The IRB has refused or repeatedly failed to comply with any of the regulations set forth in this part, and

(2) The noncompliance adversely affects the rights or welfare of the human subjects in a clinical investigation.

(c) If the Commissioner determines that disqualification is appropriate, the Commissioner will issue an order that explains the basis for the determination and that prescribes any actions to be taken with regard to ongoing clinical research conducted under the review of the IRB. The Food and Drug Administration will send notice of the disqualification to the IRB and the parent institution. Other parties with a direct interest, such as sponsors and clinical investigators, may also be sent a notice of the disqualification. In addition, the agency may elect to publish a notice of its action in theFederal Register.

(d) The Food and Drug Administration will not approve an application for a research permit for a clinical investigation that is to be under the review of a disqualified IRB or that is to be conducted at a disqualified institution, and it may refuse to consider in support of a marketing permit the data from a clinical investigation that was reviewed by a disqualified IRB as conducted at a disqualified institution, unless the IRB or the parent institution is reinstated as provided in 56.123.

Sec. 56.122 Public disclosure of information regarding revocation.

A determination that the Food and Drug Administration has disqualified an institution and the administrative record regarding that determination are disclosable to the public under part 20.

Sec. 56.123 Reinstatement of an IRB or an institution.

An IRB or an institution may be reinstated if the Commissioner determines, upon an evaluation of a written submission from the IRB or institution that explains the corrective action that the institution or IRB plans to take, that the IRB or institution has provided adequate assurance that it will operate in compliance with the standards set forth in this part. Notification of reinstatement shall be provided to all persons notified under 56.121(c).

Sec. 56.124 Actions alternative or additional to disqualification.

Disqualification of an IRB or of an institution is independent of, and neither in lieu of nor a precondition to, other proceedings or actions authorized by the act. The Food and Drug Administration may, at any time, through the Department of Justice institute any appropriate judicial proceedings (civil or criminal) and any other appropriate regulatory action, in addition to or in lieu of, and before, at the time of, or after, disqualification. The agency may also refer pertinent matters to another Federal, State, or local government agency for any action that that agency determines to be appropriate.

Authority: 21 U.S.C. 321, 343, 346, 346a, 348, 350a, 350b, 351, 352, 353, 355, 360, 360c-360f, 360h-360j, 371, 379e, 381; 42 U.S.C. 216, 241, 262, 263b-263n.

Source: 46 FR 8975, Jan. 27, 1981, unless otherwise noted.

Part 56

Part 58: Good Laboratory Practice for Nonclinical Laboratory Studies

[Code of Federal Regulations]

[Title 21, Volume 1]

[Revised as of April 1, 2009]

[CITE: 21CFR58]

Title 21--Food and Drugs

Chapter I--Food and Drug Administration

Department of Health and Human Services

Subchapter A--General

Part 58 Good Laboratory Practice for Nonclinical Laboratory Studies[1]

Subpart A--General Provisions

Sec. 58.1 Scope.

(a) This part prescribes good laboratory practices for conducting nonclinical laboratory studies that support or are intended to support applications for research or marketing permits for products regulated by the Food and Drug Administration, including food and color additives, animal food additives, human and animal drugs, medical devices for human use, biological products, and electronic products. Compliance with this part is intended to assure the quality and integrity of the safety data filed pursuant to sections 406, 408, 409, 502, 503, 505, 506, 510, 512-516, 518-520, 721, and 801 of the Federal Food, Drug, and

---

[1] Available on the FDA website at http://www.accessdata.fda.gov/scripts/cdrh/cfdocs/cfcfr/CFRSearch.cfm?CFRPart=58&showFR=1

Cosmetic Act and sections 351 and 354-360F of the Public Health Service Act.

(b) References in this part to regulatory sections of the Code of Federal Regulations are to chapter I of title 21, unless otherwise noted.

[43 FR 60013, Dec. 22, 1978, as amended at 52 FR 33779, Sept. 4, 1987; 64 FR 399, Jan. 5, 1999]

Sec. 58.3 Definitions.

As used in this part, the following terms shall have the meanings specified:

(a) *Act* means the Federal Food, Drug, and Cosmetic Act, as amended (secs. 201-902, 52 Stat. 1040et seq., as amended (21 U.S.C. 321-392)).

(b) *Test article* means any food additive, color additive, drug, biological product, electronic product, medical device for human use, or any other article subject to regulation under the act or under sections 351 and 354-360F of the Public Health Service Act.

(c) *Control article* means any food additive, color additive, drug, biological product, electronic product, medical device for human use, or any article other than a test article, feed, or water that is administered to the test system in the course of a nonclinical laboratory study for the purpose of establishing a basis for comparison with the test article.

(d) *Nonclinical laboratory study* means in vivo or in vitro experiments in which test articles are studied prospectively in test systems under laboratory conditions to determine their safety. The term does not include studies utilizing human subjects or clinical studies or field trials in animals. The term does not include basic exploratory studies carried out to determine whether a test article has any potential utility or to determine physical or chemical characteristics of a test article.

(e) *Application for research or marketing permit* includes:

(1) A color additive petition, described in part 71.

(2) A food additive petition, described in parts 171 and 571.

(3) Data and information regarding a substance submitted as part of the procedures for establishing that a substance is generally recognized as safe for use, which use results or may reasonably be expected to result, directly or indirectly, in its becoming a component or otherwise affecting the characteristics of any food, described in 170.35 and 570.35.

(4) Data and information regarding a food additive submitted as part of the procedures regarding food additives permitted to be used on an interim basis pending additional study, described in 180.1.

(5) Aninvestigational new drug application, described in part 312 of this chapter.

(6) Anew drug application, described in part 314.

(7) Data and information regarding an over-the-counter drug for human use, submitted as part of the procedures for classifying such drugs as generally recognized as safe and effective and not misbranded, described in part 330.

(8) Data and information about a substance submitted as part of the procedures for establishing a tolerance for unavoidable contaminants in food and food-packaging materials, described in parts 109 and 509.

(9) [Reserved]

(10) A Notice of Claimed Investigational Exemption for a New Animal Drug, described in part 511.

(11) A new animal drug application, described in part 514.

(12) [Reserved]

(13) An application for a biologics license, described in part 601 of this chapter.

(14) An application for an investigational device exemption, described in part 812.

(15) An Application for Premarket Approval of a Medical Device, described in section 515 of the act.

(16) A Product Development Protocol for a Medical Device, described in section 515 of the act.

(17) Data and information regarding a medical device submitted as part of the procedures for classifying such devices, described in part 860.

Part 58

(18) Data and information regarding a medical device submitted as part of the procedures for establishing, amending, or repealing a performance standard for such devices, described in part 861.

(19) Data and information regarding an electronic product submitted as part of the procedures for obtaining an exemption from notification of a radiation safety defect or failure of compliance with a radiation safety performance standard, described in subpart D of part 1003.

(20) Data and information regarding an electronic product submitted as part of the procedures for establishing, amending, or repealing a standard for such product, described in section 358 of the Public Health Service Act.

(21) Data and information regarding an electronic product submitted as part of the procedures for obtaining a variance from any electronic product performance standard as described in 1010.4.

(22) Data and information regarding an electronic product submitted as part of the procedures for granting, amending, or extending an exemption from any electronic product performance standard, as described in 1010.5.

(23) A premarket notification for a food contact substance, described in part 170, subpart D, of this chapter.

(f) *Sponsor* means:

(1) A person who initiates and supports, by provision of financial or other resources, a nonclinical laboratory study;

(2) A person who submits a nonclinical study to the Food and Drug Administration in support of an application for a research or marketing permit; or

(3) A testing facility, if it both initiates and actually conducts the study.

(g) *Testing facility* means a person who actually conducts a nonclinical laboratory study, i.e., actually uses the test article in a test system. Testing facility includes any establishment required to register under section 510 of the act that conducts nonclinical laboratory studies and any consulting laboratory described in section 704 of the act that conducts such studies. Testing facility encompasses only those operational units that are being or have been used to conduct nonclinical laboratory studies.

(h) *Person* includes an individual, partnership, corporation, association, scientific or academic establishment, government agency, or organizational unit thereof, and any other legal entity.

(i) Test system means any animal, plant, microorganism, or subparts thereof to which the test or control article is administered or added for study. Test system also includes appropriate groups or components of the system not treated with the test or control articles.

(j) *Specimen* means any material derived from a test system for examination or analysis.

(k) *Raw data* means any laboratory worksheets, records, memoranda, notes, or exact copies thereof, that are the result of original observations and activities of a nonclinical laboratory study and are necessary for the reconstruction and evaluation of the report of that study. In the event that exact transcripts of raw data have been prepared (e.g., tapes which have been transcribed verbatim, dated, and verified accurate by signature), the exact copy or exact transcript may be substituted for the original source as raw data. Raw data may include photographs, microfilm or microfiche copies, computer printouts, magnetic media, including dictated observations, and recorded data from automated instruments.

(l) *Quality assurance unit* means any person or organizational element, except the study director, designated by testing facility management to perform the duties relating to quality assurance of nonclinical laboratory studies.

(m) *Study director* means the individual responsible for the overall conduct of a nonclinical laboratory study.

(n) *Batch* means a specific quantity or lot of a test or control article that has been characterized according to 58.105(a).

(o) *Study initiation date* means the date the protocol is signed by the study director.

(p) *Study completion date* means the date the final report is signed by the study director.

Part 58

[43 FR 60013, Dec. 22, 1978, as amended at 52 FR 33779, Sept. 4, 1987; 54 FR 9039, Mar. 3, 1989; 64 FR 56448, Oct. 20, 1999; 67 FR 35729, May 21, 2002]

Sec. 58.10 Applicability to studies performed under grants and contracts.

When a sponsor conducting a nonclinical laboratory study intended to be submitted to or reviewed by the Food and Drug Administration utilizes the services of a consulting laboratory, contractor, or grantee to perform an analysis or other service, it shall notify the consulting laboratory, contractor, or grantee that the service is part of a nonclinical laboratory study that must be conducted in compliance with the provisions of this part.

Sec. 58.15 Inspection of a testing facility.

(a) A testing facility shall permit an authorized employee of the Food and Drug Administration, at reasonable times and in a reasonable manner, to inspect the facility and to inspect (and in the case of records also to copy) all records and specimens required to be maintained regarding studies within the scope of this part. The records inspection and copying requirements shall not apply to quality assurance unit records of findings and problems, or to actions recommended and taken.

(b) The Food and Drug Administration will not consider a nonclinical laboratory study in support of an application for a research or marketing permit if the testing facility refuses to permit inspection. The determination that a nonclinical laboratory study will not be considered in support of an application for a research or marketing permit does not, however, relieve the applicant for such a permit of any obligation under any applicable statute or regulation to submit the results of the study to the Food and Drug Administration.

Subpart B--Organization and Personnel

Sec. 58.29 Personnel.

(a) Each individual engaged in the conduct of or responsible for the supervision of a nonclinical laboratory study shall have education, training, and experience, or combination thereof, to enable that individual to perform the assigned functions.

(b) Each testing facility shall maintain a current summary of training and experience and job description for each individual engaged in or supervising the conduct of a nonclinical laboratory study.

(c) There shall be a sufficient number of personnel for the timely and proper conduct of the study according to the protocol.

(d) Personnel shall take necessary personal sanitation and health precautions designed to avoid contamination of test and control articles and test systems.

(e) Personnel engaged in a nonclinical laboratory study shall wear clothing appropriate for the duties they perform. Such clothing shall be changed as often as necessary to prevent microbiological, radiological, or chemical contamination of test systems and test and control articles.

(f) Any individual found at any time to have an illness that may adversely affect the quality and integrity of the nonclinical laboratory study shall be excluded from direct contact with test systems, test and control articles and any other operation or function that may adversely affect the study until the condition is corrected. All personnel shall be instructed to report to their immediate supervisors any health or medical conditions that may reasonably be considered to have an adverse effect on a nonclinical laboratory study.

Sec. 58.31 Testing facility management.

For each nonclinical laboratory study, testing facility management shall:

(a) Designate a study director as described in 58.33, before the study is initiated.

(b) Replace the study director promptly if it becomes necessary to do so during the conduct of a study.

(c) Assure that there is a quality assurance unit as described in 58.35.

(d) Assure that test and control articles or mixtures have been appropriately tested for identity, strength, purity, stability, and uniformity, as applicable.

Part 58

(e) Assure that personnel, resources, facilities, equipment, materials, and methodologies are available as scheduled.

(f) Assure that personnel clearly understand the functions they are to perform.

(g) Assure that any deviations from these regulations reported by the quality assurance unit are communicated to the study director and corrective actions are taken and documented.

[43 FR 60013, Dec. 22, 1978, as amended at 52 FR 33780, Sept. 4, 1987]

Sec. 58.33 Study director.

For each nonclinical laboratory study, a scientist or other professional of appropriate education, training, and experience, or combination thereof, shall be identified as the study director. The study director has overall responsibility for the technical conduct of the study, as well as for the interpretation, analysis, documentation and reporting of results, and represents the single point of study control. The study director shall assure that:

(a) The protocol, including any change, is approved as provided by 58.120 and is followed.

(b) All experimental data, including observations of unanticipated responses of the test system are accurately recorded and verified.

(c) Unforeseen circumstances that may affect the quality and integrity of the nonclinical laboratory study are noted when they occur, and corrective action is taken and documented.

(d) Test systems are as specified in the protocol.

(e) All applicable good laboratory practice regulations are followed.

(f) All raw data, documentation, protocols, specimens, and final reports are transferred to the archives during or at the close of the study.

[43 FR 60013, Dec. 22, 1978; 44 FR 17657, Mar. 23, 1979]

Sec. 58.35 Quality assurance unit.

(a) A testing facility shall have a quality assurance unit which shall be responsible for monitoring each study to assure management that the facilities, equipment, personnel, methods, practices, records, and controls are in conformance with the regulations in this part. For any given study, the quality assurance unit shall be entirely separate from and independent of the personnel engaged in the direction and conduct of that study.

(b) The quality assurance unit shall:

(1) Maintain a copy of a master schedule sheet of all nonclinical laboratory studies conducted at the testing facility indexed by test article and containing the test system, nature of study, date study was initiated, current status of each study, identity of the sponsor, and name of the study director.

(2) Maintain copies of all protocols pertaining to all nonclinical laboratory studies for which the unit is responsible.

(3) Inspect each nonclinical laboratory study at intervals adequate to assure the integrity of the study and maintain written and properly signed records of each periodic inspection showing the date of the inspection, the study inspected, the phase or segment of the study inspected, the person performing the inspection, findings and problems, action recommended and taken to resolve existing problems, and any scheduled date for reinspection. Any problems found during the course of an inspection which are likely to affect study integrity shall be brought to the attention of the study director and management immediately.

(4) Periodically submit to management and the study director written status reports on each study, noting any problems and the corrective actions taken.

(5) Determine that no deviations from approved protocols or standard operating procedures were made without proper authorization and documentation.

(6) Review the final study report to assure that such report accurately describes the methods and standard operating procedures, and that the reported results accurately reflect the raw data of the nonclinical laboratory study.

Part 58

(7) Prepare and sign a statement to be included with the final study report which shall specify the dates inspections were made and findings reported to management and to the study director.

(c) The responsibilities and procedures applicable to the quality assurance unit, the records maintained by the quality assurance unit, and the method of indexing such records shall be in writing and shall be maintained. These items including inspection dates, the study inspected, the phase or segment of the study inspected, and the name of the individual performing the inspection shall be made available for inspection to authorized employees of the Food and Drug Administration.

(d) A designated representative of the Food and Drug Administration shall have access to the written procedures established for the inspection and may request testing facility management to certify that inspections are being implemented, performed, documented, and followed-up in accordance with this paragraph.

[43 FR 60013, Dec. 22, 1978, as amended at 52 FR 33780, Sept. 4, 1987; 67 FR 9585, Mar. 4, 2002]

Subpart C--Facilities

Sec. 58.41 General.

Each testing facility shall be of suitable size and construction to facilitate the proper conduct of nonclinical laboratory studies. It shall be designed so that there is a degree of separation that will prevent any function or activity from having an adverse effect on the study.

[52 FR 33780, Sept. 4, 1987]

Sec. 58.43 Animal care facilities.

(a) A testing facility shall have a sufficient number of animal rooms or areas, as needed, to assure proper: (1) Separation of species or test systems, (2) isolation of individual projects, (3) quarantine of animals, and (4) routine or specialized housing of animals.

(b) A testing facility shall have a number of animal rooms or areas separate from those described in paragraph (a) of this section to ensure isolation of studies being done with test systems or test and control articles known to be biohazardous, including volatile substances, aerosols, radioactive materials, and infectious agents.

(c) Separate areas shall be provided, as appropriate, for the diagnosis, treatment, and control of laboratory animal diseases. These areas shall provide effective isolation for the housing of animals either known or suspected of being diseased, or of being carriers of disease, from other animals.

(d) When animals are housed, facilities shall exist for the collection and disposal of all animal waste and refuse or for safe sanitary storage of waste before removal from the testing facility. Disposal facilities shall be so provided and operated as to minimize vermin infestation, odors, disease hazards, and environmental contamination.

[43 FR 60013, Dec. 22, 1978, as amended at 52 FR 33780, Sept. 4, 1987]

Sec. 58.45 Animal supply facilities.

There shall be storage areas, as needed, for feed, bedding, supplies, and equipment. Storage areas for feed and bedding shall be separated from areas housing the test systems and shall be protected against infestation or contamination. Perishable supplies shall be preserved by appropriate means.

[43 FR 60013, Dec. 22, 1978, as amended at 52 FR 33780, Sept. 4, 1987]

Sec. 58.47 Facilities for handling test and control articles.

(a) As necessary to prevent contamination or mixups, there shall be separate areas for:

(1) Receipt and storage of the test and control articles.

(2) Mixing of the test and control articles with a carrier, e.g., feed.

(3) Storage of the test and control article mixtures.

(b) Storage areas for the test and/or control article and test and control mixtures shall be separate from areas housing the test systems and shall be adequate to preserve the identity, strength, purity, and stability of the articles and mixtures.

Sec. 58.49 Laboratory operation areas.

Separate laboratory space shall be provided, as needed, for the performance of the routine and specialized procedures required by nonclinical laboratory studies.

[52 FR 33780, Sept. 4, 1987]

Sec. 58.51 Specimen and data storage facilities.

Space shall be provided for archives, limited to access by authorized personnel only, for the storage and retrieval of all raw data and specimens from completed studies.

Subpart D--Equipment

Sec. 58.61 Equipment design.

Equipment used in the generation, measurement, or assessment of data and equipment used for facility environmental control shall be of appropriate design and adequate capacity to function according to the protocol and shall be suitably located for operation, inspection, cleaning, and maintenance.

[52 FR 33780, Sept. 4, 1987]

Sec. 58.63 Maintenance and calibration of equipment.

(a) Equipment shall be adequately inspected, cleaned, and maintained. Equipment used for the generation, measurement, or assessment of data shall be adequately tested, calibrated and/or standardized.

(b) The written standard operating procedures required under 58.81(b)(11) shall set forth in sufficient detail the methods, materials, and schedules to be used in the routine inspection, cleaning, maintenance, testing, calibration, and/or standardization of equipment, and shall specify, when appropriate, remedial action to be taken in the event of failure or malfunction of equipment. The written standard operating procedures shall designate the person responsible for the performance of each operation.

(c) Written records shall be maintained of all inspection, maintenance, testing, calibrating and/or standardizing operations. These records, containing the date of the operation, shall describe whether the maintenance operations were routine and followed the written standard operating procedures. Written records shall be kept of nonroutine repairs performed on equipment as a result of failure and malfunction. Such records shall document the nature of the defect, how and when the defect was discovered, and any remedial action taken in response to the defect.

[43 FR 60013, Dec. 22, 1978, as amended at 52 FR 33780, Sept. 4, 1987; 67 FR 9585, Mar. 4, 2002]

Subpart E--Testing Facilities Operation

Sec. 58.81 Standard operating procedures.

(a) A testing facility shall have standard operating procedures in writing setting forth nonclinical laboratory study methods that management is satisfied are adequate to insure the quality and integrity of the data generated in the course of a study. All deviations in a study from standard operating procedures shall be authorized by the study director and shall be documented in the raw data. Significant changes in established standard operating procedures shall be properly authorized in writing by management.

(b) Standard operating procedures shall be established for, but not limited to, the following:

(1) Animal room preparation.

(2) Animal care.

(3) Receipt, identification, storage, handling, mixing, and method of sampling of the test and control articles.

(4) Test system observations.

(5) Laboratory tests.

(6) Handling of animals found moribund or dead during study.

(7) Necropsy of animals or postmortem examination of animals.

(8) Collection and identification of specimens.

(9) Histopathology.

(10) Data handling, storage, and retrieval.

(11) Maintenance and calibration of equipment.

Part 58

(12) Transfer, proper placement, and identification of animals.

(c) Each laboratory area shall have immediately available laboratory manuals and standard operating procedures relative to the laboratory procedures being performed. Published literature may be used as a supplement to standard operating procedures.

(d) A historical file of standard operating procedures, and all revisions thereof, including the dates of such revisions, shall be maintained.

[43 FR 60013, Dec. 22, 1978, as amended at 52 FR 33780, Sept. 4, 1987]

Sec. 58.83 Reagents and solutions.

All reagents and solutions in the laboratory areas shall be labeled to indicate identity, titer or concentration, storage requirements, and expiration date. Deteriorated or outdated reagents and solutions shall not be used.

Sec. 58.90 Animal care.

(a) There shall be standard operating procedures for the housing, feeding, handling, and care of animals.

(b) All newly received animals from outside sources shall be isolated and their health status shall be evaluated in accordance with acceptable veterinary medical practice.

(c) At the initiation of a nonclinical laboratory study, animals shall be free of any disease or condition that might interfere with the purpose or conduct of the study. If, during the course of the study, the animals contract such a disease or condition, the diseased animals shall be isolated, if necessary. These animals may be treated for disease or signs of disease provided that such treatment does not interfere with the study. The diagnosis, authorizations of treatment, description of treatment, and each date of treatment shall be documented and shall be retained.

(d) Warm-blooded animals, excluding suckling rodents, used in laboratory procedures that require manipulations and observations over an extended period of time or in studies that require the animals to be removed from and returned to their home cages for any reason (e.g., cage cleaning, treatment, etc.), shall receive appropriate identification. All information needed to specifically identify each animal within an animal-housing unit shall appear on the outside of that unit.

(e) Animals of different species shall be housed in separate rooms when necessary. Animals of the same species, but used in different studies, should not ordinarily be housed in the same room when inadvertent exposure to control or test articles or animal mixup could affect the outcome of either study. If such mixed housing is necessary, adequate differentiation by space and identification shall be made.

(f) Animal cages, racks and accessory equipment shall be cleaned and sanitized at appropriate intervals.

(g) Feed and water used for the animals shall be analyzed periodically to ensure that contaminants known to be capable of interfering with the study and reasonably expected to be present in such feed or water are not present at levels above those specified in the protocol. Documentation of such analyses shall be maintained as raw data.

(h) Bedding used in animal cages or pens shall not interfere with the purpose or conduct of the study and shall be changed as often as necessary to keep the animals dry and clean.

(i) If any pest control materials are used, the use shall be documented. Cleaning and pest control materials that interfere with the study shall not be used.

[43 FR 60013, Dec. 22, 1978, as amended at 52 FR 33780, Sept. 4, 1987; 54 FR 15924, Apr. 20, 1989; 56 FR 32088, July 15, 1991; 67 FR 9585, Mar. 4, 2002]

Subpart F--Test and Control Articles

Sec. 58.105 Test and control article characterization.

(a) The identity, strength, purity, and composition or other characteristics which will appropriately define the test or control article shall be determined for each batch and shall be documented. Methods of synthesis, fabrication, or derivation of the test and control articles shall be documented by the sponsor or the testing facility. In those cases where marketed products are used as control articles, such products will be characterized by their labeling.

Part 58

(b) The stability of each test or control article shall be determined by the testing facility or by the sponsor either: (1) Before study initiation, or (2) concomitantly according to written standard operating procedures, which provide for periodic analysis of each batch.

(c) Each storage container for a test or control article shall be labeled by name, chemical abstract number or code number, batch number, expiration date, if any, and, where appropriate, storage conditions necessary to maintain the identity, strength, purity, and composition of the test or control article. Storage containers shall be assigned to a particular test article for the duration of the study.

(d) For studies of more than 4 weeks' duration, reserve samples from each batch of test and control articles shall be retained for the period of time provided by 58.195.

[43 FR 60013, Dec. 22, 1978, as amended at 52 FR 33781, Sept. 4, 1987; 67 FR 9585, Mar. 4, 2002]

Sec. 58.107 Test and control article handling.

Procedures shall be established for a system for the handling of the test and control articles to ensure that:

(a) There is proper storage.

(b) Distribution is made in a manner designed to preclude the possibility of contamination, deterioration, or damage.

(c) Proper identification is maintained throughout the distribution process.

(d) The receipt and distribution of each batch is documented. Such documentation shall include the date and quantity of each batch distributed or returned.

Sec. 58.113 Mixtures of articles with carriers.

(a) For each test or control article that is mixed with a carrier, tests by appropriate analytical methods shall be conducted:

(1) To determine the uniformity of the mixture and to determine, periodically, the concentration of the test or control article in the mixture.

(2) To determine the stability of the test and control articles in the mixture as required by the conditions of the study either:

    (i) Before study initiation, or

    (ii) Concomitantly according to written standard operating procedures which provide for periodic analysis of the test and control articles in the mixture.

(b) [Reserved]

(c) Where any of the components of the test or control article carrier mixture has an expiration date, that date shall be clearly shown on the container. If more than one component has an expiration date, the earliest date shall be shown.

[43 FR 60013, Dec. 22, 1978, as amended at 45 FR 24865, Apr. 11, 1980; 52 FR 33781, Sept. 4, 1987]

Subpart G--Protocol for and Conduct of a Nonclinical Laboratory Study

Sec. 58.120 Protocol.

(a) Each study shall have an approved written protocol that clearly indicates the objectives and all methods for the conduct of the study. The protocol shall contain, as applicable, the following information:

(1) A descriptive title and statement of the purpose of the study.

(2) Identification of the test and control articles by name, chemical abstract number, or code number.

(3) The name of the sponsor and the name and address of the testing facility at which the study is being conducted.

(4) The number, body weight range, sex, source of supply, species, strain, substrain, and age of the test system.

(5) The procedure for identification of the test system.

(6) A description of the experimental design, including the methods for the control of bias.

(7) A description and/or identification of the diet used in the study as well as solvents, emulsifiers, and/or other materials used to solubilize or suspend the test or control articles

Part 58

before mixing with the carrier. The description shall include specifications for acceptable levels of contaminants that are reasonably expected to be present in the dietary materials and are known to be capable of interfering with the purpose or conduct of the study if present at levels greater than established by the specifications.

(8) Each dosage level, expressed in milligrams per kilogram of body weight or other appropriate units, of the test or control article to be administered and the method and frequency of administration.

(9) The type and frequency of tests, analyses, and measurements to be made.

(10) The records to be maintained.

(11) The date of approval of the protocol by the sponsor and the dated signature of the study director.

(12) A statement of the proposed statistical methods to be used.

(b) All changes in or revisions of an approved protocol and the reasons therefore shall be documented, signed by the study director, dated, and maintained with the protocol.

[43 FR 60013, Dec. 22, 1978, as amended at 52 FR 33781, Sept. 4, 1987; 67 FR 9585, Mar. 4, 2002]

Sec. 58.130 Conduct of a nonclinical laboratory study.

(a) The nonclinical laboratory study shall be conducted in accordance with the protocol.

(b) The test systems shall be monitored in conformity with the protocol.

(c) Specimens shall be identified by test system, study, nature, and date of collection. This information shall be located on the specimen container or shall accompany the specimen in a manner that precludes error in the recording and storage of data.

(d) Records of gross findings for a specimen from postmortem observations should be available to a pathologist when examining that specimen histopathologically.

(e) All data generated during the conduct of a nonclinical laboratory study, except those that are generated by automated data collection systems, shall be recorded directly, promptly, and legibly in ink. All data entries shall be dated on the date of entry and signed or initialed by the person entering the data. Any change in entries shall be made so as not to obscure the original entry, shall indicate the reason for such change, and shall be dated and signed or identified at the time of the change. In automated data collection systems, the individual responsible for direct data input shall be identified at the time of data input. Any change in automated data entries shall be made so as not to obscure the original entry, shall indicate the reason for change, shall be dated, and the responsible individual shall be identified.

[43 FR 60013, Dec. 22, 1978, as amended at 52 FR 33781, Sept. 4, 1987; 67 FR 9585, Mar. 4, 2002]

Subparts H-I [Reserved]

Subpart J--Records and Reports

Sec. 58.185 Reporting of nonclinical laboratory study results.

(a) A final report shall be prepared for each nonclinical laboratory study and shall include, but not necessarily be limited to, the following:

  (1) Name and address of the facility performing the study and the dates on which the study was initiated and completed.

  (2) Objectives and procedures stated in the approved protocol, including any changes in the original protocol.

  (3) Statistical methods employed for analyzing the data.

  (4) The test and control articles identified by name, chemical abstracts number or code number, strength, purity, and composition or other appropriate characteristics.

  (5) Stability of the test and control articles under the conditions of administration.

  (6) A description of the methods used.

  (7) A description of the test system used. Where applicable, the final report shall include the number of animals used, sex,

Part 58

body weight range, source of supply, species, strain and substrain, age, and procedure used for identification.

(8) A description of the dosage, dosage regimen, route of administration, and duration.

(9) A description of all cirmcumstances that may have affected the quality or integrity of the data.

(10) The name of the study director, the names of other scientists or professionals, and the names of all supervisory personnel, involved in the study.

(11) A description of the transformations, calculations, or operations performed on the data, a summary and analysis of the data, and a statement of the conclusions drawn from the analysis.

(12) The signed and dated reports of each of the individual scientists or other professionals involved in the study.

(13) The locations where all specimens, raw data, and the final report are to be stored.

(14) The statement prepared and signed by the quality assurance unit as described in 58.35(b)(7).

(b) The final report shall be signed and dated by the study director.

(c) Corrections or additions to a final report shall be in the form of an amendment by the study director. The amendment shall clearly identify that part of the final report that is being added to or corrected and the reasons for the correction or addition, and shall be signed and dated by the person responsible.

[43 FR 60013, Dec. 22, 1978, as amended at 52 FR 33781, Sept. 4, 1987]

Sec. 58.190 Storage and retrieval of records and data.

(a) All raw data, documentation, protocols, final reports, and specimens (except those specimens obtained from mutagenicity tests and wet specimens of blood, urine, feces, and biological fluids) generated as a result of a nonclinical laboratory study shall be retained.

(b) There shall be archives for orderly storage and expedient retrieval of all raw data, documentation, protocols, specimens, and interim and final reports. Conditions of storage shall minimize deterioration of the documents or specimens in accordance with the requirements for the time period of their retention and the nature of the documents or specimens. A testing facility may contract with commercial archives to provide a repository for all material to be retained. Raw data and specimens may be retained elsewhere provided that the archives have specific reference to those other locations.

(c) An individual shall be identified as responsible for the archives.

(d) Only authorized personnel shall enter the archives.

(e) Material retained or referred to in the archives shall be indexed to permit expedient retrieval.

[43 FR 60013, Dec. 22, 1978, as amended at 52 FR 33781, Sept. 4, 1987; 67 FR 9585, Mar. 4, 2002]

Sec. 58.195 Retention of records.

(a) Record retention requirements set forth in this section do not supersede the record retention requirements of any other regulations in this chapter.

(b) Except as provided in paragraph (c) of this section, documentation records, raw data and specimens pertaining to a nonclinical laboratory study and required to be made by this part shall be retained in the archive(s) for whichever of the following periods is shortest:

(1) A period of at least 2 years following the date on which an application for a research or marketing permit, in support of which the results of the nonclinical laboratory study were submitted, is approved by the Food and Drug Administration. This requirement does not apply to studies supporting investigational new drug applications (IND's) or applications for investigational device exemptions (IDE's), records of which shall be governed by the provisions of paragraph (b)(2) of this section.

(2) A period of at least 5 years following the date on which the results of the nonclinical laboratory study are submitted to the Food and Drug Administration in support of an application for a research or marketing permit.

Part 58

(3) In other situations (e.g., where the nonclinical laboratory study does not result in the submission of the study in support of an application for a research or marketing permit), a period of at least 2 years following the date on which the study is completed, terminated, or discontinued.

(c) Wet specimens (except those specimens obtained from mutagenicity tests and wet specimens of blood, urine, feces, and biological fluids), samples of test or control articles, and specially prepared material, which are relatively fragile and differ markedly in stability and quality during storage, shall be retained only as long as the quality of the preparation affords evaluation. In no case shall retention be required for longer periods than those set forth in paragraphs (a) and (b) of this section.

(d) The master schedule sheet, copies of protocols, and records of quality assurance inspections, as required by 58.35(c) shall be maintained by the quality assurance unit as an easily accessible system of records for the period of time specified in paragraphs (a) and (b) of this section.

(e) Summaries of training and experience and job descriptions required to be maintained by 58.29(b) may be retained along with all other testing facility employment records for the length of time specified in paragraphs (a) and (b) of this section.

(f) Records and reports of the maintenance and calibration and inspection of equipment, as required by 58.63(b) and (c), shall be retained for the length of time specified in paragraph (b) of this section.

(g) Records required by this part may be retained either as original records or as true copies such as photocopies, microfilm, microfiche, or other accurate reproductions of the original records.

(h) If a facility conducting nonclinical testing goes out of business, all raw data, documentation, and other material specified in this section shall be transferred to the archives of the sponsor of the study. The Food and Drug Administration shall be notified in writing of such a transfer.

[43 FR 60013, Dec. 22, 1978, as amended at 52 FR 33781, Sept. 4, 1987; 54 FR 9039, Mar. 3, 1989]

Subpart K--Disqualification of Testing Facilities

Sec. 58.200 Purpose.

(a) The purposes of disqualification are:

(1) To permit the exclusion from consideration of completed studies that were conducted by a testing facility which has failed to comply with the requirements of the good laboratory practice regulations until it can be adequately demonstrated that such noncompliance did not occur during, or did not affect the validity or acceptability of data generated by, a particular study; and

(2) To exclude from consideration all studies completed after the date of disqualification until the facility can satisfy the Commissioner that it will conduct studies in compliance with such regulations.

(b) The determination that a nonclinical laboratory study may not be considered in support of an application for a research or marketing permit does not, however, relieve the applicant for such a permit of any obligation under any other applicable regulation to submit the results of the study to the Food and Drug Administration.

Sec. 58.202 Grounds for disqualification.

The Commissioner may disqualify a testing facility upon finding all of the following:

(a) The testing facility failed to comply with one or more of the regulations set forth in this part (or any other regulations regarding such facilities in this chapter);

(b) The noncompliance adversely affected the validity of the nonclinical laboratory studies; and

(c) Other lesser regulatory actions (e.g., warnings or rejection of individual studies) have not been or will probably not be adequate to achieve compliance with the good laboratory practice regulations.

Part 58

Sec. 58.204 Notice of and opportunity for hearing on proposed disqualification.

(a) Whenever the Commissioner has information indicating that grounds exist under 58.202 which in his opinion justify disqualification of a testing facility, he may issue to the testing facility a written notice proposing that the facility be disqualified.

(b) A hearing on the disqualification shall be conducted in accordance with the requirements for a regulatory hearing set forth in part 16 of this chapter.

Sec. 58.206 Final order on disqualification.

(a) If the Commissioner, after the regulatory hearing, or after the time for requesting a hearing expires without a request being made, upon an evaulation of the administrative record of the disqualification proceeding, makes the findings required in 58.202, he shall issue a final order disqualifying the facility. Such order shall include a statement of the basis for that determination. Upon issuing a final order, the Commissioner shall notify (with a copy of the order) the testing facility of the action.

(b) If the Commissioner, after a regulatory hearing or after the time for requesting a hearing expires without a request being made, upon an evaluation of the administrative record of the disqualification proceeding, does not make the findings required in 58.202, he shall issue a final order terminating the disqualification proceeding. Such order shall include a statement of the basis for that determination. Upon issuing a final order the Commissioner shall notify the testing facility and provide a copy of the order.

Sec. 58.210 Actions upon disqualification.

(a) Once a testing facility has been disqualified, each application for a research or marketing permit, whether approved or not, containing or relying upon any nonclinical laboratory study conducted by the disqualified testing facility may be examined to determine whether such study was or would be essential to a decision. If it is determined that a study was or would be essential, the Food and Drug Administration shall also determine whether the study is acceptable, notwithstanding the disqualification of the facility. Any study done by a testing facility before or after disqualification may be presumed to be unacceptable, and the person relying on the study may be required to establish that the study was not affected by the circumstances that led to the disqualification, e.g., by submitting validating information. If the study is then determined to be unacceptable, such data will be eliminated from consideration in support of the application; and such elimination may serve as new information justifying the termination or withdrawal of approval of the application.

(b) No nonclinical laboratory study begun by a testing facility after the date of the facility's disqualification shall be considered in support of any application for a research or marketing permit, unless the facility has been reinstated under 58.219. The determination that a study may not be considered in support of an application for a research or marketing permit does not, however, relieve the applicant for such a permit of any obligation under any other applicable regulation to submit the results of the study to the Food and Drug Administration.

[43 FR 60013, Dec. 22, 1978, as amended at 59 FR 13200, Mar. 21, 1994]

Sec. 58.213 Public disclosure of information regarding disqualification.

(a) Upon issuance of a final order disqualifying a testing facility under 58.206(a), the Commissioner may notify all or any interested persons. Such notice may be given at the discretion of the Commissioner whenever he believes that such disclosure would further the public interest or would promote compliance with the good laboratory practice regulations set forth in this part. Such notice, if given, shall include a copy of the final order issued under 58.206(a) and shall state that the disqualification constitutes a determination by the Food and Drug Administration that nonclinical laboratory studies performed by the facility will not be considered by the Food and Drug Administration in support of any application for a research or marketing permit. If such notice is sent to another Federal Government agency, the Food and Drug Administration will recommend that the agency also consider whether or not it should accept nonclinical laboratory studies performed by the testing facility. If such notice is sent to any other person, it shall state that it is given because of the relationship between the testing facility and the person being notified and that the Food and Drug Administration is not advising or recommending that any action be taken by the person notified.

Part 58

(b) A determination that a testing facility has been disqualified and the administrative record regarding such determination are disclosable to the public under part 20 of this chapter.

Sec. 58.215 Alternative or additional actions to disqualification.

(a) Disqualification of a testing facility under this subpart is independent of, and neither in lieu of nor a precondition to, other proceedings or actions authorized by the act. The Food and Drug Administration may, at any time, institute against a testing facility and/or against the sponsor of a nonclinical laboratory study that has been submitted to the Food and Drug Administration any appropriate judicial proceedings (civil or criminal) and any other appropriate regulatory action, in addition to or in lieu of, and prior to, simultaneously with, or subsequent to, disqualification. The Food and Drug Administration may also refer the matter to another Federal, State, or local government law enforcement or regulatory agency for such action as that agency deems appropriate.

(b) The Food and Drug Administration may refuse to consider any particular nonclinical laboratory study in support of an application for a research or marketing permit, if it finds that the study was not conducted in accordance with the good laboratory practice regulations set forth in this part, without disqualifying the testing facility that conducted the study or undertaking other regulatory action.

Sec. 58.217 Suspension or termination of a testing facility by a sponsor.

Termination of a testing facility by a sponsor is independent of, and neither in lieu of nor a precondition to, proceedings or actions authorized by this subpart. If a sponsor terminates or suspends a testing facility from further participation in a nonclinical laboratory study that is being conducted as part of any application for a research or marketing permit that has been submitted to any Center of the Food and Drug Administration (whether approved or not), it shall notify that Center in writing within 15 working days of the action; the notice shall include a statement of the reasons for such action. Suspension or termination of a testing facility by a sponsor does not relieve it of any obligation under any other applicable regulation to submit the results of the study to the Food and Drug Administration.

[43 FR FR 60013, Dec. 22, 1978, as amended at 50 FR 8995, Mar. 6, 1985]

Sec. 58.219 Reinstatement of a disqualified testing facility.

A testing facility that has been disqualified may be reinstated as an acceptable source of nonclinical laboratory studies to be submitted to the Food and Drug Administration if the Commissioner determines, upon an evaluation of the submission of the testing facility, that the facility can adequately assure that it will conduct future nonclinical laboratory studies in compliance with the good laboratory practice regulations set forth in this part and, if any studies are currently being conducted, that the quality and integrity of such studies have not been seriously compromised. A disqualified testing facility that wishes to be so reinstated shall present in writing to the Commissioner reasons why it believes it should be reinstated and a detailed description of the corrective actions it has taken or intends to take to assure that the acts or omissions which led to its disqualification will not recur. The Commissioner may condition reinstatement upon the testing facility being found in compliance with the good laboratory practice regulations upon an inspection. If a testing facility is reinstated, the Commissioner shall so notify the testing facility and all organizations and persons who were notified, under 58.213 of the disqualification of the testing facility. A determination that a testing facility has been reinstated is disclosable to the public under part 20 of this chapter.

Authority: 21 U.S.C. 342, 346, 346a, 348, 351, 352, 353, 355, 360, 360b-360f, 360h-360j, 371, 379e, 381; 42 U.S.C. 216, 262, 263b-263n.

Source: 43 FR 60013, Dec. 22, 1978, unless otherwise noted.

Part 58

Part 210: Current Good Manufacturing Practice In Manufacturing, Processing, Packing, or Holding of Drugs; General

[Code of Federal Regulations]

[Title 21, Volume 4]

[Revised as of April 1, 2009]

[CITE: 21CFR210]

Title 21--Food and Drugs

Chapter I--Food and Drug Administration

Department of Health and Human Services

Subchapter C--Drugs: General

Part 210 Current Good Manufacturing Practice In Manufacturing, Processing, Packing, or Holding of Drugs; General[1]

Sec. 210.1 Status of current good manufacturing practice regulations.

(a) The regulations set forth in this part and in parts 211 through 226 of this chapter contain the minimum current good manufacturing practice for methods to be used in, and the facilities or controls to be used for, the manufacture, processing, packing, or holding of a drug to assure that such drug meets the requirements of the act as

---

[1] Available on the FDA website at http://www.accessdata.fda.gov/scripts/cdrh/cfdocs/cfCFR/CFRSearch.cfm?CFRPart=210&showFR=1

to safety, and has the identity and strength and meets the quality and purity characteristics that it purports or is represented to possess.

(b) The failure to comply with any regulation set forth in this part and in parts 211 through 226 of this chapter in the manufacture, processing, packing, or holding of a drug shall render such drug to be adulterated under section 501(a)(2)(B) of the act and such drug, as well as the person who is responsible for the failure to comply, shall be subject to regulatory action.

(c) Owners and operators of establishments engaged in the recovery, donor screening, testing (including donor testing), processing, storage, labeling, packaging, or distribution of human cells, tissues, and cellular and tissue-based products (HCT/Ps), as defined in 1271.3(d) of this chapter, that are drugs (subject to review under an application submitted under section 505 of the act or under a biological product license application under section 351 of the Public Health Service Act), are subject to the donor-eligibility and applicable current good tissue practice procedures set forth in part 1271 subparts C and D of this chapter, in addition to the regulations in this part and in parts 211 through 226 of this chapter. Failure to comply with any applicable regulation set forth in this part, in parts 211 through 226 of this chapter, in part 1271 subpart C of this chapter, or in part 1271 subpart D of this chapter with respect to the manufacture, processing, packing or holding of a drug, renders an HCT/P adulterated under section 501(a)(2)(B) of the act. Such HCT/P, as well as the person who is responsible for the failure to comply, is subject to regulatory action.

Link to an amendment published at 74 FR 65431, Dec. 10, 2009.

[43 FR 45076, Sept, 29, 1978, as amended at 69 FR 29828, May 25, 2004]

Sec. 210.2 Applicability of current good manufacturing practice regulations.

(a) The regulations in this part and in parts 211 through 226 of this chapter as they may pertain to a drug; in parts 600 through 680 of this chapter as they may pertain to a biological product for human use; and in part 1271 of this chapter as they are applicable to a human cell, tissue, or cellular or tissue-based product (HCT/P) that is a drug (subject to review under an application submitted under section 505 of the act or under a biological product license application under section 351 of the Public Health Service Act); shall be considered to supplement, not supersede, each other, unless the regulations explicitly provide otherwise. In the event of a conflict between applicable regulations in this part and in other parts of this chapter, the regulation specifically applicable to the drug product in question shall supersede the more general.

(b) If a person engages in only some operations subject to the regulations in this part, in parts 211 through 226 of this chapter, in parts 600 through 680 of this chapter, and in part 1271 of this chapter, and not in others, that person need only comply with those regulations applicable to the operations in which he or she is engaged.

(c) An investigational drug for use in a phase 1 study, as described in 312.21(a) of this chapter, is subject to the statutory requirements set forth in 21 U.S.C. 351(a)(2)(B). The production of such drug is exempt from compliance with the regulations in part 211 of this chapter. However, this exemption does not apply to an investigational drug for use in a phase 1 study once the investigational drug has been made available for use by or for the sponsor in a phase 2 or phase 3 study, as described in 312.21(b) and (c) of this chapter, or the drug has been lawfully marketed. If the investigational drug has been made available in a phase 2 or phase 3 study or the drug has been lawfully marketed, the drug for use in the phase 1 study must comply with part 211.

Link to an amendment published at 74 FR 65431, Dec. 10, 2009.

[69 FR 29828, May 25, 2004, as amended at 73 FR 40462, July 15, 2008]

Sec. 210.3 Definitions.

(a) The definitions and interpretations contained in section 201 of the act shall be applicable to such terms when used in this part and in parts 211 through 226 of this chapter.

(b) The following definitions of terms apply to this part and to parts 211 through 226 of this chapter.

Part 210

(1) **Act** means the Federal Food, Drug, and Cosmetic Act, as amended (21 U.S.C. 301et seq.).

(2) **Batch** means a specific quantity of a drug or other material that is intended to have uniform character and quality, within specified limits, and is produced according to a single manufacturing order during the same cycle of manufacture.

(3) **Component** means any ingredient intended for use in the manufacture of a drug product, including those that may not appear in such drug product.

(4) **Drug product** means a finished dosage form, for example, tablet, capsule, solution, etc., that contains an active drug ingredient generally, but not necessarily, in association with inactive ingredients. The term also includes a finished dosage form that does not contain an active ingredient but is intended to be used as a placebo.

(5) **Fiber** means any particulate contaminant with a length at least three times greater than its width.

(6) **Nonfiber releasing filter** means any filter, which after appropriate pretreatment such as washing or flushing, will not release fibers into the component or drug product that is being filtered.

(7) **Active ingredient** means any component that is intended to furnish pharmacological activity or other direct effect in the diagnosis, cure, mitigation, treatment, or prevention of disease, or to affect the structure or any function of the body of man or other animals. The term includes those components that may undergo chemical change in the manufacture of the drug product and be present in the drug product in a modified form intended to furnish the specified activity or effect.

(8) **Inactive ingredient** means any component other than anactive ingredient.

(9) **In-process material** means any material fabricated, compounded, blended, or derived by chemical reaction that is produced for, and used in, the preparation of the drug product.

(10) **Lot** means a batch, or a specific identified portion of a batch, having uniform character and quality within specified limits; or, in the case of a drug product produced by continuous

process, it is a specific identified amount produced in a unit of time or quantity in a manner that assures its having uniform character and quality within specified limits.

(11) *Lot number, control number, or batch number* means any distinctive combination of letters, numbers, or symbols, or any combination of them, from which the complete history of the manufacture, processing, packing, holding, and distribution of a batch or lot of drug product or other material can be determined.

(12) *Manufacture, processing, packing, or holding of a drug product* includes packaging and labeling operations, testing, and quality control of drug products.

(13) The term *medicated feed* means any Type B or Type C medicated feed as defined in 558.3 of this chapter. The feed contains one or more drugs as defined in section 201(g) of the act. The manufacture of medicated feeds is subject to the requirements of part 225 of this chapter.

(14) The term *medicated premix* means a Type A medicated article as defined in 558.3 of this chapter. The article contains one or more drugs as defined in section 201(g) of the act. The manufacture of medicated premixes is subject to the requirements of part 226 of this chapter.

(15) *Quality control unit* means any person or organizational element designated by the firm to be responsible for the duties relating to quality control.

(16) *Strength* means:

(i) The concentration of the drug substance (for example, weight/weight, weight/volume, or unit dose/volume basis), and/or

(ii) The potency, that is, the therapeutic activity of the drug product as indicated by appropriate laboratory tests or by adequately developed and controlled clinical data (expressed, for example, in terms of units by reference to a standard).

(17) *Theoretical yield* means the quantity that would be produced at any appropriate phase of manufacture, processing, or packing of a particular drug product, based upon the quantity of components to be used, in the absence of any loss or error in actual production.

Part 210

---

(18) **Actual yield** means the quantity that is actually produced at any appropriate phase of manufacture, processing, or packing of a particular drug product.

(19) **Percentage of theoretical yield** means the ratio of the actual yield (at any appropriate phase of manufacture, processing, or packing of a particular drug product) to the theoretical yield (at the same phase), stated as a percentage.

(20) **Acceptance criteria** means the product specifications and acceptance/rejection criteria, such as acceptable quality level and unacceptable quality level, with an associated sampling plan, that are necessary for making a decision to accept or reject a lot or batch (or any other convenient subgroups of manufactured units).

(21) **Representative sample** means a sample that consists of a number of units that are drawn based on rational criteria such as random sampling and intended to assure that the sample accurately portrays the material being sampled.

(22) **Gang-printed labeling** means labeling derived from a sheet of material on which more than one item of labeling is printed.

Link to an amendment published at 74 FR 65431, Dec. 10, 2009.

[43 FR 45076, Sept. 29, 1978, as amended at 51 FR 7389, Mar. 3, 1986; 58 FR 41353, Aug. 3, 1993; 73 FR 51931, Sept. 8, 2008]

Authority: 21 U.S.C. 321, 351, 352, 355, 360b, 371, 374; 42 U.S.C. 216, 262, 263a, 264.

Source: 43 FR 45076, Sept, 29, 1978, unless otherwise noted.

Part 312: Investigational New Drug Application

[Code of Federal Regulations]

[Title 21, Volume 5]

[Revised as of April 1, 2009]

[CITE: 21CFR312]

Title 21--Food and Drugs

Chapter I--Food and Drug Administration

Department of Health and Human Services

Subchapter D--Drugs for Human Use

Part 312 Investigational New Drug Application[1]

Subpart A--General Provisions

Sec. 312.1 Scope.

(a) This part contains procedures and requirements governing the use of investigational new drugs, including procedures and requirements for the submission to, and review by, the Food and Drug Administration of investigational new drug applications (IND's). An investigational new drug for which an IND is in effect in accordance with this part is exempt from the premarketing approval requirements that are otherwise applicable and may be shipped lawfully for the purpose of conducting clinical investigations of that drug.

---

[1] Available on the FDA website at http://www.accessdata.fda.gov/scripts/cdrh/cfdocs/cfCFR/CFRSearch.cfm?CFRPart=312&showFR=1

(b) References in this part to regulations in the Code of Federal Regulations are to chapter I of title 21, unless otherwise noted.

Sec. 312.2 Applicability.

(a) Applicability. Except as provided in this section, this part applies to all clinical investigations of products that are subject to section 505 of the Federal Food, Drug, and Cosmetic Act or to the licensing provisions of the Public Health Service Act (58 Stat. 632, as amended (42 U.S.C. 201et seq.)).

(b) Exemptions.

(1) The clinical investigation of a drug product that is lawfully marketed in the United States is exempt from the requirements of this part if all the following apply:

(i) The investigation is not intended to be reported to FDA as a well-controlled study in support of a new indication for use nor intended to be used to support any other significant change in the labeling for the drug;

(ii) If the drug that is undergoing investigation is lawfully marketed as a prescription drug product, the investigation is not intended to support a significant change in the advertising for the product;

(iii) The investigation does not involve a route of administration or dosage level or use in a patient population or other factor that significantly increases the risks (or decreases the acceptability of the risks) associated with the use of the drug product;

(iv) The investigation is conducted in compliance with the requirements for institutional review set forth in part 56 and with the requirements for informed consent set forth in part 50; and

(v) The investigation is conducted in compliance with the requirements of 312.7.

(2)(i) A clinical investigation involving an in vitro diagnostic biological product listed in paragraph (b)(2)(ii) of this section is exempt from the requirements of this part if (a) it is intended to be used in a diagnostic procedure that confirms the diagnosis made by another, medically established, diagnostic product or procedure and (b) it is shipped in compliance with 312.160.

(ii) In accordance with paragraph (b)(2)(i) of this section, the following products are exempt from the requirements of this part: (a) blood grouping serum; (b) reagent red blood cells; and (c) anti-human globulin.

(3) A drug intended solely for tests in vitro or in laboratory research animals is exempt from the requirements of this part if shipped in accordance with 312.160.

(4) FDA will not accept an application for an investigation that is exempt under the provisions of paragraph (b)(1) of this section.

(5) A clinical investigation involving use of a placebo is exempt from the requirements of this part if the investigation does not otherwise require submission of an IND.

(6) A clinical investigation involving an exception from informed consent under 50.24 of this chapter is not exempt from the requirements of this part.

(c) Bioavailability studies. The applicability of this part to in vivo bioavailability studies in humans is subject to the provisions of 320.31.

(d) Unlabeled indication. This part does not apply to the use in the practice of medicine for an unlabeled indication of a new drug product approved under part 314 or of a licensed biological product.

(e) Guidance. FDA may, on its own initiative, issue guidance on the applicability of this part to particular investigational uses of drugs. On request, FDA will advise on the applicability of this part to a planned clinical investigation.

[52 FR 8831, Mar. 19, 1987, as amended at 61 FR 51529, Oct. 2, 1996; 64 FR 401, Jan. 5, 1999]

Sec. 312.3 Definitions and interpretations.

(a) The definitions and interpretations of terms contained in section 201 of the Act apply to those terms when used in this part:

(b) The following definitions of terms also apply to this part:

Act means the Federal Food, Drug, and Cosmetic Act (secs. 201-902, 52 Stat. 1040et seq., as amended (21 U.S.C. 301-392)).

Clinical investigation means any experiment in which a drug is administered or dispensed to, or used involving, one or more human subjects. For the purposes of this part, an experiment is any use of a drug except for the use of a marketed drug in the course of medical practice.

Contract research organization means a person that assumes, as an independent contractor with the sponsor, one or more of the obligations of a sponsor, e.g., design of a protocol, selection or monitoring of investigations, evaluation of reports, and preparation of materials to be submitted to the Food and Drug Administration.

FDA means the Food and Drug Administration.

IND means an investigational new drug application. For purposes of this part, "IND" is synonymous with "Notice of Claimed Investigational Exemption for a New Drug."

Independent ethics committee (IEC) means a review panel that is responsible for ensuring the protection of the rights, safety, and well-being of human subjects involved in a clinical investigation and is adequately constituted to provide assurance of that protection. An institutional review board (IRB), as defined in 56.102(g) of this chapter and subject to the requirements of part 56 of this chapter, is one type of IEC.

Investigational new drug means a new drug or biological drug that is used in a clinical investigation. The term also includes a biological product that is used in vitro for diagnostic purposes. The terms "investigational drug" and "investigational new drug" are deemed to be synonymous for purposes of this part.

Investigator means an individual who actually conducts a clinical investigation (i.e. , under whose immediate direction the drug is administered or dispensed to a subject). In the event an investigation is conducted by a team of individuals, the investigator is the responsible leader of the team. "Subinvestigator" includes any other individual member of that team.

Marketing application means an application for a new drug submitted under section 505(b) of the act or a biologics license application for a biological product submitted under the Public Health Service Act.

Sponsor means a person who takes responsibility for and initiates a clinical investigation. The sponsor may be an individual or pharmaceutical company, governmental agency, academic institution, private organization, or other organization. The sponsor does not actually conduct the investigation unless the sponsor is a sponsor-investigator. A person other than an individual that uses one or more of its own employees to conduct an investigation that it has initiated is a sponsor, not a sponsor-investigator, and the employees are investigators.

Sponsor-Investigator means an individual who both initiates and conducts an investigation, and under whose immediate direction the investigational drug is administered or dispensed. The term does not include any person other than an individual. The requirements applicable to a sponsor-investigator under this part include both those applicable to an investigator and a sponsor.

Subject means a human who participates in an investigation, either as a recipient of the investigational new drug or as a control. A subject may be a healthy human or a patient with a disease.

[52 FR 8831, Mar. 19, 1987, as amended at 64 FR 401, Jan. 5, 1999; 64 FR 56449, Oct. 20, 1999; 73 FR 22815, Apr. 28, 2008]

Sec. 312.6 Labeling of an investigational new drug.

(a) The immediate package of an investigational new drug intended for human use shall bear a label with the statement "Caution: New Drug--Limited by Federal (or United States) law to investigational use."

(b) The label or labeling of an investigational new drug shall not bear any statement that is false or misleading in any particular and shall not represent that the investigational new drug is safe or effective for the purposes for which it is being investigated.

(c) The appropriate FDA Center Director, according to the procedures set forth in 201.26 or 610.68 of this chapter, may grant an exception or alternative to the provision in paragraph (a) of this section, to the extent that this provision is not explicitly required by statute, for specified lots, batches, or other units of a human drug product that is or will be included in the Strategic National Stockpile.

[52 FR 8831, Mar. 19, 1987, as amended at 72 FR 73599, Dec. 28, 2007]

Sec. 312.7 Promotion of investigational drugs.

(a) Promotion of an investigational new drug. A sponsor or investigator, or any person acting on behalf of a sponsor or investigator, shall not represent in a promotional context that an investigational new drug is safe or effective for the purposes for which it is under investigation or otherwise promote the drug. This provision is not intended to restrict the full exchange of scientific information concerning the drug, including dissemination of scientific findings in scientific or lay media. Rather, its intent is to restrict promotional claims of safety or effectiveness of the drug for a use for which it is under investigation and to preclude commercialization of the drug before it is approved for commercial distribution.

(b) Commercial distribution of an investigational new drug. A sponsor or investigator shall not commercially distribute or test market an investigational new drug.

(c) Prolonging an investigation. A sponsor shall not unduly prolong an investigation after finding that the results of the investigation appear to establish sufficient data to support a marketing application.

[52 FR 8831, Mar. 19, 1987, as amended at 52 FR 19476, May 22, 1987; 67 FR 9585, Mar. 4, 2002; 74 FR 40899, Aug. 13, 2009]

Sec. 312.8 Charging for investigational drugs under an IND.

(a) General criteria for charging.

(1) A sponsor must meet the applicable requirements in paragraph (b) of this section for charging in a clinical trial or paragraph (c) of this section for charging for expanded access to an investigational drug for treatment use under subpart I of this part, except that sponsors need not fulfill the requirements in this section to charge for an approved drug

obtained from another entity not affiliated with the sponsor for use as part of the clinical trial evaluation (e.g., in a clinical trial of a new use of the approved drug, for use of the approved drug as an active control).

(2) A sponsor must justify the amount to be charged in accordance with paragraph (d) of this section.

(3) A sponsor must obtain prior written authorization from FDA to charge for an investigational drug.

(4) FDA will withdraw authorization to charge if it determines that charging is interfering with the development of a drug for marketing approval or that the criteria for the authorization are no longer being met.

(b) Charging in a clinical trial –

(1) Charging for a sponsor's drug. A sponsor who wishes to charge for its investigational drug, including investigational use of its approved drug, must:

(i) Provide evidence that the drug has a potential clinical benefit that, if demonstrated in the clinical investigations, would provide a significant advantage over available products in the diagnosis, treatment, mitigation, or prevention of a disease or condition;

(ii) Demonstrate that the data to be obtained from the clinical trial would be essential to establishing that the drug is effective or safe for the purpose of obtaining initial approval of a drug, or would support a significant change in the labeling of an approved drug (e.g., new indication, inclusion of comparative safety information); and

(iii) Demonstrate that the clinical trial could not be conducted without charging because the cost of the drug is extraordinary to the sponsor. The cost may be extraordinary due to manufacturing complexity, scarcity of a natural resource, the large quantity of drug needed (e.g., due to the size or duration of the trial), or some combination of these or other extraordinary circumstances (e.g., resources available to a sponsor).

(2) Duration of charging in a clinical trial. Unless FDA specifies a shorter period, charging may continue for the length of the clinical trial.

(c) Charging for expanded access to investigational drug for treatment use.

    (1) A sponsor who wishes to charge for expanded access to an investigational drug for treatment use under subpart I of this part must provide reasonable assurance that charging will not interfere with developing the drug for marketing approval.

    (2) For expanded access under 312.320 (treatment IND or treatment protocol), such assurance must include:

        (i) Evidence of sufficient enrollment in any ongoing clinical trial(s) needed for marketing approval to reasonably assure FDA that the trial(s) will be successfully completed as planned;

        (ii) Evidence of adequate progress in the development of the drug for marketing approval; and

        (iii) Information submitted under the general investigational plan (312.23(a)(3)(iv)) specifying the drug development milestones the sponsor plans to meet in the next year.

    (3) The authorization to charge is limited to the number of patients authorized to receive the drug under the treatment use, if there is a limitation.

    (4) Unless FDA specifies a shorter period, charging for expanded access to an investigational drug for treatment use under subpart I of this part may continue for 1 year from the time of FDA authorization. A sponsor may request that FDA reauthorize charging for additional periods.

(d) Costs recoverable when charging for an investigational drug.

    (1) A sponsor may recover only the direct costs of making its investigational drug available.

        (i) Direct costs are costs incurred by a sponsor that can be specifically and exclusively attributed to providing the drug for the investigational use for which FDA has authorized cost recovery. Direct costs include costs per unit to manufacture the drug (e.g., raw materials, labor, and nonreusable supplies and equipment used to manufacture the quantity of drug needed for the use for which charging is authorized) or costs to acquire the drug from another manufacturing source, and direct costs to ship and handle (e.g., store) the drug.

Part 312

(ii) Indirect costs include costs incurred primarily to produce the drug for commercial sale (e.g., costs for facilities and equipment used to manufacture the supply of investigational drug, but that are primarily intended to produce large quantities of drug for eventual commercial sale) and research and development, administrative, labor, or other costs that would be incurred even if the clinical trial or treatment use for which charging is authorized did not occur.

(2) For expanded access to an investigational drug for treatment use under 312.315 (intermediate-size patient populations) and 312.320 (treatment IND or treatment protocol), in addition to the direct costs described in paragraph (d)(1)(i) of this section, a sponsor may recover the costs of monitoring the expanded access IND or protocol, complying with IND reporting requirements, and other administrative costs directly associated with the expanded access IND.

(3) To support its calculation for cost recovery, a sponsor must provide supporting documentation to show that the calculation is consistent with the requirements of paragraphs (d)(1) and, if applicable, (d)(2) of this section. The documentation must be accompanied by a statement that an independent certified public accountant has reviewed and approved the calculations.

[74 FR 40899, Aug. 13, 2009]

Sec. 312.10 Waivers.

(a) A sponsor may request FDA to waive applicable requirement under this part. A waiver request may be submitted either in an IND or in an information amendment to an IND. In an emergency, a request may be made by telephone or other rapid communication means. A waiver request is required to contain at least one of the following:

(1) An explanation why the sponsor's compliance with the requirement is unnecessary or cannot be achieved;

(2) A description of an alternative submission or course of action that satisfies the purpose of the requirement; or

(3) Other information justifying a waiver.

(b) FDA may grant a waiver if it finds that the sponsor's noncompliance would not pose a significant and unreasonable risk to human subjects of the investigation and that one of the following is met:

(1) The sponsor's compliance with the requirement is unnecessary for the agency to evaluate the application, or compliance cannot be achieved;

(2) The sponsor's proposed alternative satisfies the requirement; or

(3) The applicant's submission otherwise justifies a waiver.

[52 FR 8831, Mar. 19, 1987, as amended at 52 FR 23031, June 17, 1987; 67 FR 9585, Mar. 4, 2002]

Subpart B--Investigational New Drug Application (IND)

Sec. 312.20 Requirement for an IND.

(a) A sponsor shall submit an IND to FDA if the sponsor intends to conduct a clinical investigation with an investigational new drug that is subject to 312.2(a).

(b) A sponsor shall not begin a clinical investigation subject to 312.2(a) until the investigation is subject to an IND which is in effect in accordance with 312.40.

(c) A sponsor shall submit a separate IND for any clinical investigation involving an exception from informed consent under 50.24 of this chapter. Such a clinical investigation is not permitted to proceed without the prior written authorization from FDA. FDA shall provide a written determination 30 days after FDA receives the IND or earlier.

[52 FR 8831, Mar. 19, 1987, as amended at 61 FR 51529, Oct. 2, 1996; 62 FR 32479, June 16, 1997]

Sec. 312.21 Phases of an investigation.

An IND may be submitted for one or more phases of an investigation. The clinical investigation of a previously untested drug is generally divided into three phases. Although in general the phases are conducted sequentially, they may overlap. These three phases of an investigation are a follows:

(a) Phase 1.

    (1) Phase 1 includes the initial introduction of an investigational new drug into humans. Phase 1 studies are typically closely monitored and may be conducted in patients or normal volunteer subjects. These studies are designed to determine the metabolism and pharmacologic actions of the drug in humans, the side effects associated with increasing doses, and, if possible, to gain early evidence on effectiveness. During Phase 1, sufficient information about the drug's pharmacokinetics and pharmacological effects should be obtained to permit the design of well-controlled, scientifically valid, Phase 2 studies. The total number of subjects and patients included in Phase 1 studies varies with the drug, but is generally in the range of 20 to 80.

    (2) Phase 1 studies also include studies of drug metabolism, structure-activity relationships, and mechanism of action in humans, as well as studies in which investigational drugs are used as research tools to explore biological phenomena or disease processes.

(b) Phase 2. Phase 2 includes the controlled clinical studies conducted to evaluate the effectiveness of the drug for a particular indication or indications in patients with the disease or condition under study and to determine the common short-term side effects and risks associated with the drug. Phase 2 studies are typically well controlled, closely monitored, and conducted in a relatively small number of patients, usually involving no more than several hundred subjects.

(c) Phase 3. Phase 3 studies are expanded controlled and uncontrolled trials. They are performed after preliminary evidence suggesting effectiveness of the drug has been obtained, and are intended to gather the additional information about effectiveness and safety that is needed to evaluate the overall benefit-risk relationship of the drug and to provide an adequate basis for physician labeling. Phase 3 studies usually include from several hundred to several thousand subjects.

Sec. 312.22 General principles of the IND submission.

(a) FDA's primary objectives in reviewing an IND are, in all phases of the investigation, to assure the safety and rights of subjects, and, in Phase 2 and 3, to help assure that the quality of the scientific evaluation of drugs is adequate to permit an evaluation of the drug's effectiveness and safety. Therefore, although FDA's review of Phase 1 submissions will focus on assessing the safety of Phase 1 investigations, FDA's review of Phases 2 and 3 submissions will also include an assessment of the scientific quality of the clinical investigations and the likelihood that the investigations will yield data capable of meeting statutory standards for marketing approval.

(b) The amount of information on a particular drug that must be submitted in an IND to assure the accomplishment of the objectives described in paragraph (a) of this section depends upon such factors as the novelty of the drug, the extent to which it has been studied previously, the known or suspected risks, and the developmental phase of the drug.

(c) The central focus of the initial IND submission should be on the general investigational plan and the protocols for specific human studies. Subsequent amendments to the IND that contain new or revised protocols should build logically on previous submissions and should be supported by additional information, including the results of animal toxicology studies or other human studies as appropriate. Annual reports to the IND should serve as the focus for reporting the status of studies being conducted under the IND and should update the general investigational plan for the coming year.

(d) The IND format set forth in 312.23 should be followed routinely by sponsors in the interest of fostering an efficient review of applications. Sponsors are expected to exercise considerable discretion, however, regarding the content of information submitted in each section, depending upon the kind of drug being studied and the nature of the available information. Section 312.23 outlines the information needed for a commercially sponsored IND for a new molecular entity. A sponsor-investigator who uses, as a research tool, an investigational new drug that is already subject to a manufacturer's IND or marketing application should follow the same general format, but ordinarily may, if authorized by the manufacturer, refer to the manufacturer's IND or marketing application in providing the technical information supporting the proposed clinical investigation. A sponsor-investigator who uses an investigational drug not subject to a manufacturer's IND or marketing application is ordinarily required to submit all technical information supporting the IND, unless such information may be referenced from the scientific literature.

Sec. 312.23 IND content and format.

(a) A sponsor who intends to conduct a clinical investigation subject to this part shall submit an "Investigational New Drug Application" (IND) including, in the following order:

  (1) Cover sheet (Form FDA-1571). A cover sheet for the application containing the following:

   (i) The name, address, and telephone number of the sponsor, the date of the application, and the name of the investigational new drug.

   (ii) Identification of the phase or phases of the clinical investigation to be conducted.

   (iii) A commitment not to begin clinical investigations until an IND covering the investigations is in effect.

   (iv) A commitment that an Institutional Review Board (IRB) that complies with the requirements set forth in part 56 will be responsible for the initial and continuing review and approval of each of the studies in the proposed clinical investigation and that the investigator will report to the IRB proposed changes in the research activity in accordance with the requirements of part 56.

   (v) A commitment to conduct the investigation in accordance with all other applicable regulatory requirements.

   (vi) The name and title of the person responsible for monitoring the conduct and progress of the clinical investigations.

   (vii) The name(s) and title(s) of the person(s) responsible under 312.32 for review and evaluation of information relevant to the safety of the drug.

(viii) If a sponsor has transferred any obligations for the conduct of any clinical study to a contract research organization, a statement containing the name and address of the contract research organization, identification of the clinical study, and a listing of the obligations transferred. If all obligations governing the conduct of the study have been transferred, a general statement of this transfer--in lieu of a listing of the specific obligations transferred--may be submitted.

(ix) The signature of the sponsor or the sponsor's authorized representative. If the person signing the application does not reside or have a place of business within the United States, the IND is required to contain the name and address of, and be countersigned by, an attorney, agent, or other authorized official who resides or maintains a place of business within the United States.

(2) A table of contents.

(3) Introductory statement and general investigational plan. (i) A brief introductory statement giving the name of the drug and all active ingredients, the drug's pharmacological class, the structural formula of the drug (if known), the formulation of the dosage form(s) to be used, the route of administration, and the broad objectives and planned duration of the proposed clinical investigation(s).

(ii) A brief summary of previous human experience with the drug, with reference to other IND's if pertinent, and to investigational or marketing experience in other countries that may be relevant to the safety of the proposed clinical investigation(s).

(iii) If the drug has been withdrawn from investigation or marketing in any country for any reason related to safety or effectiveness, identification of the country(ies) where the drug was withdrawn and the reasons for the withdrawal.

(iv) A brief description of the overall plan for investigating the drug product for the following year. The plan should include the following: (a) The rationale for the drug or the research study; (b) the indication(s) to be studied; (c) the general approach to be followed in evaluating the drug; (d) the kinds of clinical trials to be conducted in the first year following the submission (if plans are not developed for the entire year, the sponsor should so indicate); (e) the estimated number of patients to be given the drug in those studies; and (f) any risks of particular severity or seriousness anticipated on the basis of the toxicological data in animals or prior studies in humans with the drug or related drugs.

(4) [Reserved]

(5) Investigator's brochure. If required under 312.55, a copy of the investigator's brochure, containing the following information:

    (i) A brief description of the drug substance and the formulation, including the structural formula, if known.

    (ii) A summary of the pharmacological and toxicological effects of the drug in animals and, to the extent known, in humans.

    (iii) A summary of the pharmacokinetics and biological disposition of the drug in animals and, if known, in humans.

    (iv) A summary of information relating to safety and effectiveness in humans obtained from prior clinical studies. (Reprints of published articles on such studies may be appended when useful.)

    (v) A description of possible risks and side effects to be anticipated on the basis of prior experience with the drug under investigation or with related drugs, and of precautions or special monitoring to be done as part of the investigational use of the drug.

(6) Protocols.

    (i) A protocol for each planned study. (Protocols for studies not submitted initially in the IND should be submitted in accordance with 312.30(a).) In general, protocols for Phase 1 studies may be less detailed and more flexible than protocols for Phase 2 and 3 studies. Phase 1 protocols should be directed primarily at providing an outline of the investigation--an estimate of the number of patients to be involved, a description of safety exclusions, and a description of the dosing plan including duration, dose, or method to be used in determining dose--and should specify in detail only those elements of the study that are critical to safety, such as necessary monitoring of vital signs and blood chemistries. Modifications of the experimental design of Phase 1 studies that do not affect critical safety assessments are required to be reported to FDA only in the annual report.

(ii) In Phases 2 and 3, detailed protocols describing all aspects of the study should be submitted. A protocol for a Phase 2 or 3 investigation should be designed in such a way that, if the sponsor anticipates that some deviation from the study design may become necessary as the investigation progresses, alternatives or contingencies to provide for such deviation are built into the protocols at the outset. For example, a protocol for a controlled short-term study might include a plan for an early crossover of nonresponders to an alternative therapy.

(iii) A protocol is required to contain the following, with the specific elements and detail of the protocol reflecting the above distinctions depending on the phase of study:

(a) A statement of the objectives and purpose of the study.

(b) The name and address and a statement of the qualifications (curriculum vitae or other statement of qualifications) of each investigator, and the name of each subinvestigator (e.g., research fellow, resident) working under the supervision of the investigator; the name and address of the research facilities to be used; and the name and address of each reviewing Institutional Review Board.

(c) The criteria for patient selection and for exclusion of patients and an estimate of the number of patients to be studied.

(d) A description of the design of the study, including the kind of control group to be used, if any, and a description of methods to be used to minimize bias on the part of subjects, investigators, and analysts.

(e) The method for determining the dose(s) to be administered, the planned maximum dosage, and the duration of individual patient exposure to the drug.

(f) A description of the observations and measurements to be made to fulfill the objectives of the study.

(g) A description of clinical procedures, laboratory tests, or other measures to be taken to monitor the effects of the drug in human subjects and to minimize risk.

(7) Chemistry, manufacturing, and control information.

(i) As appropriate for the particular investigations covered by the IND, a section describing the composition, manufacture, and control of the drug substance and the drug product. Although in each phase of the investigation sufficient information is required to be submitted to assure the proper identification, quality, purity, and strength of the investigational drug, the amount of information needed to make that assurance will vary with the phase of the investigation, the proposed duration of the investigation, the dosage form, and the amount of information otherwise available. FDA recognizes that modifications to the method of preparation of the new drug substance and dosage form and changes in the dosage form itself are likely as the investigation progresses. Therefore, the emphasis in an initial Phase 1 submission should generally be placed on the identification and control of the raw materials and the new drug substance. Final specifications for the drug substance and drug product are not expected until the end of the investigational process.

(ii) It should be emphasized that the amount of information to be submitted depends upon the scope of the proposed clinical investigation. For example, although stability data are required in all phases of the IND to demonstrate that the new drug substance and drug product are within acceptable chemical and physical limits for the planned duration of the proposed clinical investigation, if very short-term tests are proposed, the supporting stability data can be correspondingly limited.

(iii) As drug development proceeds and as the scale or production is changed from the pilot-scale production appropriate for the limited initial clinical investigations to the larger-scale production needed for expanded clinical trials, the sponsor should submit information amendments to supplement the initial information submitted on the chemistry, manufacturing, and control processes with information appropriate to the expanded scope of the investigation.

(iv) Reflecting the distinctions described in this paragraph (a)(7), and based on the phase(s) to be studied, the submission is required to contain the following:

(a) Drug substance. A description of the drug substance, including its physical, chemical, or biological characteristics; the name and address of its manufacturer; the general method of preparation of the drug substance; the acceptable limits and analytical methods used to assure the identity, strength, quality, and purity of the drug substance; and information sufficient to support stability of the drug substance during the toxicological studies and the planned clinical studies. Reference to the current edition of the United States Pharmacopeia--National Formulary may satisfy relevant requirements in this paragraph.

(b) Drug product. A list of all components, which may include reasonable alternatives for inactive compounds, used in the manufacture of the investigational drug product, including both those components intended to appear in the drug product and those which may not appear but which are used in the manufacturing process, and, where applicable, the quantitative composition of the investigational drug product, including any reasonable variations that may be expected during the investigational stage; the name and address of the drug product manufacturer; a brief general description of the manufacturing and packaging procedure as appropriate for the product; the acceptable limits and analytical methods used to assure the identity, strength, quality, and purity of the drug product; and information sufficient to assure the product's stability during the planned clinical studies. Reference to the current edition of the United States Pharmacopeia--National Formulary may satisfy certain requirements in this paragraph.

(c) A brief general description of the composition, manufacture, and control of any placebo used in a controlled clinical trial.

(d) Labeling. A copy of all labels and labeling to be provided to each investigator.

(e) Environmental analysis requirements. A claim for categorical exclusion under 25.30 or 25.31 or an environmental assessment under 25.40.

(8) Pharmacology and toxicology information. Adequate information about pharmacological and toxicological studies of the drug involving laboratory animals or in vitro, on the basis of which the sponsor has concluded that it is reasonably safe to conduct the proposed clinical investigations. The kind, duration, and scope of animal and other tests required varies with the duration and nature of the proposed clinical investigations. Guidance documents are available from FDA that describe ways in which these requirements may be met. Such information is required to include the identification and qualifications of the individuals who evaluated the results of such studies and concluded that it is reasonably safe to begin the proposed investigations and a statement of where the investigations were conducted and where the records are available for inspection. As drug development proceeds, the sponsor is required to submit informational amendments, as appropriate, with additional information pertinent to safety.

(i) Pharmacology and drug disposition. A section describing the pharmacological effects and mechanism(s) of action of the drug in animals, and information on the absorption, distribution, metabolism, and excretion of the drug, if known.

(ii) Toxicology.

(a) An integrated summary of the toxicological effects of the drug in animals and in vitro. Depending on the nature of the drug and the phase of the investigation, the description is to include the results of acute, subacute, and chronic toxicity tests; tests of the drug's effects on reproduction and the developing fetus; any special toxicity test related to the drug's particular mode of administration or conditions of use (e.g., inhalation, dermal, or ocular toxicology); and any in vitro studies intended to evaluate drug toxicity.

(b) For each toxicology study that is intended primarily to support the safety of the proposed clinical investigation, a full tabulation of data suitable for detailed review.

(iii) For each nonclinical laboratory study subject to the good laboratory practice regulations under part 58, a statement that the study was conducted in compliance with the good laboratory practice regulations in part 58, or, if the study was not conducted in compliance with those regulations, a brief statement of the reason for the noncompliance.

(9) Previous human experience with the investigational drug. A summary of previous human experience known to the applicant, if any, with the investigational drug. The information is required to include the following:

(i) If the investigational drug has been investigated or marketed previously, either in the United States or other countries, detailed information about such experience that is relevant to the safety of the proposed investigation or to the investigation's rationale. If the drug has been the subject of controlled trials, detailed information on such trials that is relevant to an assessment of the drug's effectiveness for the proposed investigational use(s) should also be provided. Any published material that is relevant to the safety of the proposed investigation or to an assessment of the drug's effectiveness for its proposed investigational use should be provided in full. Published material that is less directly relevant may be supplied by a bibliography.

(ii) If the drug is a combination of drugs previously investigated or marketed, the information required under paragraph (a)(9)(i) of this section should be provided for each active drug component. However, if any component in such combination is subject to an approved marketing application or is otherwise lawfully marketed in the United States, the sponsor is not required to submit published material concerning that active drug component unless such material relates directly to the proposed investigational use (including publications relevant to component-component interaction).

(iii) If the drug has been marketed outside the United States, a list of the countries in which the drug has been marketed and a list of the countries in which the drug has been withdrawn from marketing for reasons potentially related to safety or effectiveness.

(10) Additional information. In certain applications, as described below, information on special topics may be needed. Such information shall be submitted in this section as follows:

    (i) Drug dependence and abuse potential. If the drug is a psychotropic substance or otherwise has abuse potential, a section describing relevant clinical studies and experience and studies in test animals.

    (ii) Radioactive drugs. If the drug is a radioactive drug, sufficient data from animal or human studies to allow a reasonable calculation of radiation-absorbed dose to the whole body and critical organs upon administration to a human subject. Phase 1 studies of radioactive drugs must include studies which will obtain sufficient data for dosimetry calculations.

    (iii) Pediatric studies. Plans for assessing pediatric safety and effectiveness.

    (iv) Other information. A brief statement of any other information that would aid evaluation of the proposed clinical investigations with respect to their safety or their design and potential as controlled clinical trials to support marketing of the drug.

(11) Relevant information. If requested by FDA, any other relevant information needed for review of the application.

(b) Information previously submitted. The sponsor ordinarily is not required to resubmit information previously submitted, but may incorporate the information by reference. A reference to information submitted previously must identify the file by name, reference number, volume, and page number where the information can be found. A reference to information submitted to the agency by a person other than the sponsor is required to contain a written statement that authorizes the reference and that is signed by the person who submitted the information.

(c) Material in a foreign language. The sponsor shall submit an accurate and complete English translation of each part of the IND that is not in English. The sponsor shall also submit a copy of each original literature publication for which an English translation is submitted.

(d) Number of copies. The sponsor shall submit an original and two copies of all submissions to the IND file, including the original submission and all amendments and reports.

(e) Numbering of IND submissions. Each submission relating to an IND is required to be numbered serially using a single, three-digit serial number. The initial IND is required to be numbered 000; each subsequent submission (e.g., amendment, report, or correspondence) is required to be numbered chronologically in sequence.

(f) Identification of exception from informed consent. If the investigation involves an exception from informed consent under 50.24 of this chapter, the sponsor shall prominently identify on the cover sheet that the investigation is subject to the requirements in 50.24 of this chapter.

[52 FR 8831, Mar. 19, 1987, as amended at 52 FR 23031, June 17, 1987; 53 FR 1918, Jan. 25, 1988; 61 FR 51529, Oct. 2, 1996; 62 FR 40599, July 29, 1997; 63 FR 66669, Dec. 2, 1998; 65 FR 56479, Sept. 19, 2000; 67 FR 9585, Mar. 4, 2002]

Sec. 312.30 Protocol amendments.

Once an IND is in effect, a sponsor shall amend it as needed to ensure that the clinical investigations are conducted according to protocols included in the application. This section sets forth the provisions under which new protocols may be submitted and changes in previously submitted protocols may be made. Whenever a sponsor intends to conduct a clinical investigation with an exception from informed consent for emergency research as set forth in 50.24 of this chapter, the sponsor shall submit a separate IND for such investigation.

(a) New protocol. Whenever a sponsor intends to conduct a study that is not covered by a protocol already contained in the IND, the sponsor shall submit to FDA a protocol amendment containing the protocol for the study. Such study may begin provided two conditions are met: (1) The sponsor has submitted the protocol to FDA for its review; and (2) the protocol has been approved by the Institutional Review Board (IRB) with responsibility for review and approval of the study in accordance with the requirements of part 56. The sponsor may comply with these two conditions in either order.

(b) Changes in a protocol.

    (1) A sponsor shall submit a protocol amendment describing any change in a Phase 1 protocol that significantly affects the safety of subjects or any change in a Phase 2 or 3 protocol that significantly affects the safety of subjects, the scope of the investigation, or the scientific quality of the study. Examples of changes requiring an amendment under this paragraph include:

        (i) Any increase in drug dosage or duration of exposure of individual subjects to the drug beyond that in the current protocol, or any significant increase in the number of subjects under study.

        (ii) Any significant change in the design of a protocol (such as the addition or dropping of a control group).

        (iii) The addition of a new test or procedure that is intended to improve monitoring for, or reduce the risk of, a side effect or adverse event; or the dropping of a test intended to monitor safety.

    (2)(i) A protocol change under paragraph (b)(1) of this section may be made provided two conditions are met:

        (a) The sponsor has submitted the change to FDA for its review; and

        (b) The change has been approved by the IRB with responsibility for review and approval of the study. The sponsor may comply with these two conditions in either order.

      (ii) Notwithstanding paragraph (b)(2)(i) of this section, a protocol change intended to eliminate an apparent immediate hazard to subjects may be implemented immediately provided FDA is subsequently notified by protocol amendment and the reviewing IRB is notified in accordance with 56.104(c).

(c) New investigator. A sponsor shall submit a protocol amendment when a new investigator is added to carry out a previously submitted protocol, except that a protocol amendment is not required when a licensed practitioner is added in the case of a treatment protocol under 312.315 or 312.320. Once the investigator is added to the study, the investigational drug may be shipped to the investigator and the investigator may begin participating in the study. The sponsor shall notify FDA of the new investigator within 30 days of the investigator being added.

(d) Content and format. A protocol amendment is required to be prominently identified as such (i.e. , "Protocol Amendment: New Protocol", "Protocol Amendment: Change in Protocol", or "Protocol Amendment: New Investigator"), and to contain the following:

(1)(i) In the case of a new protocol, a copy of the new protocol and a brief description of the most clinically significant differences between it and previous protocols.

(ii) In the case of a change in protocol, a brief description of the change and reference (date and number) to the submission that contained the protocol.

(iii) In the case of a new investigator, the investigator's name, the qualifications to conduct the investigation, reference to the previously submitted protocol, and all additional information about the investigator's study as is required under 312.23(a)(6)(iii)(b).

(2) Reference, if necessary, to specific technical information in the IND or in a concurrently submitted information amendment to the IND that the sponsor relies on to support any clinically significant change in the new or amended protocol. If the reference is made to supporting information already in the IND, the sponsor shall identify by name, reference number, volume, and page number the location of the information.

(3) If the sponsor desires FDA to comment on the submission, a request for such comment and the specific questions FDA's response should address.

(e) When submitted. A sponsor shall submit a protocol amendment for a new protocol or a change in protocol before its implementation. Protocol amendments to add a new investigator or to provide additional information about investigators may be grouped and submitted at 30-day intervals. When several submissions of new protocols or protocol changes are anticipated during a short period, the sponsor is encouraged, to the extent feasible, to include these all in a single submission.

[52 FR 8831, Mar. 19, 1987, as amended at 52 FR 23031, June 17, 1987; 53 FR 1918, Jan. 25, 1988; 61 FR 51530, Oct. 2, 1996; 67 FR 9585, Mar. 4, 2002; 74 FR 40942, Aug. 13, 2009]

Sec. 312.31 Information amendments.

(a) Requirement for information amendment. A sponsor shall report in an information amendment essential information on the IND that is not within the scope of a protocol amendment, IND safety reports, or annual report. Examples of information requiring an information amendment include:

    (1) New toxicology, chemistry, or other technical information; or

    (2) A report regarding the discontinuance of a clinical investigation.

(b) Content and format of an information amendment. An information amendment is required to bear prominent identification of its contents (e.g., "Information Amendment: Chemistry, Manufacturing, and Control", "Information Amendment: Pharmacology-Toxicology", "Information Amendment: Clinical"), and to contain the following:

    (1) A statement of the nature and purpose of the amendment.

    (2) An organized submission of the data in a format appropriate for scientific review.

    (3) If the sponsor desires FDA to comment on an information amendment, a request for such comment.

(c) When submitted. Information amendments to the IND should be submitted as necessary but, to the extent feasible, not more than every 30 days.

[52 FR 8831, Mar. 19, 1987, as amended at 52 FR 23031, June 17, 1987; 53 FR 1918, Jan. 25, 1988; 67 FR 9585, Mar. 4, 2002]

Sec. 312.32 IND safety reports.

(a) Definitions. The following definitions of terms apply to this section:

Associated with the use of the drug. There is a reasonable possibility that the experience may have been caused by the drug.

Disability. A substantial disruption of a person's ability to conduct normal life functions.

Life-threatening adverse drug experience. Any adverse drug experience that places the patient or subject, in the view of the investigator, at immediate risk of death from the reaction as it occurred,i.e. , it does not include a reaction that, had it occurred in a more severe form, might have caused death.

Serious adverse drug experience : Any adverse drug experience occurring at any dose that results in any of the following outcomes: Death, a life-threatening adverse drug experience, inpatient hospitalization or prolongation of existing hospitalization, a persistent or significant disability/incapacity, or a congenital anomaly/birth defect. Important medical events that may not result in death, be life-threatening, or require hospitalization may be considered a serious adverse drug experience when, based upon appropriate medical judgment, they may jeopardize the patient or subject and may require medical or surgical intervention to prevent one of the outcomes listed in this definition. Examples of such medical events include allergic bronchospasm requiring intensive treatment in an emergency room or at home, blood dyscrasias or convulsions that do not result in inpatient hospitalization, or the development of drug dependency or drug abuse.

Unexpected adverse drug experience : Any adverse drug experience, the specificity or severity of which is not consistent with the current investigator brochure; or, if an investigator brochure is not required or available, the specificity or severity of which is not consistent with the risk information described in the general investigational plan or elsewhere in the current application, as amended. For example, under this definition, hepatic necrosis would be unexpected (by virtue of greater severity) if the investigator brochure only referred to elevated hepatic enzymes or hepatitis. Similarly, cerebral thromboembolism and cerebral vasculitis would be unexpected (by virtue of greater specificity) if the investigator brochure only listed cerebral vascular accidents. "Unexpected," as used in this definition, refers to an adverse drug experience that has not been previously observed (e.g., included in the investigator brochure) rather than from the perspective of such experience not being anticipated from the pharmacological properties of the pharmaceutical product.

(b) Review of safety information. The sponsor shall promptly review all information relevant to the safety of the drug obtained or otherwise received by the sponsor from any source, foreign or domestic, including information derived from any clinical or epidemiological investigations, animal investigations, commercial marketing experience, reports in the scientific literature, and unpublished scientific papers, as well as reports from foreign regulatory authorities that have not already been previously reported to the agency by the sponsor.

(c) IND safety reports –

    (1) Written reports –

        (i) The sponsor shall notify FDA and all participating investigators in a written IND safety report of:

            (A) Any adverse experience associated with the use of the drug that is both serious and unexpected; or

            (B) Any finding from tests in laboratory animals that suggests a significant risk for human subjects including reports of mutagenicity, teratogenicity, or carcinogenicity. Each notification shall be made as soon as possible and in no event later than 15 calendar days after the sponsor's initial receipt of the information. Each written notification may be submitted on FDA Form 3500A or in a narrative format (foreign events may be submitted either on an FDA Form 3500A or, if preferred, on a CIOMS I form; reports from animal or epidemiological studies shall be submitted in a narrative format) and shall bear prominent identification of its contents,i.e. , "IND Safety Report." Each written notification to FDA shall be transmitted to the FDA new drug review division in the Center for Drug Evaluation and Research or the product review division in the Center for Biologics Evaluation and Research that has responsibility for review of the IND. If FDA determines that additional data are needed, the agency may require further data to be submitted.

(ii) In each written IND safety report, the sponsor shall identify all safety reports previously filed with the IND concerning a similar adverse experience, and shall analyze the significance of the adverse experience in light of the previous, similar reports.

(2) Telephone and facsimile transmission safety reports. The sponsor shall also notify FDA by telephone or by facsimile transmission of any unexpected fatal or life-threatening experience associated with the use of the drug as soon as possible but in no event later than 7 calendar days after the sponsor's initial receipt of the information. Each telephone call or facsimile transmission to FDA shall be transmitted to the FDA new drug review division in the Center for Drug Evaluation and Research or the product review division in the Center for Biologics Evaluation and Research that has responsibility for review of the IND.

(3) Reporting format or frequency. FDA may request a sponsor to submit IND safety reports in a format or at a frequency different than that required under this paragraph. The sponsor may also propose and adopt a different reporting format or frequency if the change is agreed to in advance by the director of the new drug review division in the Center for Drug Evaluation and Research or the director of the products review division in the Center for Biologics Evaluation and Research which is responsible for review of the IND.

(4) A sponsor of a clinical study of a marketed drug is not required to make a safety report for any adverse experience associated with use of the drug that is not from the clinical study itself.

(d) Followup.

(1) The sponsor shall promptly investigate all safety information received by it.

(2) Followup information to a safety report shall be submitted as soon as the relevant information is available.

(3) If the results of a sponsor's investigation show that an adverse drug experience not initially determined to be reportable under paragraph (c) of this section is so reportable, the sponsor shall report such experience in a written safety report as soon as possible, but in no event later than 15 calendar days after the determination is made.

(4) Results of a sponsor's investigation of other safety information shall be submitted, as appropriate, in an information amendment or annual report.

(e) Disclaimer. A safety report or other information submitted by a sponsor under this part (and any release by FDA of that report or information) does not necessarily reflect a conclusion by the sponsor or FDA that the report or information constitutes an admission that the drug caused or contributed to an adverse experience. A sponsor need not admit, and may deny, that the report or information submitted by the sponsor constitutes an admission that the drug caused or contributed to an adverse experience.

[52 FR 8831, Mar. 19, 1987, as amended at 52 FR 23031, June 17, 1987; 55 FR 11579, Mar. 29, 1990; 62 FR 52250, Oct. 7, 1997; 67 FR 9585, Mar. 4, 2002]

Sec. 312.33 Annual reports.

A sponsor shall within 60 days of the anniversary date that the IND went into effect, submit a brief report of the progress of the investigation that includes:

(a) Individual study information. A brief summary of the status of each study in progress and each study completed during the previous year. The summary is required to include the following information for each study:

(1) The title of the study (with any appropriate study identifiers such as protocol number), its purpose, a brief statement identifying the patient population, and a statement as to whether the study is completed.

(2) The total number of subjects initially planned for inclusion in the study; the number entered into the study to date, tabulated by age group, gender, and race; the number whose participation in the study was completed as planned; and the number who dropped out of the study for any reason.

(3) If the study has been completed, or if interim results are known, a brief description of any available study results.

(b) Summary information. Information obtained during the previous year's clinical and nonclinical investigations, including:

(1) A narrative or tabular summary showing the most frequent and most serious adverse experiences by body system.

(2) A summary of all IND safety reports submitted during the past year.

(3) A list of subjects who died during participation in the investigation, with the cause of death for each subject.

(4) A list of subjects who dropped out during the course of the investigation in association with any adverse experience, whether or not thought to be drug related.

(5) A brief description of what, if anything, was obtained that is pertinent to an understanding of the drug's actions, including, for example, information about dose response, information from controlled trials, and information about bioavailability.

(6) A list of the preclinical studies (including animal studies) completed or in progress during the past year and a summary of the major preclinical findings.

(7) A summary of any significant manufacturing or microbiological changes made during the past year.

(c) A description of the general investigational plan for the coming year to replace that submitted 1 year earlier. The general investigational plan shall contain the information required under 312.23(a)(3)(iv).

(d) If the investigator brochure has been revised, a description of the revision and a copy of the new brochure.

(e) A description of any significant Phase 1 protocol modifications made during the previous year and not previously reported to the IND in a protocol amendment.

(f) A brief summary of significant foreign marketing developments with the drug during the past year, such as approval of marketing in any country or withdrawal or suspension from marketing in any country.

(g) If desired by the sponsor, a log of any outstanding business with respect to the IND for which the sponsor requests or expects a reply, comment, or meeting.

[52 FR 8831, Mar. 19, 1987, as amended at 52 FR 23031, June 17, 1987; 63 FR 6862, Feb. 11, 1998; 67 FR 9585, Mar. 4, 2002]

Sec. 312.38 Withdrawal of an IND.

(a) At any time a sponsor may withdraw an effective IND without prejudice.

(b) If an IND is withdrawn, FDA shall be so notified, all clinical investigations conducted under the IND shall be ended, all current investigators notified, and all stocks of the drug returned to the sponsor or otherwise disposed of at the request of the sponsor in accordance with 312.59.

(c) If an IND is withdrawn because of a safety reason, the sponsor shall promptly so inform FDA, all participating investigators, and all reviewing Institutional Review Boards, together with the reasons for such withdrawal.

[52 FR 8831, Mar. 19, 1987, as amended at 52 FR 23031, June 17, 1987; 67 FR 9586, Mar. 4, 2002]

Subpart C--Administrative Actions

Sec. 312.40 General requirements for use of an investigational new drug in a clinical investigation.

(a) An investigational new drug may be used in a clinical investigation if the following conditions are met:

(1) The sponsor of the investigation submits an IND for the drug to FDA; the IND is in effect under paragraph (b) of this section; and the sponsor complies with all applicable requirements in this part and parts 50 and 56 with respect to the conduct of the clinical investigations; and

(2) Each participating investigator conducts his or her investigation in compliance with the requirements of this part and parts 50 and 56.

(b) An IND goes into effect:

(1) Thirty days after FDA receives the IND, unless FDA notifies the sponsor that the investigations described in the IND are subject to a clinical hold under 312.42; or

Part 312

(2) On earlier notification by FDA that the clinical investigations in the IND may begin. FDA will notify the sponsor in writing of the date it receives the IND.

(c) A sponsor may ship an investigational new drug to investigators named in the IND:

(1) Thirty days after FDA receives the IND; or

(2) On earlier FDA authorization to ship the drug.

(d) An investigator may not administer an investigational new drug to human subjects until the IND goes into effect under paragraph (b) of this section.

Sec. 312.41 Comment and advice on an IND.

(a) FDA may at any time during the course of the investigation communicate with the sponsor orally or in writing about deficiencies in the IND or about FDA's need for more data or information.

(b) On the sponsor's request, FDA will provide advice on specific matters relating to an IND. Examples of such advice may include advice on the adequacy of technical data to support an investigational plan, on the design of a clinical trial, and on whether proposed investigations are likely to produce the data and information that is needed to meet requirements for a marketing application.

(c) Unless the communication is accompanied by a clinical hold order under 312.42, FDA communications with a sponsor under this section are solely advisory and do not require any modification in the planned or ongoing clinical investigations or response to the agency.

[52 FR 8831, Mar. 19, 1987, as amended at 52 FR 23031, June 17, 1987; 67 FR 9586, Mar. 4, 2002]

Sec. 312.42 Clinical holds and requests for modification.

(a) General. A clinical hold is an order issued by FDA to the sponsor to delay a proposed clinical investigation or to suspend an ongoing investigation. The clinical hold order may apply to one or more of the investigations covered by an IND. When a proposed study is placed on clinical hold, subjects may not be given the investigational drug. When an ongoing study is placed on clinical hold, no new subjects may be recruited to the study and placed on the investigational drug; patients already in the study should be taken off therapy involving the investigational drug unless specifically permitted by FDA in the interest of patient safety.

(b) Grounds for imposition of clinical hold –

    (1) Clinical hold of a Phase 1 study under an IND. FDA may place a proposed or ongoing Phase 1 investigation on clinical hold if it finds that:

        (i) Human subjects are or would be exposed to an unreasonable and significant risk of illness or injury;

        (ii) The clinical investigators named in the IND are not qualified by reason of their scientific training and experience to conduct the investigation described in the IND;

        (iii) The investigator brochure is misleading, erroneous, or materially incomplete; or

        (iv) The IND does not contain sufficient information required under 312.23 to assess the risks to subjects of the proposed studies.

        (v) The IND is for the study of an investigational drug intended to treat a life-threatening disease or condition that affects both genders, and men or women with reproductive potential who have the disease or condition being studied are excluded from eligibility because of a risk or potential risk from use of the investigational drug of reproductive toxicity (i.e. , affecting reproductive organs) or developmental toxicity (i.e. , affecting potential offspring). The phrase "women with reproductive potential" does not include pregnant women. For purposes of this paragraph, "life-threatening illnesses or diseases" are defined as "diseases or conditions where the likelihood of death is high unless the course of the disease is interrupted." The clinical hold would not apply under this paragraph to clinical studies conducted:

           (A) Under special circumstances, such as studies pertinent only to one gender (e.g., studies evaluating the excretion of a drug in semen or the effects on menstrual function);

Part 312

(B) Only in men or women, as long as a study that does not exclude members of the other gender with reproductive potential is being conducted concurrently, has been conducted, or will take place within a reasonable time agreed upon by the agency; or

(C) Only in subjects who do not suffer from the disease or condition for which the drug is being studied.

(2) Clinical hold of a Phase 2 or 3 study under an IND. FDA may place a proposed or ongoing Phase 2 or 3 investigation on clinical hold if it finds that:

(i) Any of the conditions in paragraphs (b)(1)(i) through (b)(1)(v) of this section apply; or

(ii) The plan or protocol for the investigation is clearly deficient in design to meet its stated objectives.

(3) Clinical hold of an expanded access IND or expanded access protocol. FDA may place an expanded access IND or expanded access protocol on clinical hold under the following conditions:

(i) Final use. FDA may place a proposed expanded access IND or treatment use protocol on clinical hold if it is determined that:

(A) The pertinent criteria in subpart I of this part for permitting the expanded access use to begin are not satisfied; or

(B) The expanded access IND or expanded access protocol does not comply with the requirements for expanded access submissions in subpart I of this part.

(ii) Ongoing use. FDA may place an ongoing expanded access IND or expanded access protocol on clinical hold if it is determined that the pertinent criteria in subpart I of this part for permitting the expanded access are no longer satisfied.

(4) Clinical hold of any study that is not designed to be adequate and well-controlled. FDA may place a proposed or ongoing investigation that is not designed to be adequate and well-controlled on clinical hold if it finds that:

(i) Any of the conditions in paragraph (b)(1) or (b)(2) of this section apply; or

(ii) There is reasonable evidence the investigation that is not designed to be adequate and well-controlled is impeding enrollment in, or otherwise interfering with the conduct or completion of, a study that is designed to be an adequate and well-controlled investigation of the same or another investigational drug; or

(iii) Insufficient quantities of the investigational drug exist to adequately conduct both the investigation that is not designed to be adequate and well-controlled and the investigations that are designed to be adequate and well-controlled; or

(iv) The drug has been studied in one or more adequate and well-controlled investigations that strongly suggest lack of effectiveness; or

(v) Another drug under investigation or approved for the same indication and available to the same patient population has demonstrated a better potential benefit/risk balance; or

(vi) The drug has received marketing approval for the same indication in the same patient population; or

(vii) The sponsor of the study that is designed to be an adequate and well-controlled investigation is not actively pursuing marketing approval of the investigational drug with due diligence; or

(viii) The Commissioner determines that it would not be in the public interest for the study to be conducted or continued. FDA ordinarily intends that clinical holds under paragraphs (b)(4)(ii), (b)(4)(iii) and (b)(4)(v) of this section would only apply to additional enrollment in nonconcurrently controlled trials rather than eliminating continued access to individuals already receiving the investigational drug.

(5) Clinical hold of any investigation involving an exception from informed consent under 50.24 of this chapter. FDA may place a proposed or ongoing investigation involving an exception from informed consent under 50.24 of this chapter on clinical hold if it is determined that:

    (i) Any of the conditions in paragraphs (b)(1) or (b)(2) of this section apply; or

    (ii) The pertinent criteria in 50.24 of this chapter for such an investigation to begin or continue are not submitted or not satisfied.

(6) Clinical hold of any investigation involving an exception from informed consent under 50.23(d) of this chapter. FDA may place a proposed or ongoing investigation involving an exception from informed consent under 50.23(d) of this chapter on clinical hold if it is determined that:

    (i) Any of the conditions in paragraphs (b)(1) or (b)(2) of this section apply; or

    (ii) A determination by the President to waive the prior consent requirement for the administration of an investigational new drug has not been made.

(c) Discussion of deficiency. Whenever FDA concludes that a deficiency exists in a clinical investigation that may be grounds for the imposition of clinical hold FDA will, unless patients are exposed to immediate and serious risk, attempt to discuss and satisfactorily resolve the matter with the sponsor before issuing the clinical hold order.

(d) Imposition of clinical hold. The clinical hold order may be made by telephone or other means of rapid communication or in writing. The clinical hold order will identify the studies under the IND to which the hold applies, and will briefly explain the basis for the action. The clinical hold order will be made by or on behalf of the Division Director with responsibility for review of the IND. As soon as possible, and no more than 30 days after imposition of the clinical hold, the Division Director will provide the sponsor a written explanation of the basis for the hold.

(e) Resumption of clinical investigations. An investigation may only resume after FDA (usually the Division Director, or the Director's designee, with responsibility for review of the IND) has notified the sponsor that the investigation may proceed. Resumption of the affected investigation(s) will be authorized when the sponsor corrects the deficiency(ies) previously cited or otherwise satisfies the agency that the investigation(s) can proceed. FDA may notify a sponsor of its determination regarding the clinical hold by telephone or other means of rapid communication. If a sponsor of an IND that has been placed on clinical hold requests in writing that the clinical hold be removed and submits a complete response to the issue(s) identified in the clinical hold order, FDA shall respond in writing to the sponsor within 30-calendar days of receipt of the request and the complete response. FDA's response will either remove or maintain the clinical hold, and will state the reasons for such determination. Notwithstanding the 30-calendar day response time, a sponsor may not proceed with a clinical trial on which a clinical hold has been imposed until the sponsor has been notified by FDA that the hold has been lifted.

(f) Appeal. If the sponsor disagrees with the reasons cited for the clinical hold, the sponsor may request reconsideration of the decision in accordance with 312.48.

(g) Conversion of IND on clinical hold to inactive status. If all investigations covered by an IND remain on clinical hold for 1 year or more, the IND may be placed on inactive status by FDA under 312.45.

[52 FR 8831, Mar. 19, 1987, as amended at 52 FR 19477, May 22, 1987; 57 FR 13249, Apr. 15, 1992; 61 FR 51530, Oct. 2, 1996; 63 FR 68678, Dec. 14, 1998; 64 FR 54189, Oct. 5, 1999; 65 FR 34971, June 1, 2000; 74 FR 40942, Aug. 13, 2009]

Sec. 312.44 Termination.

(a) General. This section describes the procedures under which FDA may terminate an IND. If an IND is terminated, the sponsor shall end all clinical investigations conducted under the IND and recall or otherwise provide for the disposition of all unused supplies of the drug. A termination action may be based on deficiencies in the IND or in the conduct of an investigation under an IND. Except as provided in paragraph (d) of this section, a termination shall be preceded by a proposal to terminate by FDA and an opportunity for the sponsor to respond. FDA will, in general, only initiate an action under this section after first attempting to resolve differences informally or, when appropriate, through the clinical hold procedures described in 312.42.

(b) Grounds for termination –

(1) Phase 1. FDA may propose to terminate an IND during Phase 1 if it finds that:

(i) Human subjects would be exposed to an unreasonable and significant risk of illness or unjury.

(ii) The IND does not contain sufficient information required under 312.23 to assess the safety to subjects of the clinical investigations.

(iii) The methods, facilities, and controls used for the manufacturing, processing, and packing of the investigational drug are inadequate to establish and maintain appropriate standards of identity, strength, quality, and purity as needed for subject safety.

(iv) The clinical investigations are being conducted in a manner substantially different than that described in the protocols submitted in the IND.

(v) The drug is being promoted or distributed for commercial purposes not justified by the requirements of the investigation or permitted by 312.7.

(vi) The IND, or any amendment or report to the IND, contains an untrue statement of a material fact or omits material information required by this part.

(vii) The sponsor fails promptly to investigate and inform the Food and Drug Administration and all investigators of serious and unexpected adverse experiences in accordance with 312.32 or fails to make any other report required under this part.

(viii) The sponsor fails to submit an accurate annual report of the investigations in accordance with 312.33.

(ix) The sponsor fails to comply with any other applicable requirement of this part, part 50, or part 56.

(x) The IND has remained on inactive status for 5 years or more.

(xi) The sponsor fails to delay a proposed investigation under the IND or to suspend an ongoing investigation that has been placed on clinical hold under 312.42(b)(4).

(2) Phase 2 or 3. FDA may propose to terminate an IND during Phase 2 or Phase 3 if FDA finds that:

(i) Any of the conditions in paragraphs (b)(1)(i) through (b)(1)(xi) of this section apply; or

(ii) The investigational plan or protocol(s) is not reasonable as a bona fide scientific plan to determine whether or not the drug is safe and effective for use; or

(iii) There is convincing evidence that the drug is not effective for the purpose for which it is being investigated.

(3) FDA may propose to terminate a treatment IND if it finds that:

(i) Any of the conditions in paragraphs (b)(1)(i) through (x) of this section apply; or

(ii) Any of the conditions in 312.42(b)(3) apply.

(c) Opportunity for sponsor response. (1) If FDA proposes to terminate an IND, FDA will notify the sponsor in writing, and invite correction or explanation within a period of 30 days.

(2) On such notification, the sponsor may provide a written explanation or correction or may request a conference with FDA to provide the requested explanation or correction. If the sponsor does not respond to the notification within the allocated time, the IND shall be terminated.

(3) If the sponsor responds but FDA does not accept the explanation or correction submitted, FDA shall inform the sponsor in writing of the reason for the nonacceptance and provide the sponsor with an opportunity for a regulatory hearing before FDA under part 16 on the question of whether the IND should be terminated. The sponsor's request for a regulatory hearing must be made within 10 days of the sponsor's receipt of FDA's notification of nonacceptance.

(d) Immediate termination of IND. Notwithstanding paragraphs (a) through (c) of this section, if at any time FDA concludes that continuation of the investigation presents an immediate and substantial danger to the health of individuals, the agency shall immediately, by written notice to the sponsor from the Director of the Center for Drug Evaluation and Research or the Director of the Center for Biologics Evaluation and Research, terminate the IND. An IND so terminated is subject to reinstatement by the Director on the basis of additional submissions that eliminate such danger. If an IND is terminated under this paragraph, the agency will afford the sponsor an opportunity for a regulatory hearing under part 16 on the question of whether the IND should be reinstated.

[52 FR 8831, Mar. 19, 1987, as amended at 52 FR 23031, June 17, 1987; 55 FR 11579, Mar. 29, 1990; 57 FR 13249, Apr. 15, 1992; 67 FR 9586, Mar. 4, 2002]

Sec. 312.45 Inactive status.

(a) If no subjects are entered into clinical studies for a period of 2 years or more under an IND, or if all investigations under an IND remain on clinical hold for 1 year or more, the IND may be placed by FDA on inactive status. This action may be taken by FDA either on request of the sponsor or on FDA's own initiative. If FDA seeks to act on its own initiative under this section, it shall first notify the sponsor in writing of the proposed inactive status. Upon receipt of such notification, the sponsor shall have 30 days to respond as to why the IND should continue to remain active.

(b) If an IND is placed on inactive status, all investigators shall be so notified and all stocks of the drug shall be returned or otherwise disposed of in accordance with 312.59.

(c) A sponsor is not required to submit annual reports to an IND on inactive status. An inactive IND is, however, still in effect for purposes of the public disclosure of data and information under 312.130.

(d) A sponsor who intends to resume clinical investigation under an IND placed on inactive status shall submit a protocol amendment under 312.30 containing the proposed general investigational plan for the coming year and appropriate protocols. If the protocol amendment relies on information previously submitted, the plan shall reference such information. Additional information supporting the proposed investigation, if any, shall be submitted in an information amendment. Notwithstanding the provisions of 312.30, clinical investigations under an IND on inactive status may only resume (1) 30 days after FDA receives the protocol amendment, unless FDA notifies the sponsor that the investigations described in the amendment are subject to a clinical hold under 312.42, or (2) on earlier notification by FDA that the clinical investigations described in the protocol amendment may begin.

(e) An IND that remains on inactive status for 5 years or more may be terminated under 312.44.

[52 FR 8831, Mar. 19, 1987, as amended at 52 FR 23031, June 17, 1987; 67 FR 9586, Mar. 4, 2002]

Sec. 312.47 Meetings.

(a) General. Meetings between a sponsor and the agency are frequently useful in resolving questions and issues raised during the course of a clinical investigation. FDA encourages such meetings to the extent that they aid in the evaluation of the drug and in the solution of scientific problems concerning the drug, to the extent that FDA's resources permit. The general principle underlying the conduct of such meetings is that there should be free, full, and open communication about any scientific or medical question that may arise during the clinical investigation. These meetings shall be conducted and documented in accordance with part 10.

(b) "End-of-Phase 2" meetings and meetings held before submission of a marketing application. At specific times during the drug investigation process, meetings between FDA and a sponsor can be especially helpful in minimizing wasteful expenditures of time and money and thus in speeding the drug development and evaluation process. In particular, FDA has found that meetings at the end of Phase 2 of an investigation (end-of-Phase 2 meetings) are of considerable assistance in planning later studies and that meetings held near completion of Phase 3 and before submission of a marketing application ("pre-NDA" meetings) are helpful in developing methods of presentation and submission of data in the marketing application that facilitate review and allow timely FDA response.

(1) End-of-Phase 2 meetings –

(i) Purpose. The purpose of an end-of-phase 2 meeting is to determine the safety of proceeding to Phase 3, to evaluate the Phase 3 plan and protocols and the adequacy of current studies and plans to assess pediatric safety and effectiveness, and to identify any additional information necessary to support a marketing application for the uses under investigation.

(ii) Eligibility for meeting. While the end-of-Phase 2 meeting is designed primarily for IND's involving new molecular entities or major new uses of marketed drugs, a sponsor of any IND may request and obtain an end-of-Phase 2 meeting.

(iii) Timing. To be most useful to the sponsor, end-of-Phase 2 meetings should be held before major commitments of effort and resources to specific Phase 3 tests are made. The scheduling of an end-of-Phase 2 meeting is not, however, intended to delay the transition of an investigation from Phase 2 to Phase 3.

(iv) Advance information. At least 1 month in advance of an end-of-Phase 2 meeting, the sponsor should submit background information on the sponsor's plan for Phase 3, including summaries of the Phase 1 and 2 investigations, the specific protocols for Phase 3 clinical studies, plans for any additional nonclinical studies, plans for pediatric studies, including a time line for protocol finalization, enrollment, completion, and data analysis, or information to support any planned request for waiver or deferral of pediatric studies, and, if available, tentative labeling for the drug. The recommended contents of such a submission are described more fully in FDA Staff Manual Guide 4850.7 that is publicly available under FDA's public information regulations in part 20.

(v) Conduct of meeting. Arrangements for an end-of-Phase 2 meeting are to be made with the division in FDA's Center for Drug Evaluation and Research or the Center for Biologics Evaluation and Research which is responsible for review of the IND. The meeting will be scheduled by FDA at a time convenient to both FDA and the sponsor. Both the sponsor and FDA may bring consultants to the meeting. The meeting should be directed primarily at establishing agreement between FDA and the sponsor of the overall plan for Phase 3 and the objectives and design of particular studies. The adequacy of the technical information to support Phase 3 studies and/or a marketing application may also be discussed. FDA will also provide its best judgment, at that time, of the pediatric studies that will be required for the drug product and whether their submission will be deferred until after approval. Agreements reached at the meeting on these matters will be recorded in minutes of the conference that will be taken by FDA in accordance with 10.65 and provided to the sponsor. The minutes along with any other written material provided to the sponsor will serve as a permanent record of any agreements reached. Barring a significant scientific development that requires otherwise, studies conducted in accordance with the agreement shall be presumed to be sufficient in objective and design for the purpose of obtaining marketing approval for the drug.

(2) "Pre-NDA" and "pre-BLA" meetings. FDA has found that delays associated with the initial review of a marketing application may be reduced by exchanges of information about a proposed marketing application. The primary purpose of this kind of exchange is to uncover any major unresolved problems, to identify those studies that the sponsor is relying on as adequate and well-controlled to establish the drug's effectiveness, to identify the status of ongoing or needed studies adequate to assess pediatric safety and effectiveness, to acquaint FDA reviewers with the general information to be submitted in the marketing application (including technical information), to discuss appropriate methods for statistical analysis of the data, and to discuss the best approach to the presentation and formatting of data in the marketing application. Arrangements for such a meeting are to be initiated by the sponsor with the division responsible for review of the IND. To permit FDA to provide the sponsor with the most useful advice on preparing a marketing application, the sponsor should submit to FDA's reviewing division at least 1 month in advance of the meeting the following information:

(i) A brief summary of the clinical studies to be submitted in the application.

(ii) A proposed format for organizing the submission, including methods for presenting the data.

(iii) Information on the status of needed or ongoing pediatric studies.

(iv) Any other information for discussion at the meeting.

[52 FR 8831, Mar. 19, 1987, as amended at 52 FR 23031, June 17, 1987; 55 FR 11580, Mar. 29, 1990; 63 FR 66669, Dec. 2, 1998; 67 FR 9586, Mar. 4, 2002]

Sec. 312.48 Dispute resolution.

(a) General. The Food and Drug Administration is committed to resolving differences between sponsors and FDA reviewing divisions with respect to requirements for IND's as quickly and amicably as possible through the cooperative exchange of information and views.

(b) Administrative and procedural issues. When administrative or procedural disputes arise, the sponsor should first attempt to resolve the matter with the division in FDA's Center for Drug Evaluation and Research or Center for Biologics Evaluation and Research which is responsible for review of the IND, beginning with the consumer safety officer assigned to the application. If the dispute is not resolved, the sponsor may raise the matter with the person designated as ombudsman, whose function shall be to investigate what has happened and to facilitate a timely and equitable resolution. Appropriate issues to raise with the ombudsman include resolving difficulties in scheduling meetings and obtaining timely replies to inquiries. Further details on this procedure are contained in FDA Staff Manual Guide 4820.7 that is publicly available under FDA's public information regulations in part 20.

(c) Scientific and medical disputes. (1) When scientific or medical disputes arise during the drug investigation process, sponsors should discuss the matter directly with the responsible reviewing officials. If necessary, sponsors may request a meeting with the appropriate reviewing officials and management representatives in order to seek a resolution. Requests for such meetings shall be directed to the director of the division in FDA's Center for Drug Evaluation and Research or Center for Biologics Evaluation and Research which is responsible for review of the IND. FDA will make every attempt to grant requests for meetings that involve important issues and that can be scheduled at mutually convenient times.

(2) The "end-of-Phase 2" and "pre-NDA" meetings described in 312.47(b) will also provide a timely forum for discussing and resolving scientific and medical issues on which the sponsor disagrees with the agency.

(3) In requesting a meeting designed to resolve a scientific or medical dispute, applicants may suggest that FDA seek the advice of

outside experts, in which case FDA may, in its discretion, invite to the meeting one or more of its advisory committee members or other consultants, as designated by the agency. Applicants may rely on, and may bring to any meeting, their own consultants. For major scientific and medical policy issues not resolved by informal meetings, FDA may refer the matter to one of its standing advisory committees for its consideration and recommendations.

[52 FR 8831, Mar. 19, 1987, as amended at 55 FR 11580, Mar. 29, 1990]

Subpart D--Responsibilities of Sponsors and Investigators

Sec. 312.50 General responsibilities of sponsors.

Sponsors are responsibile for selecting qualified investigators, providing them with the information they need to conduct an investigation properly, ensuring proper monitoring of the investigation(s), ensuring that the investigation(s) is conducted in accordance with the general investigational plan and protocols contained in the IND, maintaining an effective IND with respect to the investigations, and ensuring that FDA and all participating investigators are promptly informed of significant new adverse effects or risks with respect to the drug. Additional specific responsibilities of sponsors are described elsewhere in this part.

Sec. 312.52 Transfer of obligations to a contract research organization.

(a) A sponsor may transfer responsibility for any or all of the obligations set forth in this part to a contract research organization. Any such transfer shall be described in writing. If not all obligations are transferred, the writing is required to describe each of the obligations being assumed by the contract research organization. If all obligations are transferred, a general statement that all obligations have been transferred is acceptable. Any obligation not covered by the written description shall be deemed not to have been transferred.

(b) A contract research organization that assumes any obligation of a sponsor shall comply with the specific regulations in this chapter applicable to this obligation and shall be subject to the same regulatory action as a sponsor for failure to comply with any obligation assumed under these regulations. Thus, all references to "sponsor" in this part apply to a contract research organization to the extent that it assumes one or more obligations of the sponsor.

Sec. 312.53 Selecting investigators and monitors.

(a) Selecting investigators. A sponsor shall select only investigators qualified by training and experience as appropriate experts to investigate the drug.

(b) Control of drug. A sponsor shall ship investigational new drugs only to investigators participating in the investigation.

(c) Obtaining information from the investigator. Before permitting an investigator to begin participation in an investigation, the sponsor shall obtain the following:

(1) A signed investigator statement (Form FDA-1572) containing:

(i) The name and address of the investigator;

(ii) The name and code number, if any, of the protocol(s) in the IND identifying the study(ies) to be conducted by the investigator;

(iii) The name and address of any medical school, hospital, or other research facility where the clinical investigation(s) will be conducted;

(iv) The name and address of any clinical laboratory facilities to be used in the study;

(v) The name and address of the IRB that is responsible for review and approval of the study(ies);

(vi) A commitment by the investigator that he or she:

(a) Will conduct the study(ies) in accordance with the relevant, current protocol(s) and will only make changes in a protocol after notifying the sponsor, except when necessary to protect the safety, the rights, or welfare of subjects;

(b) Will comply with all requirements regarding the obligations of clinical investigators and all other pertinent requirements in this part;

(c) Will personally conduct or supervise the described investigation(s);

(d) Will inform any potential subjects that the drugs are being used for investigational purposes and will ensure that the requirements relating to obtaining informed consent (21 CFR part 50) and institutional review board review and approval (21 CFR part 56) are met;

(e) Will report to the sponsor adverse experiences that occur in the course of the investigation(s) in accordance with 312.64;

(f) Has read and understands the information in the investigator's brochure, including the potential risks and side effects of the drug; and

(g) Will ensure that all associates, colleagues, and employees assisting in the conduct of the study(ies) are informed about their obligations in meeting the above commitments.

(vii) A commitment by the investigator that, for an investigation subject to an institutional review requirement under part 56, an IRB that complies with the requirements of that part will be responsible for the initial and continuing review and approval of the clinical investigation and that the investigator will promptly report to the IRB all changes in the research activity and all unanticipated problems involving risks to human subjects or others, and will not make any changes in the research without IRB approval, except where necessary to eliminate apparent immediate hazards to the human subjects.

(viii) A list of the names of the subinvestigators (e.g., research fellows, residents) who will be assisting the investigator in the conduct of the investigation(s).

(2) Curriculum vitae. A curriculum vitae or other statement of qualifications of the investigator showing the education, training, and experience that qualifies the investigator as an

Part 312

expert in the clinical investigation of the drug for the use under investigation.

(3) Clinical protocol.

(i) For Phase 1 investigations, a general outline of the planned investigation including the estimated duration of the study and the maximum number of subjects that will be involved.

(ii) For Phase 2 or 3 investigations, an outline of the study protocol including an approximation of the number of subjects to be treated with the drug and the number to be employed as controls, if any; the clinical uses to be investigated; characteristics of subjects by age, sex, and condition; the kind of clinical observations and laboratory tests to be conducted; the estimated duration of the study; and copies or a description of case report forms to be used.

(4) Financial disclosure information. Sufficient accurate financial information to allow the sponsor to submit complete and accurate certification or disclosure statements required under part 54 of this chapter. The sponsor shall obtain a commitment from the clinical investigator to promptly update this information if any relevant changes occur during the course of the investigation and for 1 year following the completion of the study.

(d) Selecting monitors. A sponsor shall select a monitor qualified by training and experience to monitor the progress of the investigation.

[52 FR 8831, Mar. 19, 1987, as amended at 52 FR 23031, June 17, 1987; 61 FR 57280, Nov. 5, 1996; 63 FR 5252, Feb. 2, 1998; 67 FR 9586, Mar. 4, 2002]

Sec. 312.54 Emergency research under 50.24 of this chapter.

(a) The sponsor shall monitor the progress of all investigations involving an exception from informed consent under 50.24 of this chapter. When the sponsor receives from the IRB information concerning the public disclosures required by 50.24(a)(7)(ii) and (a)(7)(iii) of this chapter, the sponsor promptly shall submit to the IND file and to Docket Number 95S-0158 in the Division of Dockets Management (HFA-305), Food and Drug Administration, 5630 Fishers Lane, rm. 1061, Rockville, MD

20852, copies of the information that was disclosed, identified by the IND number.

(b) The sponsor also shall monitor such investigations to identify when an IRB determines that it cannot approve the research because it does not meet the criteria in the exception in 50.24(a) of this chapter or because of other relevant ethical concerns. The sponsor promptly shall provide this information in writing to FDA, investigators who are asked to participate in this or a substantially equivalent clinical investigation, and other IRB's that are asked to review this or a substantially equivalent investigation.

[61 FR 51530, Oct. 2, 1996, as amended at 68 FR 24879, May 9, 2003]

Sec. 312.55 Informing investigators.

(a) Before the investigation begins, a sponsor (other than a sponsor-investigator) shall give each participating clinical investigator an investigator brochure containing the information described in 312.23(a)(5).

(b) The sponsor shall, as the overall investigation proceeds, keep each participating investigator informed of new observations discovered by or reported to the sponsor on the drug, particularly with respect to adverse effects and safe use. Such information may be distributed to investigators by means of periodically revised investigator brochures, reprints or published studies, reports or letters to clinical investigators, or other appropriate means. Important safety information is required to be relayed to investigators in accordance with 312.32.

[52 FR 8831, Mar. 19, 1987, as amended at 52 FR 23031, June 17, 1987; 67 FR 9586, Mar. 4, 2002]

Sec. 312.56 Review of ongoing investigations.

(a) The sponsor shall monitor the progress of all clinical investigations being conducted under its IND.

(b) A sponsor who discovers that an investigator is not complying with the signed agreement (Form FDA-1572), the general investigational plan, or the requirements of this part or other applicable parts shall promptly either secure compliance or discontinue shipments of the investigational new drug to the

Part 312

investigator and end the investigator's participation in the investigation. If the investigator's participation in the investigation is ended, the sponsor shall require that the investigator dispose of or return the investigational drug in accordance with the requirements of 312.59 and shall notify FDA.

(c) The sponsor shall review and evaluate the evidence relating to the safety and effectiveness of the drug as it is obtained from the investigator. The sponsors shall make such reports to FDA regarding information relevant to the safety of the drug as are required under 312.32. The sponsor shall make annual reports on the progress of the investigation in accordance with 312.33.

(d) A sponsor who determines that its investigational drug presents an unreasonable and significant risk to subjects shall discontinue those investigations that present the risk, notify FDA, all institutional review boards, and all investigators who have at any time participated in the investigation of the discontinuance, assure the disposition of all stocks of the drug outstanding as required by 312.59, and furnish FDA with a full report of the sponsor's actions. The sponsor shall discontinue the investigation as soon as possible, and in no event later than 5 working days after making the determination that the investigation should be discontinued. Upon request, FDA will confer with a sponsor on the need to discontinue an investigation.

[52 FR 8831, Mar. 19, 1987, as amended at 52 FR 23031, June 17, 1987; 67 FR 9586, Mar. 4, 2002]

Sec. 312.57 Recordkeeping and record retention.

(a) A sponsor shall maintain adequate records showing the receipt, shipment, or other disposition of the investigational drug. These records are required to include, as appropriate, the name of the investigator to whom the drug is shipped, and the date, quantity, and batch or code mark of each such shipment.

(b) A sponsor shall maintain complete and accurate records showing any financial interest in 54.4(a)(3)(i), (a)(3)(ii), (a)(3)(iii), and (a)(3)(iv) of this chapter paid to clinical investigators by the sponsor of the covered study. A sponsor shall also maintain complete and accurate records concerning all other financial interests of investigators subject to part 54 of this chapter.

(c) A sponsor shall retain the records and reports required by this part for 2 years after a marketing application is approved for the drug; or, if an application is not approved for the drug, until 2 years after shipment and delivery of the drug for investigational use is discontinued and FDA has been so notified.

(d) A sponsor shall retain reserve samples of any test article and reference standard identified in, and used in any of the bioequivalence or bioavailability studies described in, 320.38 or 320.63 of this chapter, and release the reserve samples to FDA upon request, in accordance with, and for the period specified in 320.38.

[52 FR 8831, Mar. 19, 1987, as amended at 52 FR 23031, June 17, 1987; 58 FR 25926, Apr. 28, 1993; 63 FR 5252, Feb. 2, 1998; 67 FR 9586, Mar. 4, 2002]

Sec. 312.58 Inspection of sponsor's records and reports.

(a) FDA inspection. A sponsor shall upon request from any properly authorized officer or employee of the Food and Drug Administration, at reasonable times, permit such officer or employee to have access to and copy and verify any records and reports relating to a clinical investigation conducted under this part. Upon written request by FDA, the sponsor shall submit the records or reports (or copies of them) to FDA. The sponsor shall discontinue shipments of the drug to any investigator who has failed to maintain or make available records or reports of the investigation as required by this part.

(b) Controlled substances. If an investigational new drug is a substance listed in any schedule of the Controlled Substances Act (21 U.S.C. 801; 21 CFR part 1308), records concerning shipment, delivery, receipt, and disposition of the drug, which are required to be kept under this part or other applicable parts of this chapter shall, upon the request of a properly authorized employee of the Drug Enforcement Administration of the U.S. Department of Justice, be made available by the investigator or sponsor to whom the request is made, for inspection and copying. In addition, the sponsor shall assure that adequate precautions are taken, including storage of the investigational drug in a securely locked, substantially constructed cabinet, or other securely locked, substantially constructed enclosure, access to which is limited, to prevent theft or diversion of the substance into illegal channels of distribution.

Sec. 312.59 Disposition of unused supply of investigational drug.

The sponsor shall assure the return of all unused supplies of the investigational drug from each individual investigator whose participation in the investigation is discontinued or terminated. The sponsor may authorize alternative disposition of unused supplies of the investigational drug provided this alternative disposition does not expose humans to risks from the drug. The sponsor shall maintain written records of any disposition of the drug in accordance with 312.57.

[52 FR 8831, Mar. 19, 1987, as amended at 52 FR 23031, June 17, 1987; 67 FR 9586, Mar. 4, 2002]

Sec. 312.60 General responsibilities of investigators.

An investigator is responsible for ensuring that an investigation is conducted according to the signed investigator statement, the investigational plan, and applicable regulations; for protecting the rights, safety, and welfare of subjects under the investigator's care; and for the control of drugs under investigation. An investigator shall, in accordance with the provisions of part 50 of this chapter, obtain the informed consent of each human subject to whom the drug is administered, except as provided in 50.23 or 50.24 of this chapter. Additional specific responsibilities of clinical investigators are set forth in this part and in parts 50 and 56 of this chapter.

[52 FR 8831, Mar. 19, 1987, as amended at 61 FR 51530, Oct. 2, 1996]

Sec. 312.61 Control of the investigational drug.

An investigator shall administer the drug only to subjects under the investigator's personal supervision or under the supervision of a subinvestigator responsible to the investigator. The investigator shall not supply the investigational drug to any person not authorized under this part to receive it.

Sec. 312.62 Investigator recordkeeping and record retention.

(a) Disposition of drug. An investigator is required to maintain adequate records of the disposition of the drug, including dates, quantity, and use by subjects. If the investigation is terminated, suspended, discontinued, or completed, the investigator shall return the unused supplies of the drug to the sponsor, or otherwise provide for disposition of the unused supplies of the drug under 312.59.

(b) Case histories. An investigator is required to prepare and maintain adequate and accurate case histories that record all observations and other data pertinent to the investigation on each individual administered the investigational drug or employed as a control in the investigation. Case histories include the case report forms and supporting data including, for example, signed and dated consent forms and medical records including, for example, progress notes of the physician, the individual's hospital chart(s), and the nurses' notes. The case history for each individual shall document that informed consent was obtained prior to participation in the study.

(c) Record retention. An investigator shall retain records required to be maintained under this part for a period of 2 years following the date a marketing application is approved for the drug for the indication for which it is being investigated; or, if no application is to be filed or if the application is not approved for such indication, until 2 years after the investigation is discontinued and FDA is notified.

[52 FR 8831, Mar. 19, 1987, as amended at 52 FR 23031, June 17, 1987; 61 FR 57280, Nov. 5, 1996; 67 FR 9586, Mar. 4, 2002]

Sec. 312.64 Investigator reports.

(a) Progress reports. The investigator shall furnish all reports to the sponsor of the drug who is responsible for collecting and evaluating the results obtained. The sponsor is required under 312.33 to submit annual reports to FDA on the progress of the clinical investigations.

(b) Safety reports. An investigator shall promptly report to the sponsor any adverse effect that may reasonably be regarded as caused by, or probably caused by, the drug. If the adverse effect is alarming, the investigator shall report the adverse effect immediately.

(c) Final report. An investigator shall provide the sponsor with an adequate report shortly after completion of the investigator's participation in the investigation.

(d) Financial disclosure reports. The clinical investigator shall provide the sponsor with sufficient accurate financial information to allow an applicant to submit complete and accurate certification or disclosure statements as required under part 54 of this chapter. The clinical investigator shall promptly update this information if any relevant changes occur during the course of the investigation and for 1 year following the completion of the study.

[52 FR 8831, Mar. 19, 1987, as amended at 52 FR 23031, June 17, 1987; 63 FR 5252, Feb. 2, 1998; 67 FR 9586, Mar. 4, 2002]

Sec. 312.66 Assurance of IRB review.

An investigator shall assure that an IRB that complies with the requirements set forth in part 56 will be responsible for the initial and continuing review and approval of the proposed clinical study. The investigator shall also assure that he or she will promptly report to the IRB all changes in the research activity and all unanticipated problems involving risk to human subjects or others, and that he or she will not make any changes in the research without IRB approval, except where necessary to eliminate apparent immediate hazards to human subjects.

[52 FR 8831, Mar. 19, 1987, as amended at 52 FR 23031, June 17, 1987; 67 FR 9586, Mar. 4, 2002]

Sec. 312.68 Inspection of investigator's records and reports.

An investigator shall upon request from any properly authorized officer or employee of FDA, at reasonable times, permit such officer or employee to have access to, and copy and verify any records or reports made by the investigator pursuant to 312.62. The investigator is not required to divulge subject names unless the records of particular individuals require a more detailed study of the cases, or unless there is reason to believe that the records do not represent actual case studies, or do not represent actual results obtained.

Sec. 312.69 Handling of controlled substances.

If the investigational drug is subject to the Controlled Substances Act, the investigator shall take adequate precautions, including storage of the investigational drug in a securely locked, substantially constructed cabinet, or other securely locked, substantially constructed enclosure, access to which is limited, to prevent theft or diversion of the substance into illegal channels of distribution.

Sec. 312.70 Disqualification of a clinical investigator.

(a) If FDA has information indicating that an investigator (including a sponsor-investigator) has repeatedly or deliberately failed to comply with the requirements of this part, part 50, or part 56 of this chapter, or has submitted to FDA or to the sponsor false information in any required report, the Center for Drug Evaluation and Research or the Center for Biologics Evaluation and Research will furnish the investigator written notice of the matter complained of and offer the investigator an opportunity to explain the matter in writing, or, at the option of the investigator, in an informal conference. If an explanation is offered but not accepted by the Center for Drug Evaluation and Research or the Center for Biologics Evaluation and Research, the investigator will be given an opportunity for a regulatory hearing under part 16 on the question of whether the investigator is entitled to receive investigational new drugs.

(b) After evaluating all available information, including any explanation presented by the investigator, if the Commissioner determines that the investigator has repeatedly or deliberately failed to comply with the requirements of this part, part 50, or part 56 of this chapter, or has deliberately or repeatedly submitted false information to FDA or to the sponsor in any required report, the Commissioner will notify the investigator and the sponsor of any investigation in which the investigator has been named as a participant that the investigator is not entitled to receive investigational drugs. The notification will provide a statement of basis for such determination.

(c) Each IND and each approved application submitted under part 314 containing data reported by an investigator who has been determined to be ineligible to receive investigational drugs will be examined to determine whether the investigator has submitted unreliable data that are essential to the continuation of the investigation or essential to the approval of any marketing application.

(d) If the Commissioner determines, after the unreliable data submitted by the investigator are eliminated from consideration, that the data remaining are inadequate to support a conclusion that it is reasonably safe to continue the investigation, the Commissioner will notify the sponsor who shall have an opportunity for a regulatory hearing under part 16. If a danger to the public health exists, however, the Commissioner shall terminate the IND immediately and notify the sponsor of the determination. In such case, the sponsor shall have an opportunity for a regulatory hearing before FDA under part 16 on the question of whether the IND should be reinstated.

(e) If the Commissioner determines, after the unreliable data submitted by the investigator are eliminated from consideration, that the continued approval of the drug product for which the data were submitted cannot be justified, the Commissioner will proceed to withdraw approval of the drug product in accordance with the applicable provisions of the act.

(f) An investigator who has been determined to be ineligible to receive investigational drugs may be reinstated as eligible when the Commissioner determines that the investigator has presented adequate assurances that the investigator will employ investigational drugs solely in compliance with the provisions of this part and of parts 50 and 56.

[52 FR 8831, Mar. 19, 1987, as amended at 52 FR 23031, June 17, 1987; 55 FR 11580, Mar. 29, 1990; 62 FR 46876, Sept. 5, 1997; 67 FR 9586, Mar. 4, 2002]

Subpart E--Drugs Intended to Treat Life-threatening and Severely-debilitating Illnesses

Sec. 312.80 Purpose.

The purpose of this section is to establish procedures designed to expedite the development, evaluation, and marketing of new therapies intended to treat persons with life-threatening and severely-debilitating illnesses, especially where no satisfactory alternative therapy exists. As stated 314.105(c) of this chapter, while the statutory standards of safety and effectiveness apply to all drugs, the many kinds of drugs that are subject to them, and the wide range of uses for those drugs, demand flexibility in applying the standards. The Food and Drug Administration (FDA) has determined that it is appropriate to exercise the broadest flexibility in applying the statutory standards, while preserving appropriate guarantees for safety and effectiveness. These procedures reflect the recognition that physicians and patients are generally willing to accept greater risks or side effects from products that treat life-threatening and severely-debilitating illnesses, than they would accept from products that treat less serious illnesses. These procedures also reflect the recognition that the benefits of the drug need to be evaluated in light of the severity of the disease being treated. The procedure outlined in this section should be interpreted consistent with that purpose.

Sec. 312.81 Scope.

This section applies to new drug and biological products that are being studied for their safety and effectiveness in treating life-threatening or severely-debilitating diseases.

(a) For purposes of this section, the term "life-threatening" means:

    (1) Diseases or conditions where the likelihood of death is high unless the course of the disease is interrupted; and

    (2) Diseases or conditions with potentially fatal outcomes, where the end point of clinical trial analysis is survival.

(b) For purposes of this section, the term "severely debilitating" means diseases or conditions that cause major irreversible morbidity.

(c) Sponsors are encouraged to consult with FDA on the applicability of these procedures to specific products.

[53 FR 41523, Oct. 21, 1988, as amended at 64 FR 401, Jan. 5, 1999]

Sec. 312.82 Early consultation.

For products intended to treat life-threatening or severely-debilitating illnesses, sponsors may request to meet with FDA-reviewing officials early in the drug development process to review and reach agreement on the design of necessary preclinical and clinical studies. Where appropriate, FDA will invite to such meetings one or more outside expert scientific consultants or advisory committee members. To the extent FDA resources permit, agency reviewing officials will honor requests for such meetings

(a) Pre-investigational new drug (IND) meetings. Prior to the submission of the initial IND, the sponsor may request a meeting with FDA-reviewing officials. The primary purpose of this meeting is to review and reach agreement on the design of animal studies needed to initiate human testing. The meeting may also provide an opportunity for discussing the scope and design of phase 1 testing, plans for studying the drug product in pediatric populations, and the best approach for presentation and formatting of data in the IND.

(b) End-of-phase 1 meetings. When data from phase 1 clinical testing are available, the sponsor may again request a meeting with FDA-reviewing officials. The primary purpose of this meeting is to review and reach agreement on the design of phase 2 controlled clinical trials, with the goal that such testing will be adequate to provide sufficient data on the drug's safety and effectiveness to support a decision on its approvability for marketing, and to discuss the need for, as well as the design and timing of, studies of the drug in pediatric patients. For drugs for life-threatening diseases, FDA will provide its best judgment, at that time, whether pediatric studies will be required and whether their submission will be deferred until after approval. The procedures outlined in 312.47(b)(1) with respect to end-of-phase 2 conferences, including documentation of agreements reached, would also be used for end-of-phase 1 meetings.

[53 FR 41523, Oct. 21, 1988, as amended at 63 FR 66669, Dec. 2, 1998]

Sec. 312.83 Treatment protocols.

If the preliminary analysis of phase 2 test results appears promising, FDA may ask the sponsor to submit a treatment protocol to be reviewed under the procedures and criteria listed in 312.34 and 312.35. Such a treatment protocol, if requested and granted, would normally remain in effect while the complete data necessary for a marketing application are being assembled by the sponsor and reviewed by FDA (unless grounds exist for clinical hold of ongoing protocols, as provided in 312.42(b)(3)(ii)).

Sec. 312.84 Risk-benefit analysis in review of marketing applications for drugs to treat life-threatening and severely-debilitating illnesses.

(a) FDA's application of the statutory standards for marketing approval shall recognize the need for a medical risk-benefit judgment in making the final decision on approvability. As part of this evaluation, consistent with the statement of purpose in 312.80, FDA will consider whether the benefits of the drug outweigh the known and potential risks of the drug and the need to answer remaining questions about risks and benefits of the drug, taking into consideration the severity of the disease and the absence of satisfactory alternative therapy.

(b) In making decisions on whether to grant marketing approval for products that have been the subject of an end-of-phase 1 meeting under 312.82, FDA will usually seek the advice of outside expert scientific consultants or advisory committees. Upon the filing of such a marketing application under 314.101 or part 601 of this chapter, FDA will notify the members of the relevant standing advisory committee of the application's filing and its availability for review.

(c) If FDA concludes that the data presented are not sufficient for marketing approval, FDA will issue a complete response letter under 314.110 of this chapter or the biological product licensing procedures. Such letter, in describing the deficiencies in the application, will address why the results of the research design agreed to under 312.82, or in subsequent meetings, have not provided sufficient evidence for marketing approval. Such letter will also describe any recommendations made by the advisory committee regarding the application.

(d) Marketing applications submitted under the procedures contained in this section will be subject to the requirements and procedures contained in part 314 or part 600 of this chapter, as well as those in this subpart.

[53 FR 41523, Oct. 21, 1988, as amended at 73 FR 39607, July 10, 2008]

Sec. 312.85 Phase 4 studies.

Concurrent with marketing approval, FDA may seek agreement from the sponsor to conduct certain postmarketing (phase 4) studies to delineate additional information about the drug's risks, benefits, and optimal use. These studies could include, but would not be limited to, studying different doses or schedules of administration than were used in phase 2 studies, use of the drug in other patient populations or other stages of the disease, or use of the drug over a longer period of time.

Sec. 312.86 Focused FDA regulatory research.

At the discretion of the agency, FDA may undertake focused regulatory research on critical rate-limiting aspects of the preclinical, chemical/manufacturing, and clinical phases of drug development and evaluation. When initiated, FDA will undertake such research efforts as a means for meeting a public health need in facilitating the development of therapies to treat life-threatening or severely debilitating illnesses.

Sec. 312.87 Active monitoring of conduct and evaluation of clinical trials.

For drugs covered under this section, the Commissioner and other agency officials will monitor the progress of the conduct and evaluation of clinical trials and be involved in facilitating their appropriate progress.

Sec. 312.88 Safeguards for patient safety.

All of the safeguards incorporated within parts 50, 56, 312, 314, and 600 of this chapter designed to ensure the safety of clinical testing and the safety of products following marketing approval apply to drugs covered by this section. This includes the requirements for informed consent (part 50 of this chapter) and institutional review boards (part 56 of this chapter). These safeguards further include the review of animal studies prior to initial human testing (312.23), and the monitoring of adverse drug experiences through the requirements of IND safety reports (312.32), safety update reports during agency review of a marketing application (314.50 of this chapter), and postmarketing adverse reaction reporting (314.80 of this chapter).

Subpart F--Miscellaneous

Sec. 312.110 Import and export requirements.

(a) Imports. An investigational new drug offered for import into the United States complies with the requirements of this part if it is subject to an IND that is in effect for it under 312.40 and: (1) The consignee in the United States is the sponsor of the IND; (2) the consignee is a qualified investigator named in the IND; or (3) the consignee is the domestic agent of a foreign sponsor, is responsible for the control and distribution of the investigational drug, and the IND identifies the consignee and describes what, if any, actions the consignee will take with respect to the investigational drug.

(b) Exports. An investigational new drug may be exported from the United States for use in a clinical investigation under any of the following conditions:

(1) An IND is in effect for the drug under 312.40, the drug complies with the laws of the country to which it is being exported, and each person who receives the drug is an investigator in a study submitted to and allowed to proceed under the IND; or

(2) The drug has valid marketing authorization in Australia, Canada, Israel, Japan, New Zealand, Switzerland, South Africa, or in any country in the European Union or the European Economic Area, and complies with the laws of the country to which it is being exported, section 802(b)(1)(A), (f), and (g) of the act, and 1.101 of this chapter; or

(3) The drug is being exported to Australia, Canada, Israel, Japan, New Zealand, Switzerland, South Africa, or to any country in the European Union or the European Economic Area, and complies with the laws of the country to which it is being exported, the applicable provisions of section 802(c), (f), and (g) of the act, and 1.101 of this chapter. Drugs exported under this paragraph that are not the subject of an IND are exempt from the label requirement in 312.6(a); or

(4) Except as provided in paragraph (b)(5) of this section, the person exporting the drug sends a written certification to the Office of International Programs (HFG-1), Food and Drug Administration, 5600 Fishers Lane, Rockville, MD 20857, at the time the drug is first exported and maintains records documenting compliance with this paragraph. The certification shall describe the drug that is to be exported (i.e. , trade name (if any), generic name, and dosage form), identify the country or countries to which the drug is to be exported, and affirm that:

(i) The drug is intended for export;

(ii) The drug is intended for investigational use in a foreign country;

(iii) The drug meets the foreign purchaser's or consignee's specifications;

(iv) The drug is not in conflict with the importing country's laws;

(v) The outer shipping package is labeled to show that the package is intended for export from the United States;

(vi) The drug is not sold or offered for sale in the United States;

(vii) The clinical investigation will be conducted in accordance with 312.120;

(viii) The drug is manufactured, processed, packaged, and held in substantial conformity with current good manufacturing practices;

(ix) The drug is not adulterated within the meaning of section 501(a)(1), (a)(2)(A), (a)(3), (c), or (d) of the act;

(x) The drug does not present an imminent hazard to public health, either in the United States, if the drug were to be reimported, or in the foreign country; and

(xi) The drug is labeled in accordance with the foreign country's laws.

(5) In the event of a national emergency in a foreign country, where the national emergency necessitates exportation of an investigational new drug, the requirements in paragraph (b)(4) of this section apply as follows:

(i) Situations where the investigational new drug is to be stockpiled in anticipation of a national emergency. There may be instances where exportation of an investigational new drug is needed so that the drug may be stockpiled and made available for use by the importing country if and when a national emergency arises. In such cases:

(A) A person may export an investigational new drug under paragraph (b)(4) of this section without making an affirmation with respect to any one or more of paragraphs (b)(4)(i), (b)(4)(iv), (b)(4)(vi), (b)(4)(vii), (b)(4)(viii), and/or (b)(4)(ix) of this section, provided that he or she:

(1) Provides a written statement explaining why compliance with each such paragraph is not feasible or is contrary to the best interests of the individuals who may receive the investigational new drug;

(2) Provides a written statement from an authorized official of the importing country's government. The statement must attest that the official agrees with the exporter's statement made under paragraph (b)(5)(i)(A)(1) of this section; explain that the drug is to be stockpiled solely for use of the importing country in a national emergency; and describe the potential national emergency that warrants exportation of the investigational new drug under this provision; and

(3) Provides a written statement showing that the Secretary of Health and Human Services (the Secretary), or his or her designee, agrees with the findings of the authorized official of the importing country's government. Persons who wish to obtain a written statement from the Secretary should direct their requests to Secretary's Operations Center, Office of Emergency Operations and Security Programs, Office of Public Health Emergency Preparedness, Office of the Secretary, Department of Health and Human Services, 200 Independence Ave. SW., Washington, DC 20201. Requests may be also be sent by FAX: 202-619-7870 or by e-mail:HHS.SOC@hhs.gov.

(B) Exportation may not proceed until FDA has authorized exportation of the investigational new drug. FDA may deny authorization if the statements provided under paragraphs (b)(5)(i)(A)(1) or (b)(5)(i)(A)(2) of this section are inadequate or if exportation is contrary to public health.

(ii) Situations where the investigational new drug is to be used for a sudden and immediate national emergency. There may be instances where exportation of an investigational new drug is needed so that the drug may be used in a sudden and immediate national emergency that has developed or is developing. In such cases:

(A) A person may export an investigational new drug under paragraph (b)(4) of this section without making an affirmation with respect to any one or more of paragraphs (b)(4)(i), (b)(4)(iv), (b)(4)(v), (b)(4)(vi), (b)(4)(vii), (b)(4)(viii), (b)(4)(ix), and/or (b)(4)(xi), provided that he or she:

(1) Provides a written statement explaining why compliance with each such paragraph is not feasible or is contrary to the best interests of the individuals who are expected to receive the investigational new drug and

(2) Provides sufficient information from an authorized official of the importing country's government to enable the Secretary, or his or her designee, to decide whether a national emergency has developed or is developing in the importing country, whether the investigational new drug will be used solely for that national emergency, and whether prompt exportation of the investigational new drug is necessary. Persons who wish to obtain a determination from the Secretary should direct their requests to Secretary's Operations Center, Office of Emergency Operations and Security Programs, Office of Public Health Emergency Preparedness, Office of the Secretary, Department of Health and Human Services, 200 Independence Ave. SW., Washington, DC 20201. Requests may be also be sent by FAX: 202-619-7870 or by e-mail:HHS.SOC@hhs.gov.

(B) Exportation may proceed without prior FDA authorization.

(c) Limitations. Exportation under paragraph (b) of this section may not occur if:

(1) For drugs exported under paragraph (b)(1) of this section, the IND pertaining to the clinical investigation is no longer in effect;

(2) For drugs exported under paragraph (b)(2) of this section, the requirements in section 802(b)(1), (f), or (g) of the act are no longer met;

(3) For drugs exported under paragraph (b)(3) of this section, the requirements in section 802(c), (f), or (g) of the act are no longer met;

(4) For drugs exported under paragraph (b)(4) of this section, the conditions underlying the certification or the statements submitted under paragraph (b)(5) of this section are no longer met; or

(5) For any investigational new drugs under this section, the drug no longer complies with the laws of the importing country.

(d) Insulin and antibiotics. New insulin and antibiotic drug products may be exported for investigational use in accordance with section 801(e)(1) of the act without complying with this section.

[52 FR 8831, Mar. 19, 1987, as amended at 52 FR 23031, June 17, 1987; 64 FR 401, Jan. 5, 1999; 67 FR 9586, Mar. 4, 2002; 70 FR 70729, Nov. 23, 2005]

Sec. 312.120 Foreign clinical studies not conducted under an IND.

(a) Acceptance of studies.

(1) FDA will accept as support for an IND or application for marketing approval (an application under section 505 of the act or section 351 of the Public Health Service Act (the PHS Act) (42 U.S.C. 262)) a well-designed and well-conducted foreign clinical study not conducted under an IND, if the following conditions are met:

(i) The study was conducted in accordance with good clinical practice (GCP). For the purposes of this section, GCP is defined as a standard for the design, conduct, performance, monitoring, auditing, recording, analysis, and reporting of clinical trials in a way that provides assurance that the data and reported results are credible and accurate and that the rights, safety, and well-being of trial subjects are protected. GCP includes review and approval (or provision of a favorable opinion) by an independent ethics committee (IEC) before initiating a study, continuing review of an ongoing study by an IEC, and obtaining and documenting the freely given informed consent of the subject (or a subject's legally authorized representative, if the subject is unable to provide informed consent) before initiating a study. GCP does not require informed consent in life-threatening situations when the IEC reviewing the study finds, before initiation of the study, that informed consent is not feasible and either that the conditions present are consistent with those described in 50.23 or 50.24(a) of this chapter, or that the measures described in the study protocol or elsewhere will protect the rights, safety, and well-being of subjects; and

(ii) FDA is able to validate the data from the study through an onsite inspection if the agency deems it necessary.

(2) Although FDA will not accept as support for an IND or application for marketing approval a study that does not meet the conditions of paragraph (a)(1) of this section, FDA will examine data from such a study.

(3) Marketing approval of a new drug based solely on foreign clinical data is governed by 314.106 of this chapter.

(b) Supporting information. A sponsor or applicant who submits data from a foreign clinical study not conducted under an IND as support for an IND or application for marketing approval must submit to FDA, in addition to information required elsewhere in parts 312, 314, or 601 of this chapter, a description of the actions the sponsor or applicant took to ensure that the research conformed to GCP as described in paragraph (a)(1)(i) of this section. The description is not required to duplicate information already submitted in the IND or application for marketing approval. Instead, the description must provide either the following information or a cross-reference to another section of the submission where the information is located:

(1) The investigator's qualifications;

(2) A description of the research facilities;

(3) A detailed summary of the protocol and results of the study and, should FDA request, case records maintained by the investigator or additional background data such as hospital or other institutional records;

(4) A description of the drug substance and drug product used in the study, including a description of the components, formulation, specifications, and, if available, bioavailability of the specific drug product used in the clinical study;

(5) If the study is intended to support the effectiveness of a drug product, information showing that the study is adequate and well controlled under 314.126 of this chapter;

(6) The name and address of the IEC that reviewed the study and a statement that the IEC meets the definition in 312.3 of this chapter. The sponsor or applicant must maintain records supporting such statement, including records of the names and qualifications of IEC members, and make these records available for agency review upon request;

(7) A summary of the IEC's decision to approve or modify and approve the study, or to provide a favorable opinion;

(8) A description of how informed consent was obtained;

(9) A description of what incentives, if any, were provided to subjects to participate in the study;

(10) A description of how the sponsor(s) monitored the study and ensured that the study was carried out consistently with the study protocol; and

(11) A description of how investigators were trained to comply with GCP (as described in paragraph (a)(1)(i) of this section) and to conduct the study in accordance with the study protocol, and a statement on whether written commitments by investigators to comply with GCP and the protocol were obtained. Any signed written commitments by investigators must be maintained by the sponsor or applicant and made available for agency review upon request.

(c) Waivers.

(1) A sponsor or applicant may ask FDA to waive any applicable requirements under paragraphs (a)(1) and (b) of this section. A waiver request may be submitted in an IND or in an information amendment to an IND, or in an application or in an amendment or supplement to an application submitted under part 314 or 601 of this chapter. A waiver request is required to contain at least one of the following:

(i) An explanation why the sponsor's or applicant's compliance with the requirement is unnecessary or cannot be achieved;

(ii) A description of an alternative submission or course of action that satisfies the purpose of the requirement; or

(iii) Other information justifying a waiver.

(2) FDA may grant a waiver if it finds that doing so would be in the interest of the public health.

(d) Records. A sponsor or applicant must retain the records required by this section for a foreign clinical study not conducted under an IND as follows:

(1) If the study is submitted in support of an application for marketing approval, for 2 years after an agency decision on that application;

(2) If the study is submitted in support of an IND but not an application for marketing approval, for 2 years after the submission of the IND.

[73 FR 22815, Apr. 28, 2008]

Sec. 312.130 Availability for public disclosure of data and information in an IND.

(a) The existence of an investigational new drug application will not be disclosed by FDA unless it has previously been publicly disclosed or acknowledged.

(b) The availability for public disclosure of all data and information in an investigational new drug application for a new drug will be handled in accordance with the provisions established in 314.430 for the confidentiality of data and information in applications submitted in part 314. The availability for public disclosure of all data and information in an investigational new drug application for a biological product will be governed by the provisions of 601.50 and 601.51.

(c) Notwithstanding the provisions of 314.430, FDA shall disclose upon request to an individual to whom an investigational new drug has been given a copy of any IND safety report relating to the use in the individual.

(d) The availability of information required to be publicly disclosed for investigations involving an exception from informed consent under 50.24 of this chapter will be handled as follows: Persons wishing to request the publicly disclosable information in the IND that was required to be filed in Docket Number 95S-0158 in the Division of Dockets Management (HFA-305), Food and Drug Administration, 5630 Fishers Lane, rm. 1061, Rockville, MD 20852, shall submit a request under the Freedom of Information Act.

[52 FR 8831, Mar. 19, 1987. Redesignated at 53 FR 41523, Oct. 21, 1988, as amended at 61 FR 51530, Oct. 2, 1996; 64 FR 401, Jan. 5, 1999; 68 FR 24879, May 9, 2003]

Sec. 312.140 Address for correspondence.

(a) A sponsor must send an initial IND submission to the Center for Drug Evaluation and Research (CDER) or to the Center for Biologics Evaluation and Research (CBER), depending on the Center responsible for regulating the product as follows:

   (1) For drug products regulated by CDER. Send the IND submission to the Central Document Room, Center for Drug Evaluation and Research, Food and Drug Administration, 5901-B Ammendale Rd., Beltsville, MD 20705-1266; except send an IND submission for an in vivo bioavailability or bioequivalence study in humans to support an abbreviated new drug application to the Office of Generic Drugs (HFD-600), Center for Drug Evaluation and Research, Food and Drug Administration, Metro Park North VII, 7620 Standish Pl., Rockville, MD 20855.

   (2) For biological products regulated by CDER. Send the IND submission to the CDER Therapeutic Biological Products Document Room, Center for Drug Evaluation and Research, Food and Drug Administration, 12229 Wilkins Ave., Rockville, MD 20852.

   (3) For biological products regulated by CBER. Send the IND submission to the Document Control Center (HFM-99), Center for Biologics Evaluation and Research, Food and Drug Administration, 1401 Rockville Pike, suite 200N, Rockville, MD 20852-1448.

(b) On receiving the IND, the responsible Center will inform the sponsor which one of the divisions in CDER or CBER is responsible for the IND. Amendments, reports, and other correspondence relating to matters covered by the IND should be sent to the appropriate center at the address indicated in this section and marked to the attention of the responsible division. The outside wrapper of each submission shall state what is contained in the submission, for example, "IND Application", "Protocol Amendment", etc.

(c) All correspondence relating to export of an investigational drug under 312.110(b)(2) shall be submitted to the International Affairs

Staff (HFY-50), Office of Health Affairs, Food and Drug Administration, 5600 Fishers Lane, Rockville, MD 20857.

[70 FR 14981, Mar. 24, 2005, as amended at 74 FR 13113, Mar. 26, 2009; 74 FR 55771, Oct. 29, 2009; 75 FR 37295, June 29, 2010]

Sec. 312.145 Guidance documents.

(a) FDA has made available guidance documents under 10.115 of this chapter to help you to comply with certain requirements of this part.

(b) The Center for Drug Evaluation and Research (CDER) and the Center for Biologics Evaluation and Research (CBER) maintain lists of guidance documents that apply to the centers' regulations. The lists are maintained on the Internet and are published annually in theFederal Register.A request for a copy of the CDER list should be directed to the Office of Training and Communications, Division of Drug Information, Center for Drug Evaluation and Research, Food and Drug Administration, 10903 New Hampshire Ave., Silver Spring, MD 20993-0002. A request for a copy of the CBER list should be directed to the Office of Communication, Training, and Manufacturers Assistance (HFM-40), Center for Biologics Evaluation and Research, Food and Drug Administration, 1401 Rockville Pike, Rockville, MD 20852-1448.

[65 FR 56479, Sept. 19, 2000, as amended at 74 FR 13113, Mar. 26, 2009]

Subpart G--Drugs for Investigational Use in Laboratory Research Animals or In Vitro Tests

Sec. 312.160 Drugs for investigational use in laboratory research animals or in vitro tests.

(a) Authorization to ship.

(1)(i) A person may ship a drug intended solely for tests in vitro or in animals used only for laboratory research purposes if it is labeled as follows:

CAUTION: Contains a new drug for investigational use only in laboratory research animals, or for tests in vitro. Not for use in humans.

(ii) A person may ship a biological product for investigational in vitro diagnostic use that is listed in 312.2(b)(2)(ii) if it is labeled as follows:

CAUTION: Contains a biological product for investigational in vitro diagnostic tests only.

(2) A person shipping a drug under paragraph (a) of this section shall use due diligence to assure that the consignee is regularly engaged in conducting such tests and that the shipment of the new drug will actually be used for tests in vitro or in animals used only for laboratory research.

(3) A person who ships a drug under paragraph (a) of this section shall maintain adequate records showing the name and post office address of the expert to whom the drug is shipped and the date, quantity, and batch or code mark of each shipment and delivery. Records of shipments under paragraph (a)(1)(i) of this section are to be maintained for a period of 2 years after the shipment. Records and reports of data and shipments under paragraph (a)(1)(ii) of this section are to be maintained in accordance with 312.57(b). The person who ships the drug shall upon request from any properly authorized officer or employee of the Food and Drug Administration, at reasonable times, permit such officer or employee to have access to and copy and verify records required to be maintained under this section.

(b) Termination of authorization to ship. FDA may terminate authorization to ship a drug under this section if it finds that:

(1) The sponsor of the investigation has failed to comply with any of the conditions for shipment established under this section; or

(2) The continuance of the investigation is unsafe or otherwise contrary to the public interest or the drug is used for purposes other than bona fide scientific investigation. FDA will notify the person shipping the drug of its finding and invite immediate correction. If correction is not immediately made, the person shall have an opportunity for a regulatory hearing before FDA pursuant to part 16.

(c) Disposition of unused drug. The person who ships the drug under paragraph (a) of this section shall assure the return of all unused supplies of the drug from individual investigators whenever the investigation discontinues or the investigation is terminated. The person who ships the drug may authorize in writing alternative disposition of unused supplies of the drug provided this alternative disposition does not expose humans to risks from the drug, either directly or indirectly (e.g., through food-producing animals). The shipper shall maintain records of any alternative disposition.

[52 FR 8831, Mar. 19, 1987, as amended at 52 FR 23031, June 17, 1987. Redesignated at 53 FR 41523, Oct. 21, 1988; 67 FR 9586, Mar. 4, 2002]

Subpart H [Reserved]

Subpart I--Expanded Access to Investigational Drugs for Treatment Use

Sec. 312.300 General.

(a) Scope. This subpart contains the requirements for the use of investigational new drugs and approved drugs where availability is limited by a risk evaluation and mitigation strategy (REMS) when the primary purpose is to diagnose, monitor, or treat a patient's disease or condition. The aim of this subpart is to facilitate the availability of such drugs to patients with serious diseases or conditions when there is no comparable or satisfactory alternative therapy to diagnose, monitor, or treat the patient's disease or condition.

(b) Definitions. The following definitions of terms apply to this subpart:

Immediately life-threatening disease or condition means a stage of disease in which there is reasonable likelihood that death will occur within a matter of months or in which premature death is likely without early treatment.

Serious disease or condition means a disease or condition associated with morbidity that has substantial impact on day-to-day functioning. Short-lived and self-limiting morbidity will usually not be sufficient, but the morbidity need not be irreversible, provided it is persistent or recurrent. Whether a disease or condition is serious is a matter of clinical judgment, based on its impact on such factors as survival, day-to-day functioning, or the likelihood that the disease, if left untreated, will progress from a less severe condition to a more serious one.

Sec. 312.305 Requirements for all expanded access uses.

The criteria, submission requirements, safeguards, and beginning treatment information set out in this section apply to all expanded access uses described in this subpart. Additional criteria, submission requirements, and safeguards that apply to specific types of expanded access are described in 312.310 through 312.320.

(a) Criteria. FDA must determine that:

(1) The patient or patients to be treated have a serious or immediately life-threatening disease or condition, and there is no comparable or satisfactory alternative therapy to diagnose, monitor, or treat the disease or condition;

(2) The potential patient benefit justifies the potential risks of the treatment use and those potential risks are not unreasonable in the context of the disease or condition to be treated; and

(3) Providing the investigational drug for the requested use will not interfere with the initiation, conduct, or completion of clinical investigations that could support marketing approval of the expanded access use or otherwise compromise the potential development of the expanded access use.

(b) Submission.

(1) An expanded access submission is required for each type of expanded access described in this subpart. The submission may be a new IND or a protocol amendment to an existing IND. Information required for a submission may be supplied by referring to pertinent information contained in an existing IND if the sponsor of the existing IND grants a right of reference to the IND.

(2) The expanded access submission must include:

(i) A cover sheet (Form FDA 1571) meeting the requirements of 312.23(a);

(ii) The rationale for the intended use of the drug, including a list of available therapeutic options that would ordinarily be tried before resorting to the investigational drug or an explanation of why the use of the investigational drug is preferable to the use of available therapeutic options;

    (iii) The criteria for patient selection or, for an individual patient, a description of the patient's disease or condition, including recent medical history and previous treatments of the disease or condition;

    (iv) The method of administration of the drug, dose, and duration of therapy;

    (v) A description of the facility where the drug will be manufactured;

    (vi) Chemistry, manufacturing, and controls information adequate to ensure the proper identification, quality, purity, and strength of the investigational drug;

    (vii) Pharmacology and toxicology information adequate to conclude that the drug is reasonably safe at the dose and duration proposed for expanded access use (ordinarily, information that would be adequate to permit clinical testing of the drug in a population of the size expected to be treated); and

    (viii) A description of clinical procedures, laboratory tests, or other monitoring necessary to evaluate the effects of the drug and minimize its risks.

(3) The expanded access submission and its mailing cover must be plainly marked "EXPANDED ACCESS SUBMISSION." If the expanded access submission is for a treatment IND or treatment protocol, the applicable box on Form FDA 1571 must be checked.

(c) Safeguards. The responsibilities of sponsors and investigators set forth in subpart D of this part are applicable to expanded access use under this subpart as described in this paragraph.

(1) A licensed physician under whose immediate direction an investigational drug is administered or dispensed for an expanded access use under this subpart is considered aninvestigator , for purposes of this part, and must comply with the responsibilities for investigators set forth in subpart D of this part to the extent they are applicable to the expanded access use.

(2) An individual or entity that submits an expanded access IND or protocol under this subpart is considered asponsor , for purposes of this part, and must comply with the responsibilities for sponsors set forth in subpart D of this

part to the extent they are applicable to the expanded access use.

(3) A licensed physician under whose immediate direction an investigational drug is administered or dispensed, and who submits an IND for expanded access use under this subpart is considered asponsor-investigator , for purposes of this part, and must comply with the responsibilities for sponsors and investigators set forth in subpart D of this part to the extent they are applicable to the expanded access use.

(4) Investigators. In all cases of expanded access, investigators are responsible for reporting adverse drug events to the sponsor, ensuring that the informed consent requirements of part 50 of this chapter are met, ensuring that IRB review of the expanded access use is obtained in a manner consistent with the requirements of part 56 of this chapter, and maintaining accurate case histories and drug disposition records and retaining records in a manner consistent with the requirements of 312.62. Depending on the type of expanded access, other investigator responsibilities under subpart D may also apply.

(5) Sponsors. In all cases of expanded access, sponsors are responsible for submitting IND safety reports and annual reports (when the IND or protocol continues for 1 year or longer) to FDA as required by 312.32 and 312.33, ensuring that licensed physicians are qualified to administer the investigational drug for the expanded access use, providing licensed physicians with the information needed to minimize the risk and maximize the potential benefits of the investigational drug (the investigator's brochure must be provided if one exists for the drug), maintaining an effective IND for the expanded access use, and maintaining adequate drug disposition records and retaining records in a manner consistent with the requirements of 312.57. Depending on the type of expanded access, other sponsor responsibilities under subpart D may also apply.

(d) Beginning treatment –

(1) INDs. An expanded access IND goes into effect 30 days after FDA receives the IND or on earlier notification by FDA that the expanded access use may begin.

(2) Protocols. With the following exceptions, expanded access use under a protocol submitted under an existing IND may begin as described in 312.30(a).

   (i) Expanded access use under the emergency procedures described in 312.310(d) may begin when the use is authorized by the FDA reviewing official.

   (ii) Expanded access use under 312.320 may begin 30 days after FDA receives the protocol or upon earlier notification by FDA that use may begin.

(3) Clinical holds. FDA may place any expanded access IND or protocol on clinical hold as described in 312.42.

Sec. 312.310 Individual patients, including for emergency use.

Under this section, FDA may permit an investigational drug to be used for the treatment of an individual patient by a licensed physician.

(a) Criteria. The criteria in 312.305(a) must be met; and the following determinations must be made:

   (1) The physician must determine that the probable risk to the person from the investigational drug is not greater than the probable risk from the disease or condition; and

   (2) FDA must determine that the patient cannot obtain the drug under another IND or protocol.

(b) Submission. The expanded access submission must include information adequate to demonstrate that the criteria in 312.305(a) and paragraph (a) of this section have been met. The expanded access submission must meet the requirements of 312.305(b).

   (1) If the drug is the subject of an existing IND, the expanded access submission may be made by the sponsor or by a licensed physician.

   (2) A sponsor may satisfy the submission requirements by amending its existing IND to include a protocol for individual patient expanded access.

   (3) A licensed physician may satisfy the submission requirements by obtaining from the sponsor permission for FDA to refer to any information in the IND that would be needed to support the expanded access request (right of reference) and by providing any other required information not contained in

the IND (usually only the information specific to the individual patient).

(c) Safeguards.

(1) Treatment is generally limited to a single course of therapy for a specified duration unless FDA expressly authorizes multiple courses or chronic therapy.

(2) At the conclusion of treatment, the licensed physician or sponsor must provide FDA with a written summary of the results of the expanded access use, including adverse effects.

(3) FDA may require sponsors to monitor an individual patient expanded access use if the use is for an extended duration.

(4) When a significant number of similar individual patient expanded access requests have been submitted, FDA may ask the sponsor to submit an IND or protocol for the use under 312.315 or 312.320.

(d) Emergency procedures. If there is an emergency that requires the patient to be treated before a written submission can be made, FDA may authorize the expanded access use to begin without a written submission. The FDA reviewing official may authorize the emergency use by telephone.

(1) Emergency expanded access use may be requested by telephone, facsimile, or other means of electronic communications. For investigational biological drug products regulated by the Center for Biologics Evaluation and Research, the request should be directed to the Office of Communication, Outreach and Development, Center for Biologics Evaluation and Research, 301-827-1800 or 1-800-835-4709, e-mail:ocod@fda.hhs.gov. For all other investigational drugs, the request for authorization should be directed to the Division of Drug Information, Center for Drug Evaluation and Research, 301-796-3400, e-mail:druginfo@fda.hhs.gov. After normal working hours (8 a.m. to 4:30 p.m.), the request should be directed to the FDA Emergency Call Center, 866-300-4374, e-mail:emergency.operations@fda.hhs.gov.

(2) The licensed physician or sponsor must explain how the expanded access use will meet the requirements of 312.305 and 312.310 and must agree to submit an expanded access

submission within 15 working days of FDA's authorization of
the use.

[74 FR 40942, Aug. 13, 2009, as amended at 75 FR 32659, June 9, 2010]

Sec. 312.315 Intermediate-size patient populations.

Under this section, FDA may permit an investigational drug to be
used for the treatment of a patient population smaller than that typical
of a treatment IND or treatment protocol. FDA may ask a sponsor to
consolidate expanded access under this section when the agency has
received a significant number of requests for individual patient
expanded access to an investigational drug for the same use.

(a) Need for expanded access. Expanded access under this section
may be needed in the following situations:

(1) Drug not being developed. The drug is not being developed,
for example, because the disease or condition is so rare that
the sponsor is unable to recruit patients for a clinical trial.

(2) Drug being developed. The drug is being studied in a clinical
trial, but patients requesting the drug for expanded access use
are unable to participate in the trial. For example, patients
may not be able to participate in the trial because they have a
different disease or stage of disease than the one being
studied or otherwise do not meet the enrollment criteria,
because enrollment in the trial is closed, or because the trial
site is not geographically accessible.

(3) Approved or related drug.

(i) The drug is an approved drug product that is no longer
marketed for safety reasons or is unavailable through
marketing due to failure to meet the conditions of the
approved application, or

(ii) The drug contains the same active moiety as an approved
drug product that is unavailable through marketing due to
failure to meet the conditions of the approved application
or a drug shortage.

(b) Criteria. The criteria in 312.305(a) must be met; and FDA must
determine that:

(1) There is enough evidence that the drug is safe at the dose and
duration proposed for expanded access use to justify a clinical

trial of the drug in the approximate number of patients expected to receive the drug under expanded access; and

(2)   There is at least preliminary clinical evidence of effectiveness of the drug, or of a plausible pharmacologic effect of the drug to make expanded access use a reasonable therapeutic option in the anticipated patient population.

(c)   Submission. The expanded access submission must include information adequate to satisfy FDA that the criteria in 312.305(a) and paragraph (b) of this section have been met. The expanded access submission must meet the requirements of 312.305(b). In addition:

(1)   The expanded access submission must state whether the drug is being developed or is not being developed and describe the patient population to be treated.

(2)   If the drug is not being actively developed, the sponsor must explain why the drug cannot currently be developed for the expanded access use and under what circumstances the drug could be developed.

(3)   If the drug is being studied in a clinical trial, the sponsor must explain why the patients to be treated cannot be enrolled in the clinical trial and under what circumstances the sponsor would conduct a clinical trial in these patients.

(d)   Safeguards.

(1)   Upon review of the IND annual report, FDA will determine whether it is appropriate for the expanded access to continue under this section.

(i)   If the drug is not being actively developed or if the expanded access use is not being developed (but another use is being developed), FDA will consider whether it is possible to conduct a clinical study of the expanded access use.

(ii)   If the drug is being actively developed, FDA will consider whether providing the investigational drug for expanded access use is interfering with the clinical development of the drug.

(iii)   As the number of patients enrolled increases, FDA may ask the sponsor to submit an IND or protocol for the use under 312.320.

(2) The sponsor is responsible for monitoring the expanded access protocol to ensure that licensed physicians comply with the protocol and the regulations applicable to investigators.

Sec. 312.320 Treatment IND or treatment protocol.

Under this section, FDA may permit an investigational drug to be used for widespread treatment use.

(a) Criteria. The criteria in 312.305(a) must be met, and FDA must determine that:

    (1) Trial status.

        (i) The drug is being investigated in a controlled clinical trial under an IND designed to support a marketing application for the expanded access use, or

        (ii) All clinical trials of the drug have been completed; and

    (2) Marketing status. The sponsor is actively pursuing marketing approval of the drug for the expanded access use with due diligence; and

    (3) Evidence.

        (i) When the expanded access use is for a serious disease or condition, there is sufficient clinical evidence of safety and effectiveness to support the expanded access use. Such evidence would ordinarily consist of data from phase 3 trials, but could consist of compelling data from completed phase 2 trials; or

        (ii) When the expanded access use is for an immediately life-threatening disease or condition, the available scientific evidence, taken as a whole, provides a reasonable basis to conclude that the investigational drug may be effective for the expanded access use and would not expose patients to an unreasonable and significant risk of illness or injury. This evidence would ordinarily consist of clinical data from phase 3 or phase 2 trials, but could be based on more preliminary clinical evidence.

(b) Submission. The expanded access submission must include information adequate to satisfy FDA that the criteria in 312.305(a) and paragraph (a) of this section have been met. The expanded access submission must meet the requirements of 312.305(b).

(c) Safeguard. The sponsor is responsible for monitoring the treatment protocol to ensure that licensed physicians comply with the protocol and the regulations applicable to investigators.

Authority: 21 U.S.C. 321, 331, 351, 352, 353, 355, 360bbb, 371; 42 U.S.C. 262.

Source: 52 FR 8831, Mar. 19, 1987, unless otherwise noted.

Part 312

Part 314: Applications for FDA Approval to Market a New Drug

[Code of Federal Regulations]

[Title 21, Volume 5]

[Revised as of April 1, 2009]

[CITE: 21CFR314]

Title 21--Food and Drugs

Chapter I--Food and Drug Administration

Department of Health and Human Services

Subchapter D--Drugs for Human Use

Part 314 Applications for FDA Approval to Market a New Drug[1]

Subpart A--General Provisions

Sec. 314.1 Scope of this part.

(a) This part sets forth procedures and requirements for the submission to, and the review by, the Food and Drug Administration of applications and abbreviated applications to market a new drug under section 505 of the Federal Food, Drug, and Cosmetic Act, as well as amendments, supplements, and postmarketing reports to them.

(b) This part does not apply to drug products subject to licensing by FDA under the Public Health Service Act (58 Stat. 632 as amended (42 U.S.C. 201et seq.)) and subchapter F of chapter I of title 21 of the Code of Federal Regulations.

---

[1] Available on the FDA website at http://www.accessdata.fda.gov/scripts/cdrh/cfdocs/cfcfr/CFRSearch.cfm?CFRPart=314&showFR=1

(c) References in this part to regulations in the Code of Federal
Regulations are to chapter I of title 21, unless otherwise noted.

[50 FR 7493, Feb. 22, 1985, as amended at 57 FR 17981, Apr. 28, 1992; 64 FR
401, Jan. 5, 1999]

Sec. 314.2 Purpose.

The purpose of this part is to establish an efficient and thorough drug
review process in order to: (a) Facilitate the approval of drugs shown
to be safe and effective; and (b) ensure the disapproval of drugs not
shown to be safe and effective. These regulations are also intended to
establish an effective system for FDA's surveillance of marketed
drugs. These regulations shall be construed in light of these objectives.

Sec. 314.3 Definitions.

(a) The definitions and interpretations contained in section 201 of the
act apply to those terms when used in this part.

(b) The following definitions of terms apply to this part:

Abbreviated application means the application described under
314.94, including all amendments and supplements to the
application. "Abbreviated application" applies to both an
abbreviated new drug application and an abbreviated
antibiotic application.

Act means the Federal Food, Drug, and Cosmetic Act (sections
201-901 (21 U.S.C. 301-392)).

Applicant means any person who submits an application or
abbreviated application or an amendment or supplement to
them under this part to obtain FDA approval of a new drug
or an antibiotic drug and any person who owns an approved
application or abbreviated application.

Application means the application described under 314.50,
including all amendements and supplements to the
application.

505(b)(2) Application means an application submitted under
section 505(b)(1) of the act for a drug for which the
investigations described in section 505(b)(1)(A) of the act and
relied upon by the applicant for approval of the application
were not conducted by or for the applicant and for which the

applicant has not obtained a right of reference or use from the person by or for whom the investigations were conducted.

Approval letter means a written communication to an applicant from FDA approving an application or an abbreviated application.

Assess the effects of the change means to evaluate the effects of a manufacturing change on the identity, strength, quality, purity, and potency of a drug product as these factors may relate to the safety or effectiveness of the drug product.

Authorized generic drug means a listed drug, as defined in this section, that has been approved under section 505(c) of the act and is marketed, sold, or distributed directly or indirectly to retail class of trade with labeling, packaging (other than repackaging as the listed drug in blister packs, unit doses, or similar packaging for use in institutions), product code, labeler code, trade name, or trademark that differs from that of the listed drug.

Class 1 resubmission means the resubmission of an application or efficacy supplement, following receipt of a complete response letter, that contains one or more of the following: Final printed labeling, draft labeling, certain safety updates, stability updates to support provisional or final dating periods, commitments to perform postmarketing studies (including proposals for such studies), assay validation data, final release testing on the last lots used to support approval, minor reanalyses of previously submitted data, and other comparatively minor information.

Class 2 resubmission means the resubmission of an application or efficacy supplement, following receipt of a complete response letter, that includes any item not specified in the definition of "Class 1 resubmission," including any item that would require presentation to an advisory committee.

Complete response letter means a written communication to an applicant from FDA usually describing all of the deficiencies that the agency has identified in an application or abbreviated application that must be satisfactorily addressed before it can be approved.

Drug product means a finished dosage form, for example, tablet, capsule, or solution, that contains a drug substance, generally, but not necessarily, in association with one or more other ingredients.

Drug substance means an active ingredient that is intended to furnish pharmacological activity or other direct effect in the diagnosis, cure, mitigation, treatment, or prevention of disease or to affect the structure or any function of the human body, but does not include intermediates use in the synthesis of such ingredient.

Efficacy supplement means a supplement to an approved application proposing to make one or more related changes from among the following changes to product labeling:

(1) Add or modify an indication or claim;

(2) Revise the dose or dose regimen;

(3) Provide for a new route of administration;

(4) Make a comparative efficacy claim naming another drug product;

(5) Significantly alter the intended patient population;

(6) Change the marketing status from prescription to over-the-counter use;

(7) Provide for, or provide evidence of effectiveness necessary for, the traditional approval of a product originally approved under subpart H of part 314; or

(8) Incorporate other information based on at least one adequate and well-controlled clinical study.

FDA means the Food and Drug Administration.

Listed drug means a new drug product that has an effective approval under section 505(c) of the act for safety and effectiveness or under section 505(j) of the act, which has not been withdrawn or suspended under section 505(e)(1) through (e)(5) or (j)(5) of the act, and which has not been withdrawn from sale for what FDA has determined are reasons of safety or effectiveness. Listed drug status is evidenced by the drug product's identification as a drug with an effective approval in the current edition of FDA's "Approved Drug Products with Therapeutic Equivalence Evaluations" (the list) or any current supplement thereto, as a drug with an effective approval. A drug product is deemed to be a listed drug on the date of effective approval of the application or abbreviated application for that drug product.

Newly acquired information means data, analyses, or other information not previously submitted to the agency, which may include (but are not limited to) data derived from new clinical studies, reports of adverse events, or new analyses of previously submitted data (e.g., meta-analyses) if the studies, events or analyses reveal risks of a different type or greater severity or frequency than previously included in submissions to FDA.

Original application means a pending application for which FDA has never issued a complete response letter or approval letter, or an application that was submitted again after FDA had refused to file it or after it was withdrawn without being approved.

Reference listed drug means the listed drug identified by FDA as the drug product upon which an applicant relies in seeking approval of its abbreviated application.

Resubmission means submission by the applicant of all materials needed to fully address all deficiencies identified in the complete response letter. An application or abbreviated application for which FDA issued a complete response letter, but which was withdrawn before approval and later submitted again, is not a resubmission.

Right of reference or use means the authority to rely upon, and otherwise use, an investigation for the purpose of obtaining approval of an application, including the ability to make available the underlying raw data from the investigation for FDA audit, if necessary.

Specification means the quality standard (i.e. , tests, analytical procedures, and acceptance criteria) provided in an approved application to confirm the quality of drug substances, drug products, intermediates, raw materials, reagents, components, in-process materials, container closure systems, and other materials used in the production of a drug substance or drug product. For the purpose of this definition,acceptance criteria means numerical limits, ranges, or other criteria for the tests described.

The list means the list of drug products with effective approvals published in the current edition of FDA's publication

Part 314

"Approved Drug Products with Therapeutic Equivalence Evaluations" and any current supplement to the publication.

[50 FR 7493, Feb. 22, 1985, as amended at 57 FR 17981, Apr. 28, 1992; 69 FR 18763, Apr. 8, 2004; 73 FR 39607, July 10, 2008; 73 FR 49609, Aug. 22, 2008; 74 FR 37167, July 28, 2009]

Subpart B--Applications

Sec. 314.50 Content and format of an application.

Applications and supplements to approved applications are required to be submitted in the form and contain the information, as appropriate for the particular submission, required under this section. Three copies of the application are required: An archival copy, a review copy, and a field copy. An application for a new chemical entity will generally contain an application form, an index, a summary, five or six technical sections, case report tabulations of patient data, case report forms, drug samples, and labeling, including, if applicable, any Medication Guide required under part 208 of this chapter. Other applications will generally contain only some of those items, and information will be limited to that needed to support the particular submission. These include an application of the type described in section 505(b)(2) of the act, an amendment, and a supplement. The application is required to contain reports of all investigations of the drug product sponsored by the applicant, and all other information about the drug pertinent to an evaluation of the application that is received or otherwise obtained by the applicant from any source. FDA will maintain guidance documents on the format and content of applications to assist applicants in their preparation.

(a) Application form. The applicant shall submit a completed and signed application form that contains the following:

(1) The name and address of the applicant; the date of the application; the application number if previously issued (for example, if the application is a resubmission, an amendment, or a supplement); the name of the drug product, including its established, proprietary, code, and chemical names; the dosage form and strength; the route of administration; the identification numbers of all investigational new drug applications that are referenced in the application; the identification numbers of all drug master files and other applications under this part that are referenced in the

application; and the drug product's proposed indications for use.

(2) A statement whether the submission is an original submission, a 505(b)(2) application, a resubmission, or a supplement to an application under 314.70.

(3) A statement whether the applicant proposes to market the drug product as a prescription or an over-the-counter product.

(4) A check-list identifying what enclosures required under this section the applicant is submitting.

(5) The applicant, or the applicant's attorney, agent, or other authorized official shall sign the application. If the person signing the application does not reside or have a place of business within the United States, the application is required to contain the name and address of, and be countersigned by, an attorney, agent, or other authorized official who resides or maintains a place of business within the United States.

(b) Index. The archival copy of the application is required to contain a comprehensive index by volume number and page number to the summary under paragraph (c) of this section, the technical sections under paragraph (d) of this section, and the supporting information under paragraph (f) of this section.

(c) Summary.

(1) An application is required to contain a summary of the application in enough detail that the reader may gain a good general understanding of the data and information in the application, including an understanding of the quantitative aspects of the data. The summary is not required for supplements under 314.70. Resubmissions of an application should contain an updated summary, as appropriate. The summary should discuss all aspects of the application, and synthesize the information into a well-structured and unified document. The summary should be written at approximately the level of detail required for publication in, and meet the editorial standards generally applied by, refereed scientific and medical journals. In addition to the agency personnel reviewing the summary in the context of their review of the application, FDA may furnish the summary to FDA advisory committee members and agency officials whose duties require

an understanding of the application. To the extent possible, data in the summary should be presented in tabular and graphic forms. FDA has prepared a guideline under 10.90(b) that provides information about how to prepare a summary. The summary required under this paragraph may be used by FDA or the applicant to prepare the Summary Basis of Approval document for public disclosure (under 314.430(e)(2)(ii)) when the application is approved.

(2) The summary is required to contain the following information:

(i) The proposed text of the labeling, including, if applicable, any Medication Guide required under part 208 of this chapter, for the drug, with annotations to the information in the summary and technical sections of the application that support the inclusion of each statement in the labeling, and, if the application is for a prescription drug, statements describing the reasons for omitting a section or subsection of the labeling format in 201.57 of this chapter.

(ii) A statement identifying the pharmacologic class of the drug and a discussion of the scientific rationale for the drug, its intended use, and the potential clinical benefits of the drug product.

(iii) A brief description of the marketing history, if any, of the drug outside the United States, including a list of the countries in which the drug has been marketed, a list of any countries in which the drug has been withdrawn from marketing for any reason related to safety or effectiveness, and a list of countries in which applications for marketing are pending. The description is required to describe both marketing by the applicant and, if known, the marketing history of other persons.

(iv) A summary of the chemistry, manufacturing, and controls section of the application.

(v) A summary of the nonclinical pharmacology and toxicology section of the application.

(vi) A summary of the human pharmacokinetics and bioavailability section of the application.

(vii) A summary of the microbiology section of the application (for anti-infective drugs only).

(viii) A summary of the clinical data section of the application, including the results of statistical analyses of the clinical trials.

(ix) A concluding discussion that presents the benefit and risk considerations related to the drug, including a discussion of any proposed additional studies or surveillance the applicant intends to conduct postmarketing.

(d) Technical sections. The application is required to contain the technical sections described below. Each technical section is required to contain data and information in sufficient detail to permit the agency to make a knowledgeable judgment about whether to approve the application or whether grounds exist under section 505(d) of the act to refuse to approve the application. The required technical sections are as follows:

(1) Chemistry, manufacturing, and controls section. A section describing the composition, manufacture, and specification of the drug substance and the drug product, including the following:

(i) Drug substance. A full description of the drug substance including its physical and chemical characteristics and stability; the name and address of its manufacturer; the method of synthesis (or isolation) and purification of the drug substance; the process controls used during manufacture and packaging; and the specifications necessary to ensure the identity, strength, quality, and purity of the drug substance and the bioavailability of the drug products made from the substance, including, for example, tests, analytical procedures, and acceptance criteria relating to stability, sterility, particle size, and crystalline form. The application may provide additionally for the use of alternatives to meet any of these requirements, including alternative sources, process controls, and analytical procedures. Reference to the current edition of the U.S. Pharmacopeia and the National Formulary may satisfy relevant requirements in this paragraph.

(ii)(a) Drug product. A list of all components used in the manufacture of the drug product (regardless of whether they appear in the drug product) and a statement of the composition of the drug product; the specifications for each component; the name and address of each manufacturer of the drug product; a description of the manufacturing and packaging procedures and in-process controls for the drug product; the specifications necessary to ensure the identity, strength, quality, purity, potency, and bioavailability of the drug product, including, for example, tests, analytical procedures, and acceptance criteria relating to sterility, dissolution rate, container closure systems; and stability data with proposed expiration dating. The application may provide additionally for the use of alternatives to meet any of these requirements, including alternative components, manufacturing and packaging procedures, in-process controls, and analytical procedures. Reference to the current edition of the U.S. Pharmacopeia and the National Formulary may satisfy relevant requirements in this paragraph.

(b) Unless provided by paragraph (d)(1)(ii)(a) of this section, for each batch of the drug product used to conduct a bioavailability or bioequivalence study described in 320.38 or 320.63 of this chapter or used to conduct a primary stability study: The batch production record; the specification for each component and for the drug product; the names and addresses of the sources of the active and noncompendial inactive components and of the container and closure system for the drug product; the name and address of each contract facility involved in the manufacture, processing, packaging, or testing of the drug product and identification of the operation performed by each contract facility; and the results of any test performed on the components used in the manufacture of the drug product as required by 211.84(d) of this chapter and on the drug product as required by 211.165 of this chapter.

(c) The proposed or actual master production record, including a description of the equipment, to be used for the manufacture of a commercial lot of the drug product or a comparably detailed description of the production process for a representative batch of the drug product.

(iii) Environmental impact. The application is required to contain either a claim for categorical exclusion under 25.30 or 25.31 of this chapter or an environmental assessment under 25.40 of this chapter.

(iv) The applicant may, at its option, submit a complete chemistry, manufacturing, and controls section 90 to 120 days before the anticipated submission of the remainder of the application. FDA will review such early submissions as resources permit.

(v) The applicant shall include a statement certifying that the field copy of the application has been provided to the applicant's home FDA district office.

Part 314

(2) Nonclinical pharmacology and toxicology section. A section describing, with the aid of graphs and tables, animal and in vitro studies with drug, including the following:

(i) Studies of the pharmacological actions of the drug in relation to its proposed therapeutic indication and studies that otherwise define the pharmacologic properties of the drug or are pertinent to possible adverse effects.

(ii) Studies of the toxicological effects of the drug as they relate to the drug's intended clinical uses, including, as appropriate, studies assessing the drug's acute, subacute, and chronic toxicity; carcinogenicity; and studies of toxicities related to the drug's particular mode of administration or conditions of use.

(iii) Studies, as appropriate, of the effects of the drug on reproduction and on the developing fetus.

(iv) Any studies of the absorption, distribution, metabolism, and excretion of the drug in animals.

(v) For each nonclinical laboratory study subject to the good laboratory practice regulations under part 58 a statement that it was conducted in compliance with the good laboratory practice regulations in part 58, or, if the study was not conducted in compliance with those regulations, a brief statement of the reason for the noncompliance.

(3) Human pharmacokinetics and bioavailability section. A section describing the human pharmacokinetic data and human bioavailability data, or information supporting a

waiver of the submission of in vivo bioavailability data under subpart B of part 320, including the following:

(i) A description of each of the bioavailability and pharmacokinetic studies of the drug in humans performed by or on behalf of the applicant that includes a description of the analytical procedures and statistical methods used in each study and a statement with respect to each study that it either was conducted in compliance with the institutional review board regulations in part 56, or was not subject to the regulations under 56.104 or 56.105, and that it was conducted in compliance with the informed consent regulations in part 50.

(ii) If the application describes in the chemistry, manufacturing, and controls section tests, analytical procedures, and acceptance criteria needed to assure the bioavailability of the drug product or drug substance, or both, a statement in this section of the rationale for establishing the tests, analytical procedures, and acceptance criteria, including data and information supporting the rationale.

(iii) A summarizing discussion and analysis of the pharmacokinetics and metabolism of the active ingredients and the bioavailability or bioequivalence, or both, of the drug product.

(4) Microbiology section. If the drug is an anti-infective drug, a section describing the microbiology data, including the following:

(i) A description of the biochemical basis of the drug's action on microbial physiology.

(ii) A description of the antimicrobial spectra of the drug, including results of in vitro preclinical studies to demonstrate concentrations of the drug required for effective use.

(iii) A description of any known mechanisms of resistance to the drug, including results of any known epidemiologic studies to demonstrate prevalence of resistance factors.

(iv) A description of clinical microbiology laboratory procedures (for example, in vitro sensitivity discs) needed for effective use of the drug.

(5) Clinical data section. A section describing the clinical investigations of the drug, including the following:

(i) A description and analysis of each clinical pharmacology study of the drug, including a brief comparison of the results of the human studies with the animal pharmacology and toxicology data.

(ii) A description and analysis of each controlled clinical study pertinent to a proposed use of the drug, including the protocol and a description of the statistical analyses used to evaluate the study. If the study report is an interim analysis, this is to be noted and a projected completion date provided. Controlled clinical studies that have not been analyzed in detail for any reason (e.g., because they have been discontinued or are incomplete) are to be included in this section, including a copy of the protocol and a brief description of the results and status of the study.

(iii) A description of each uncontrolled clinical study, a summary of the results, and a brief statement explaining why the study is classified as uncontrolled.

(iv) A description and analysis of any other data or information relevant to an evaluation of the safety and effectiveness of the drug product obtained or otherwise received by the applicant from any source, foreign or domestic, including information derived from clinical investigations, including controlled and uncontrolled studies of uses of the drug other than those proposed in the application, commercial marketing experience, reports in the scientific literature, and unpublished scientific papers.

(v) An integrated summary of the data demonstrating substantial evidence of effectiveness for the claimed indications. Evidence is also required to support the dosage and administration section of the labeling, including support for the dosage and dose interval recommended. The effectiveness data shall be presented by gender, age, and racial subgroups and shall identify any modifications of dose or dose interval needed for specific subgroups. Effectiveness data from other subgroups of the population of patients treated, when appropriate, such as patients with renal failure or patients with

different levels of severity of the disease, also shall be
presented.

(vi) A summary and updates of safety information, as follows:

(a) The applicant shall submit an integrated summary of
all available information about the safety of the drug
product, including pertinent animal data,
demonstrated or potential adverse effects of the
drug, clinically significant drug/drug interactions,
and other safety considerations, such as data from
epidemiological studies of related drugs. The safety
data shall be presented by gender, age, and racial
subgroups. When appropriate, safety data from other
subgroups of the population of patients treated also
shall be presented, such as for patients with renal
failure or patients with different levels of severity of
the disease. A description of any statistical analyses
performed in analyzing safety data should also be
included, unless already included under paragraph
(d)(5)(ii) of this section.

(b) The applicant shall, under section 505(i) of the act,
update periodically its pending application with new
safety information learned about the drug that may
reasonably affect the statement of contraindications,
warnings, precautions, and adverse reactions in the
draft labeling and, if applicable, any Medication
Guide required under part 208 of this chapter. These
"safety update reports" are required to include the
same kinds of information (from clinical studies,
animal studies, and other sources) and are required
to be submitted in the same format as the integrated
summary in paragraph (d)(5)(vi)(a) of this section. In
addition, the reports are required to include the case
report forms for each patient who died during a
clinical study or who did not complete the study
because of an adverse event (unless this requirement
is waived). The applicant shall submit these reports
(1) 4 months after the initial submission; (2) in a
resubmission following receipt of a complete
response letter; and (3) at other times as requested
by FDA. Prior to the submission of the first such
report, applicants are encouraged to consult with

FDA regarding further details on its form and content.

(vii) If the drug has a potential for abuse, a description and analysis of studies or information related to abuse of the drug, including a proposal for scheduling under the Controlled Substances Act. A description of any studies related to overdosage is also required, including information on dialysis, antidotes, or other treatments, if known.

(viii) An integrated summary of the benefits and risks of the drug, including a discussion of why the benefits exceed the risks under the conditions stated in the labeling.

(ix) A statement with respect to each clinical study involving human subjects that it either was conducted in compliance with the institutional review board regulations in part 56, or was not subject to the regulations under 56.104 or 56.105, and that it was conducted in compliance with the informed consent regulations in part 50.

(x) If a sponsor has transferred any obligations for the conduct of any clinical study to a contract research organization, a statement containing the name and address of the contract research organization, identification of the clinical study, and a listing of the obligations transferred. If all obligations governing the conduct of the study have been transferred, a general statement of this transfer--in lieu of a listing of the specific obligations transferred--may be submitted.

(xi) If original subject records were audited or reviewed by the sponsor in the course of monitoring any clinical study to verify the accuracy of the case reports submitted to the sponsor, a list identifying each clinical study so audited or reviewed.

(6) Statistical section. A section describing the statistical evaluation of clinical data, including the following:

(i) A copy of the information submitted under paragraph (d)(5)(ii) of this section concerning the description and analysis of each controlled clinical study, and the documentation and supporting statistical analyses used in evaluating the controlled clinical studies.

(ii) A copy of the information submitted under paragraph (d)(5)(vi)(a) of this section concerning a summary of information about the safety of the drug product, and the documentation and supporting statistical analyses used in evaluating the safety information.

(7) Pediatric use section. A section describing the investigation of the drug for use in pediatric populations, including an integrated summary of the information (the clinical pharmacology studies, controlled clinical studies, or uncontrolled clinical studies, or other data or information) that is relevant to the safety and effectiveness and benefits and risks of the drug in pediatric populations for the claimed indications, a reference to the full descriptions of such studies provided under paragraphs (d)(3) and (d)(5) of this section, and information required to be submitted under 314.55.

(e) Samples and labeling.

(1) Upon request from FDA, the applicant shall submit the samples described below to the places identified in the agency's request. FDA will generally ask applicants to submit samples directly to two or more agency laboratories that will perform all necessary tests on the samples and validate the applicant's analytical procedures.

(i) Four representative samples of the following, each sample in sufficient quantity to permit FDA to perform three times each test described in the application to determine whether the drug substance and the drug product meet the specifications given in the application:

(a) The drug product proposed for marketing;

(b) The drug substance used in the drug product from which the samples of the drug product were taken; and

(c) Reference standards and blanks (except that reference standards recognized in an official compendium need not be submitted).

(ii) Samples of the finished market package, if requested by FDA.

(2) The applicant shall submit the following in the archival copy of the application:

(i) Three copies of the analytical procedures and related descriptive information contained in the chemistry, manufacturing, and controls section under paragraph (d)(1) of this section for the drug substance and the drug product that are necessary for FDA's laboratories to perform all necessary tests on the samples and to validate the applicant's analytical procedures. The related descriptive information includes a description of each sample; the proposed regulatory specifications for the drug; a detailed description of the methods of analysis; supporting data for accuracy, specificity, precision and ruggedness; and complete results of the applicant's tests on each sample.

(ii) Copies of the label and all labeling for the drug product (including, if applicable, any Medication Guide required under part 208 of this chapter) for the drug product (4 copies of draft labeling or 12 copies of final printed labeling).

(f) Case report forms and tabulations. The archival copy of the application is required to contain the following case report tabulations and case report forms:

(1) Case report tabulations. The application is required to contain tabulations of the data from each adequate and well-controlled study under 314.126 (Phase 2 and Phase 3 studies as described in 312.21 (b) and (c) of this chapter), tabulations of the data from the earliest clinical pharmacology studies (Phase 1 studies as described in 312.21(a) of this chapter), and tabulations of the safety data from other clinical studies. Routine submission of other patient data from uncontrolled studies is not required. The tabulations are required to include the data on each patient in each study, except that the applicant may delete those tabulations which the agency agrees, in advance, are not pertinent to a review of the drug's safety or effectiveness. Upon request, FDA will discuss with the applicant in a "pre-NDA" conference those tabulations that may be appropriate for such deletion. Barring unforeseen circumstances, tabulations agreed to be deleted at such a conference will not be requested during the conduct of FDA's review of the application. If such unforeseen circumstances do occur, any request for deleted tabulations will be made by the director of the FDA division responsible

for reviewing the application, in accordance with paragraph (f)(3) of this section.

(2) Case report forms. The application is required to contain copies of individual case report forms for each patient who died during a clinical study or who did not complete the study because of an adverse event, whether believed to be drug related or not, including patients receiving reference drugs or placebo. This requirement may be waived by FDA for specific studies if the case report forms are unnecessary for a proper review of the study.

(3) Additional data. The applicant shall submit to FDA additional case report forms and tabulations needed to conduct a proper review of the application, as requested by the director of the FDA division responsible for reviewing the application. The applicant's failure to submit information requested by FDA within 30 days after receipt of the request may result in the agency viewing any eventual submission as a major amendment under 314.60 and extending the review period as necessary. If desired by the applicant, the FDA division director will verify in writing any request for additional data that was made orally.

(4) Applicants are invited to meet with FDA before submitting an application to discuss the presentation and format of supporting information. If the applicant and FDA agree, the applicant may submit tabulations of patient data and case report forms in a form other than hard copy, for example, on microfiche or computer tapes.

(g) Other. The following general requirements apply to the submission of information within the summary under paragraph (c) of this section and within the technical sections under paragraph (d) of this section.

(1) The applicant ordinarily is not required to resubmit information previously submitted, but may incorporate the information by reference. A reference to information submitted previously is required to identify the file by name, reference number, volume, and page number in the agency's records where the information can be found. A reference to information submitted to the agency by a person other than the applicant is required to contain a written statement that authorizes the reference and that is signed by the person who submitted the information.

(2) The applicant shall submit an accurate and complete English translation of each part of the application that is not in English. The applicant shall submit a copy of each original literature publication for which an English translation is submitted.

(3) If an applicant who submits a new drug application under section 505(b) of the act obtains a "right of reference or use," as defined under 314.3(b), to an investigation described in clause (A) of section 505(b)(1) of the act, the applicant shall include in its application a written statement signed by the owner of the data from each such investigation that the applicant may rely on in support of the approval of its application, and provide FDA access to, the underlying raw data that provide the basis for the report of the investigation submitted in its application.

(h) Patent information. The application is required to contain the patent information described under 314.53.

(i) Patent certification –

    (1) Contents. A 505(b)(2) application is required to contain the following:

        (i) Patents claiming drug, drug product, or method of use.

            (A) Except as provided in paragraph (i)(2) of this section, a certification with respect to each patent issued by the United States Patent and Trademark Office that, in the opinion of the applicant and to the best of its knowledge, claims a drug (the drug product or drug substance that is a component of the drug product) on which investigations that are relied upon by the applicant for approval of its application were conducted or that claims an approved use for such drug and for which information is required to be filed under section 505(b) and (c) of the act and 314.53. For each such patent, the applicant shall provide the patent number and certify, in its opinion and to the best of its knowledge, one of the following circumstances:

                (1) That the patent information has not been submitted to FDA. The applicant shall entitle such a certification "Paragraph I Certification";

Part 314

(2) That the patent has expired. The applicant shall entitle such a certification "Paragraph II Certification";

(3) The date on which the patent will expire. The applicant shall entitle such a certification "Paragraph III Certification"; or

(4) That the patent is invalid, unenforceable, or will not be infringed by the manufacture, use, or sale of the drug product for which the application is submitted. The applicant shall entitle such a certification "Paragraph IV Certification". This certification shall be submitted in the following form:

I, (name of applicant), certify that Patent No. _____ (is invalid, unenforceable, or will not be infringed by the manufacture, use, or sale of) (name of proposed drug product) for which this application is submitted.

The certification shall be accompanied by a statement that the applicant will comply with the requirements under 314.52(a) with respect to providing a notice to each owner of the patent or their representatives and to the holder of the approved application for the drug product which is claimed by the patent or a use of which is claimed by the patent and with the requirements under 314.52(c) with respect to the content of the notice.

(B) If the drug on which investigations that are relied upon by the applicant were conducted is itself a licensed generic drug of a patented drug first approved under section 505(b) of the act, the appropriate patent certification under this section with respect to each patent that claims the first-approved patented drug or that claims an approved use for such a drug.

(ii) No relevant patents. If, in the opinion of the applicant and to the best of its knowledge, there are no patents described in paragraph (i)(1)(i) of this section, a certification in the following form:

In the opinion and to the best knowledge of (name of applicant), there are no patents that claim the drug or drugs on which investigations that are relied upon in this application were conducted or that claim a use of such drug or drugs.

(iii) Method of use patent.

    (A) If information that is submitted under section 505(b) or (c) of the act and 314.53 is for a method of use patent, and the labeling for the drug product for which the applicant is seeking approval does not include any indications that are covered by the use patent, a statement explaining that the method of use patent does not claim any of the proposed indications.

    (B) If the labeling of the drug product for which the applicant is seeking approval includes an indication that, according to the patent information submitted under section 505(b) or (c) of the act and 314.53 or in the opinion of the applicant, is claimed by a use patent, the applicant shall submit an applicable certification under paragraph (i)(1)(i) of this section.

(2) Method of manufacturing patent. An applicant is not required to make a certification with respect to any patent that claims only a method of manufacturing the drug product for which the applicant is seeking approval.

(3) Licensing agreements. If a 505(b)(2) application is for a drug or method of using a drug claimed by a patent and the applicant has a licensing agreement with the patent owner, the applicant shall submit a certification under paragraph (i)(1)(i)(A)(4) of this section ("Paragraph IV Certification") as to that patent and a statement that it has been granted a patent license. If the patent owner consents to an immediate effective date upon approval of the 505(b)(2) application, the application shall contain a written statement from the patent owner that it has a licensing agreement with the applicant and that it consents to an immediate effective date.

(4) Late submission of patent information. If a patent described in paragraph (i)(1)(i)(A) of this section is issued and the holder of the approved application for the patented drug does not submit the required information on the patent within 30 days of issuance of the patent, an applicant who submitted a

505(b)(2) application that, before the submission of the patent information, contained an appropriate patent certification is not required to submit an amended certification. An applicant whose 505(b)(2) application is filed after a late submission of patent information or whose 505(b)(2) application was previously filed but did not contain an appropriate patent certification at the time of the patent submission shall submit a certification under paragraph (i)(1)(i) or (i)(1)(ii) of this section or a statement under paragraph (i)(1)(iii) of this section as to that patent.

(5) Disputed patent information. If an applicant disputes the accuracy or relevance of patent information submitted to FDA, the applicant may seek a confirmation of the correctness of the patent information in accordance with the procedures under 314.53(f). Unless the patent information is withdrawn or changed, the applicant must submit an appropriate certification for each relevant patent.

(6) Amended certifications. A certification submitted under paragraphs (i)(1)(i) through (i)(1)(iii) of this section may be amended at any time before the effective date of the approval of the application. An applicant shall submit an amended certification as an amendment to a pending application or by letter to an approved application. If an applicant with a pending application voluntarily makes a patent certification for an untimely filed patent, the applicant may withdraw the patent certification for the untimely filed patent. Once an amendment or letter for the change in certification has been submitted, the application will no longer be considered to be one containing the prior certification.

(i) After finding of infringement. An applicant who has submitted a certification under paragraph (i)(1)(i)(A)(4) of this section and is sued for patent infringement within 45 days of the receipt of notice sent under 314.52 shall amend the certification if a final judgment in the action is entered finding the patent to be infringed unless the final judgment also finds the patent to be invalid. In the amended certification, the applicant shall certify under paragraph (i)(1)(i)(A)(3) of this section that the patent will expire on a specific date.

(ii) After removal of a patent from the list. If a patent is removed from the list, any applicant with a pending application (including a tentatively approved application with a delayed effective date) who has made a certification with respect to such patent shall amend its certification. The applicant shall certify under paragraph (i)(1)(ii) of this section that no patents described in paragraph (i)(1)(i) of this section claim the drug or, if other relevant patents claim the drug, shall amend the certification to refer only to those relevant patents. In the amendment, the applicant shall state the reason for the change in certification (that the patent is or has been removed from the list). A patent that is the subject of a lawsuit under 314.107(c) shall not be removed from the list until FDA determines either that no delay in effective dates of approval is required under that section as a result of the lawsuit, that the patent has expired, or that any such period of delay in effective dates of approval is ended. An applicant shall submit an amended certification as an amendment to a pending application. Once an amendment for the change has been submitted, the application will no longer be considered to be one containing a certification under paragraph (i)(1)(i)(A)(4) of this section.

(iii) Other amendments.

(A) Except as provided in paragraphs (i)(4) and (i)(6)(iii)(B) of this section, an applicant shall amend a submitted certification if, at any time before the effective date of the approval of the application, the applicant learns that the submitted certification is no longer accurate.

(B) An applicant is not required to amend a submitted certification when information on an otherwise applicable patent is submitted after the effective date of approval for the 505(b)(2) application.

(j) Claimed exclusivity. A new drug product, upon approval, may be entitled to a period of marketing exclusivity under the provisions of 314.108. If an applicant believes its drug product is entitled to a period of exclusivity, it shall submit with the new drug application prior to approval the following information:

(1) A statement that the applicant is claiming exclusivity.

(2) A reference to the appropriate paragraph under 314.108 that supports its claim.

Part 314

(3) If the applicant claims exclusivity under 314.108(b)(2), information to show that, to the best of its knowledge or belief, a drug has not previously been approved under section 505(b) of the act containing any active moiety in the drug for which the applicant is seeking approval.

(4) If the applicant claims exclusivity under 314.108(b)(4) or (b)(5), the following information to show that the application contains "new clinical investigations" that are "essential to approval of the application or supplement" and were "conducted or sponsored by the applicant:"

    (i) "New clinical investigations. " A certification that to the best of the applicant's knowledge each of the clinical investigations included in the application meets the definition of "new clinical investigation" set forth in 314.108(a).

    (ii) "Essential to approval." A list of all published studies or publicly available reports of clinical investigations known to the applicant through a literature search that are relevant to the conditions for which the applicant is seeking approval, a certification that the applicant has thoroughly searched the scientific literature and, to the best of the applicant's knowledge, the list is complete and accurate and, in the applicant's opinion, such published studies or publicly available reports do not provide a sufficient basis for the approval of the conditions for which the applicant is seeking approval without reference to the new clinical investigation(s) in the application, and an explanation as to why the studies or reports are insufficient.

    (iii) "Conducted or sponsored by." If the applicant was the sponsor named in the Form FDA-1571 for an investigational new drug application (IND) under which the new clinical investigation(s) that is essential to the approval of its application was conducted, identification of the IND by number. If the applicant was not the sponsor of the IND under which the clinical investigation(s) was conducted, a certification that the applicant or its predecessor in interest provided substantial support for the clinical investigation(s) that is essential to the approval of its application, and information supporting the certification. To demonstrate "substantial support," an applicant must either provide a certified statement from a certified public accountant that the applicant provided 50 percent or more of the cost of conducting the study or provide an explanation of why FDA should consider the applicant to have conducted or sponsored the study if the applicant's financial contribution to the study is less than 50 percent or the applicant did not sponsor the investigational new drug. A predecessor in interest is an entity, e.g., a corporation, that the applicant has taken over, merged with, or purchased, or from which the applicant has purchased all rights to the drug. Purchase of nonexclusive rights to a clinical investigation after it is completed is not sufficient to satisfy this definition.

(k) Financial certification or disclosure statement. The application shall contain a financial certification or disclosure statement or both as required by part 54 of this chapter.

(l) Format of an original application –

(1) Archival copy. The applicant must submit a complete archival copy of the application that contains the information required under paragraphs (a) through (f) of this section. FDA will maintain the archival copy during the review of the application to permit individual reviewers to refer to information that is not contained in their particular technical sections of the application, to give other agency personnel access to the application for official business, and to maintain in one place a complete copy of the application. Except as required by paragraph (l)(1)(i) of this section, applicants may submit the archival copy on paper or in electronic format provided that electronic submissions are made in accordance with part 11 of this chapter.

(i) Labeling. The content of labeling required under 201.100(d)(3) of this chapter (commonly referred to as the package insert or professional labeling), including all text, tables, and figures, must be submitted to the agency in electronic format as described in paragraph (l)(5) of this section. This requirement is in addition to the requirements of paragraph (e)(2)(ii) of this section that copies of the formatted label and all labeling be submitted. Submissions under this paragraph must be made in accordance with part 11 of this chapter, except for the requirements of 11.10(a), (c) through (h), and (k), and the corresponding requirements of 11.30.

(ii) [Reserved]

(2) Review copy. The applicant must submit a review copy of the application. Each of the technical sections, described in paragraphs (d)(1) through (d)(6) of this section, in the review copy is required to be separately bound with a copy of the application form required under paragraph (a) of this section and a copy of the summary required under paragraph (c) of this section.

(3) Field copy. The applicant must submit a field copy of the application that contains the technical section described in paragraph (d)(1) of this section, a copy of the application form required under paragraph (a) of this section, a copy of the summary required under paragraph (c) of this section, and a certification that the field copy is a true copy of the technical section described in paragraph (d)(1) of this section contained in the archival and review copies of the application.

(4) Binding folders. The applicant may obtain from FDA sufficient folders to bind the archival, the review, and the field copies of the application.

(5) Electronic format submissions. Electronic format submissions must be in a form that FDA can process, review, and archive. FDA will periodically issue guidance on how to provide the electronic submission (e.g., method of transmission, media, file formats, preparation and organization of files).

[50 FR 7493, Feb. 22, 1985]

Editorial Note: For Federal Register citations affecting 314.50, see the List of CFR Sections Affected, which appears in the Finding Aids section of the printed volume and on GPO Access.

Sec. 314.52 Notice of certification of invalidity or noninfringement of a patent.

(a) Notice of certification. For each patent which claims the drug or drugs on which investigations that are relied upon by the applicant for approval of its application were conducted or which claims a use for such drug or drugs and which the applicant certifies under 314.50(i)(1)(i)(A)(4) that a patent is invalid, unenforceable, or will not be infringed, the applicant shall send notice of such certification by registered or certified mail, return receipt requested to each of the following persons:

   (1) Each owner of the patent that is the subject of the certification or the representative designated by the owner to receive the notice. The name and address of the patent owner or its representative may be obtained from the United States Patent and Trademark Office; and

   (2) The holder of the approved application under section 505(b) of the act for each drug product which is claimed by the patent or a use of which is claimed by the patent and for which the applicant is seeking approval, or, if the application holder does not reside or maintain a place of business within the United States, the application holder's attorney, agent, or other authorized official. The name and address of the application holder or its attorney, agent, or authorized official may be obtained from the Orange Book Staff, Office of Generic Drugs, 7500 Standish Pl., Rockville, MD 20855.

   (3) This paragraph does not apply to a use patent that claims no uses for which the applicant is seeking approval.

(b) Sending the notice. The applicant shall send the notice required by paragraph (a) of this section when it receives from FDA an acknowledgment letter stating that its application has been filed. At the same time, the applicant shall amend its application to include a statement certifying that the notice has been provided to each person identified under paragraph (a) of this section and that the notice met the content requirement under paragraph (c) of this section.

(c) Content of a notice. In the notice, the applicant shall cite section 505(b)(3)(B) of the act and shall include, but not be limited to, the following information:

Part 314

(1) A statement that a 505(b)(2) application submitted by the applicant has been filed by FDA.

(2) The application number.

(3) The established name, if any, as defined in section 502(e)(3) of the act, of the proposed drug product.

(4) The active ingredient, strength, and dosage form of the proposed drug product.

(5) The patent number and expiration date, as submitted to the agency or as known to the applicant, of each patent alleged to be invalid, unenforceable, or not infringed.

(6) A detailed statement of the factual and legal basis of the applicant's opinion that the patent is not valid, unenforceable, or will not be infringed. The applicant shall include in the detailed statement:

    (i) For each claim of a patent alleged not to be infringed, a full and detailed explanation of why the claim is not infringed.

    (ii) For each claim of a patent alleged to be invalid or unenforceable, a full and detailed explanation of the grounds supporting the allegation.

(7) If the applicant does not reside or have a place of business in the United States, the name and address of an agent in the United States authorized to accept service of process for the applicant.

(d) Amendment to an application. If an application is amended to include the certification described in 314.50(i), the applicant shall send the notice required by paragraph (a) of this section at the same time that the amendment to the application is submitted to FDA.

(e) Documentation of receipt of notice. The applicant shall amend its application to document receipt of the notice required under paragraph (a) of this section by each person provided the notice. The applicant shall include a copy of the return receipt or other similar evidence of the date the notification was received. FDA will accept as adequate documentation of the date of receipt a return receipt or a letter acknowledging receipt by the person provided the notice. An applicant may rely on another form of documentation only if FDA has agreed to such documentation in advance. A copy of the notice itself need not be submitted to the agency.

(f) Approval. If the requirements of this section are met, the agency will presume the notice to be complete and sufficient, and it will count the day following the date of receipt of the notice by the patent owner or its representative and by the approved application holder as the first day of the 45-day period provided for in section 505(c)(3)(C) of the act. FDA may, if the applicant amends its application with a written statement that a later date should be used, count from such later date.

[59 FR 50362, Oct. 3, 1994, as amended at 68 FR 36703, June 18, 2003; 69 FR 11310, Mar. 10, 2004; 74 FR 9766, Mar. 6, 2009; 74 FR 36605, July 24, 2009]

Sec. 314.53 Submission of patent information.

(a) Who must submit patent information. This section applies to any applicant who submits to FDA a new drug application or an amendment to it under section 505(b) of the act and 314.50 or a supplement to an approved application under 314.70, except as provided in paragraph (d)(2) of this section.

(b) Patents for which information must be submitted and patents for which information must not be submitted –

(1) General requirements. An applicant described in paragraph (a) of this section shall submit the required information on the declaration form set forth in paragraph (c) of this section for each patent that claims the drug or a method of using the drug that is the subject of the new drug application or amendment or supplement to it and with respect to which a claim of patent infringement could reasonably be asserted if a person not licensed by the owner of the patent engaged in the manufacture, use, or sale of the drug product. For purposes of this part, such patents consist of drug substance (active ingredient) patents, drug product (formulation and composition) patents, and method-of-use patents. For patents that claim the drug substance, the applicant shall submit information only on those patents that claim the drug substance that is the subject of the pending or approved application or that claim a drug substance that is the same as the active ingredient that is the subject of the approved or pending application. For patents that claim a polymorph that

is the same as the active ingredient described in the approved or pending application, the applicant shall certify in the declaration forms that the applicant has test data, as set forth in paragraph (b)(2) of this section, demonstrating that a drug product containing the polymorph will perform the same as the drug product described in the new drug application. For patents that claim a drug product, the applicant shall submit information only on those patents that claim a drug product, as is defined in 314.3, that is described in the pending or approved application. For patents that claim a method of use, the applicant shall submit information only on those patents that claim indications or other conditions of use that are described in the pending or approved application. The applicant shall separately identify each pending or approved method of use and related patent claim. For approved applications, the applicant submitting the method-of-use patent shall identify with specificity the section of the approved labeling that corresponds to the method of use claimed by the patent submitted. Process patents, patents claiming packaging, patents claiming metabolites, and patents claiming intermediates are not covered by this section, and information on these patents must not be submitted to FDA.

(2)   Test Data for Submission of Patent Information for Patents That Claim a Polymorph. The test data, referenced in paragraph (b)(1) of this section, must include the following:

 (i)   A full description of the polymorphic form of the drug substance, including its physical and chemical characteristics and stability; the method of synthesis (or isolation) and purification of the drug substance; the process controls used during manufacture and packaging; and such specifications and analytical methods as are necessary to assure the identity, strength, quality, and purity of the polymorphic form of the drug substance;

 (ii) The executed batch record for a drug product containing the polymorphic form of the drug substance and documentation that the batch was manufactured under current good manufacturing practice requirements;

 (iii) Demonstration of bioequivalence between the executed batch of the drug product that contains the polymorphic form of the drug substance and the drug product as described in the NDA;

Part 314

(iv) A list of all components used in the manufacture of the drug product containing the polymorphic form and a statement of the composition of the drug product; a statement of the specifications and analytical methods for each component; a description of the manufacturing and packaging procedures and in-process controls for the drug product; such specifications and analytical methods as are necessary to assure the identity, strength, quality, purity, and bioavailability of the drug product, including release and stability data complying with the approved product specifications to demonstrate pharmaceutical equivalence and comparable product stability; and

(v) Comparative in vitro dissolution testing on 12 dosage units each of the executed test batch and the new drug application product.

(c) Reporting requirements –

(1) General requirements. An applicant described in paragraph (a) of this section shall submit the required patent information described in paragraph (c)(2) of this section for each patent that meets the requirements described in paragraph (b) of this section. We will not accept the patent information unless it is complete and submitted on the appropriate forms, FDA Forms 3542 or 3542a. These forms may be obtained on the Internet athttp://www.fda.gov by searching for "forms".

(2) Drug substance (active ingredient), drug product (formulation or composition), and method-of-use patents –

(i) Original Declaration. For each patent that claims a drug substance (active ingredient), drug product (formulation and composition), or method of use, the applicant shall submit FDA Form 3542a. The following information and verification is required:

(A) New drug application number;

(B) Name of new drug application sponsor;

(C) Trade name (or proposed trade name) of new drug;

(D) Active ingredient(s) of new drug;

(E) Strength(s) of new drug;

(F) Dosage form of new drug;

(G) United States patent number, issue date, and expiration date of patent submitted;

(H) The patent owner's name, full address, phone number and, if available, fax number and e-mail address;

(I) The name, full address, phone number and, if available, fax number and e-mail address of an agent or representative who resides or maintains a place of business within the United States authorized to receive notice of patent certification under sections 505(b)(3) and 505(j)(2)(B) of the act and 314.52 and 314.95 (if patent owner or new drug application applicant or holder does not reside or have a place of business within the United States);

(J) Information on whether the patent has been submitted previously for the new drug application;

(K) Information on whether the expiration date is a new expiration date if the patent had been submitted previously for listing;

(L) Information on whether the patent is a product-by-process patent in which the product claimed is novel;

(M) Information on the drug substance (active ingredient) patent including the following:

(1) Whether the patent claims the drug substance that is the active ingredient in the drug product described in the new drug application or supplement;

(2) Whether the patent claims a polymorph that is the same active ingredient that is described in the pending application or supplement;

(3) Whether the applicant has test data, described in paragraph (b)(2) of this section, demonstrating that a drug product containing the polymorph will perform the same as the drug product described in the new drug application or supplement, and a description of the polymorphic form(s) claimed by the patent for which such test data exist;

(4) Whether the patent claims only a metabolite of the active ingredient; and

(5) Whether the patent claims only an intermediate;

(N) Information on the drug product (composition/formulation) patent including the following:

(1) Whether the patent claims the drug product for which approval is being sought, as defined in 314.3; and

(2) Whether the patent claims only an intermediate;

(O) Information on each method-of-use patent including the following:

(1) Whether the patent claims one or more methods of using the drug product for which use approval is being sought and a description of each pending method of use or related indication and related patent claim of the patent being submitted; and

(2) Identification of the specific section of the proposed labeling for the drug product that corresponds to the method of use claimed by the patent submitted;

(P) Whether there are no relevant patents that claim the drug substance (active ingredient), drug product (formulation or composition) or method(s) of use, for which the applicant is seeking approval and with respect to which a claim of patent infringement could reasonably be asserted if a person not licensed by the owner of the patent engaged in the manufacture, use, or sale of the drug product;

(Q) A signed verification which states:

"The undersigned declares that this is an accurate and complete submission of patent information for the NDA, amendment or supplement pending under section 505 of the Federal Food, Drug, and Cosmetic Act. This time-sensitive patent information is submitted pursuant to 21 CFR 314.53. I attest that I am familiar with 21 CFR 314.53 and this submission complies with the requirements of the

Part 314

regulation. I verify under penalty of perjury that the foregoing is true and correct."; and

(R) Information on whether the applicant, patent owner or attorney, agent, representative or other authorized official signed the form; the name of the person; and the full address, phone number and, if available, the fax number and e-mail address.

(ii) Submission of patent information upon and after approval. Within 30 days after the date of approval of its application or supplement, the applicant shall submit FDA Form 3542 for each patent that claims the drug substance (active ingredient), drug product (formulation and composition), or approved method of use. FDA will rely only on the information submitted on this form and will not list or publish patent information if the patent declaration is incomplete or indicates the patent is not eligible for listing. Patent information must also be submitted for patents issued after the date of approval of the new drug application as required in paragraph (c)(2)(ii) of this section. As described in paragraph (d)(4) of this section, patent information must be submitted to FDA within 30 days of the date of issuance of the patent. If the applicant submits the required patent information within the 30 days, but we notify an applicant that a declaration form is incomplete or shows that the patent is not eligible for listing, the applicant must submit an acceptable declaration form within 15 days of FDA notification to be considered timely filed. The following information and verification statement is required:

(A) New drug application number;

(B) Name of new drug application sponsor;

(C) Trade name of new drug;

(D) Active ingredient(s) of new drug;

(E) Strength(s) of new drug;

(F) Dosage form of new drug;

(G) Approval date of new drug application or supplement;

(H) United States patent number, issue date, and expiration date of patent submitted;

(I) The patent owner's name, full address, phone number and, if available, fax number and e-mail address;

(J) The name, full address, phone number and, if available, fax number and e-mail address of an agent or representative who resides or maintains a place of business within the United States authorized to receive notice of patent certification under sections 505(b)(3) and 505(j)(2)(B) of the act and 314.52 and 314.95 (if patent owner or new drug application applicant or holder does not reside or have a place of business within the United States);

(K) Information on whether the patent has been submitted previously for the new drug application;

(L) Information on whether the expiration date is a new expiration date if the patent had been submitted previously for listing;

(M) Information on whether the patent is a product-by-process patent in which the product claimed is novel;

(N) Information on the drug substance (active ingredient) patent including the following:

   (1) Whether the patent claims the drug substance that is the active ingredient in the drug product described in the approved application;

   (2) Whether the patent claims a polymorph that is the same as the active ingredient that is described in the approved application;

   (3) Whether the applicant has test data, described at paragraph (b)(2) of this section, demonstrating that a drug product containing the polymorph will perform the same as the drug product described in the approved application and a description of the polymorphic form(s) claimed by the patent for which such test data exist;

   (4) Whether the patent claims only a metabolite of the active ingredient; and

   (5) Whether the patent claims only an intermediate;

(O) Information on the drug product (composition/formulation) patent including the following:

   (1) Whether the patent claims the approved drug product as defined in 314.3; and

   (2) Whether the patent claims only an intermediate;

(P) Information on each method-of-use patent including the following:

   (1) Whether the patent claims one or more approved methods of using the approved drug product and a description of each approved method of use or indication and related patent claim of the patent being submitted;

   (2) Identification of the specific section of the approved labeling for the drug product that corresponds to the method of use claimed by the patent submitted; and

   (3) The description of the patented method of use as required for publication;

(Q) Whether there are no relevant patents that claim the approved drug substance (active ingredient), the approved drug product (formulation or composition) or approved method(s) of use and with respect to which a claim of patent infringement could reasonably be asserted if a person not licensed by the owner of the patent engaged in the manufacture, use, or sale of the drug product;

(R) A signed verification which states: "The undersigned declares that this is an accurate and complete submission of patent information for the NDA, amendment or supplement approved under section 505 of the Federal Food, Drug, and Cosmetic Act. This time-sensitive patent information is submitted pursuant to 21 CFR 314.53. I attest that I am familiar with 21 CFR 314.53 and this submission complies with the requirements of the regulation. I verify under penalty of perjury that the foregoing is true and correct."; and

(S) Information on whether the applicant, patent owner or attorney, agent, representative or other authorized official signed the form; the name of the person; and the full address, phone number and, if available, the fax number and e-mail address.

(3) No relevant patents. If the applicant believes that there are no relevant patents that claim the drug substance (active ingredient), drug product (formulation or composition), or the method(s) of use for which the applicant has received approval, and with respect to which a claim of patent infringement could reasonably be asserted if a person not licensed by the owner of the patent engaged in the manufacture, use, or sale of the drug product, the applicant will verify this information in the appropriate forms, FDA Forms 3542 or 3542a.

(4) Authorized signature. The declarations required by this section shall be signed by the applicant or patent owner, or the applicant's or patent owner's attorney, agent (representative), or other authorized official.

(d) When and where to submit patent information –

(1) Original application. An applicant shall submit with its original application submitted under this part, including an application described in section 505(b)(2) of the act, the information described in paragraph (c) of this section on each drug (ingredient), drug product (formulation and composition), and method of use patent issued before the application is filed with FDA and for which patent information is required to be submitted under this section. If a patent is issued after the application is filed with FDA but before the application is approved, the applicant shall, within 30 days of the date of issuance of the patent, submit the required patent information in an amendment to the application under 314.60.

(2) Supplements.

(i) An applicant shall submit patent information required under paragraph (c) of this section for a patent that claims the drug, drug product, or method of use for which approval is sought in any of the following supplements:

(A) To change the formulation;

(B) To add a new indication or other condition of use, including a change in route of administration;

(C) To change the strength;

(D) To make any other patented change regarding the drug, drug product, or any method of use.

(ii) If the applicant submits a supplement for one of the changes listed under paragraph (d)(2)(i) of this section and existing patents for which information has already been submitted to FDA claim the changed product, the applicant shall submit a certification with the supplement identifying the patents that claim the changed product.

(iii) If the applicant submits a supplement for one of the changes listed under paragraph (d)(2)(i) of this section and no patents, including previously submitted patents, claim the changed product, it shall so certify.

(iv) The applicant shall comply with the requirements for amendment of formulation or composition and method of use patent information under paragraphs (c)(2)(ii) and (d)(3) of this section.

(3) Patent information deadline. If a patent is issued for a drug, drug product, or method of use after an application is approved, the applicant shall submit to FDA the required patent information within 30 days of the date of issuance of the patent.

(4) Copies. The applicant shall submit two copies of each submission of patent information, an archival copy and a copy for the chemistry, manufacturing, and controls section of the review copy, to the Central Document Room, Center for Drug Evaluation and Research, Food and Drug Administration, 5901-B Ammendale Rd., Beltsville, MD 20705-1266. The applicant shall submit the patent information by letter separate from, but at the same time as, submission of the supplement.

(5) Submission date. Patent information shall be considered to be submitted to FDA as of the date the information is received by the Central Document Room.

(6) Identification. Each submission of patent information, except information submitted with an original application, and its mailing cover shall bear prominent identification as to its

contents,i.e. , "Patent Information," or, if submitted after approval of an application, "Time Sensitive Patent Information."

(e) Public disclosure of patent information. FDA will publish in the list the patent number and expiration date of each patent that is required to be, and is, submitted to FDA by an applicant, and for each use patent, the approved indications or other conditions of use covered by a patent. FDA will publish such patent information upon approval of the application, or, if the patent information is submitted by the applicant after approval of an application as provided under paragraph (d)(2) of this section, as soon as possible after the submission to the agency of the patent information. Patent information submitted by the last working day of a month will be published in that month's supplement to the list. Patent information received by the agency between monthly publication of supplements to the list will be placed on public display in FDA's Freedom of Information Staff. A request for copies of the file shall be sent in writing to the Freedom of Information Staff (HFI-35), Food and Drug Administration, rm. 12A-16, 5600 Fishers Lane, Rockville, MD 20857.

(f) Correction of patent information errors. If any person disputes the accuracy or relevance of patent information submitted to the agency under this section and published by FDA in the list, or believes that an applicant has failed to submit required patent information, that person must first notify the agency in writing stating the grounds for disagreement. Such notification should be directed to the Office of Generic Drugs, OGD Document Room, Attention: Orange Book Staff, 7500 Standish Pl., Rockville, MD 20855. The agency will then request of the applicable new drug application holder that the correctness of the patent information or omission of patent information be confirmed. Unless the application holder withdraws or amends its patent information in response to FDA's request, the agency will not change the patent information in the list. If the new drug application holder does not change the patent information submitted to FDA, a 505(b)(2) application or an abbreviated new drug application under section 505(j) of the act submitted for a drug that is claimed by a patent for which information has been submitted must, despite any disagreement as to the correctness of the patent information, contain an appropriate certification for each listed patent.

[59 FR 50363, Oct. 3, 1994, as amended at 68 FR 36703, June 18, 2003; 69 FR 13473, Mar. 23, 2004; 74 FR 9766, Mar. 6, 2009; 74 FR 36605, July 24, 2009]

Part 314

Sec. 314.54 Procedure for submission of an application requiring investigations for approval of a new indication for, or other change from, a listed drug.

(a) The act does not permit approval of an abbreviated new drug application for a new indication, nor does it permit approval of other changes in a listed drug if investigations, other than bioavailability or bioequivalence studies, are essential to the approval of the change. Any person seeking approval of a drug product that represents a modification of a listed drug (e.g., a new indication or new dosage form) and for which investigations, other than bioavailability or bioequivalence studies, are essential to the approval of the changes may, except as provided in paragraph (b) of this section, submit a 505(b)(2) application. This application need contain only that information needed to support the modification(s) of the listed drug.

   (1) The applicant shall submit a complete archival copy of the application that contains the following:

      (i) The information required under 314.50(a), (b), (c), (d)(1), (d)(3), (e), and (g), except that 314.50(d)(1)(ii)(c) shall contain the proposed or actual master production record, including a description of the equipment, to be used for the manufacture of a commercial lot of the drug product.

      (ii) The information required under 314.50 (d)(2), (d)(4) (if an anti-infective drug), (d)(5), (d)(6), and (f) as needed to support the safety and effectiveness of the drug product.

      (iii) Identification of the listed drug for which FDA has made a finding of safety and effectiveness and on which finding the applicant relies in seeking approval of its proposed drug product by established name, if any, proprietary name, dosage form, strength, route of administration, name of listed drug's application holder, and listed drug's approved application number.

      (iv) If the applicant is seeking approval only for a new indication and not for the indications approved for the listed drug on which the applicant relies, a certification so stating.

      (v) Any patent information required under section 505(b)(1) of the act with respect to any patent which claims the drug for which approval is sought or a method of using such drug and to which a claim of patent infringement could reasonably be asserted if a person not licensed by the owner of the patent engaged in the manufacture, use, or sale of the drug product.

(vi) Any patent certification or statement required under section 505(b)(2) of the act with respect to any relevant patents that claim the listed drug or that claim any other drugs on which investigations relied on by the applicant for approval of the application were conducted, or that claim a use for the listed or other drug.

(vii) If the applicant believes the change for which it is seeking approval is entitled to a period of exclusivity, the information required under 314.50(j).

(2) The applicant shall submit a review copy that contains the technical sections described in 314.50(d)(1), except that 314.50(d)(1)(ii)(c) shall contain the proposed or actual master production record, including a description of the equipment, to be used for the manufacture of a commercial lot of the drug product, and paragraph (d)(3), and the technical sections described in paragraphs (d)(2), (d)(4), (d)(5), (d)(6), and (f) when needed to support the modification. Each of the technical sections in the review copy is required to be separately bound with a copy of the information required under 314.50 (a), (b), and (c) and a copy of the proposed labeling.

(3) The information required by 314.50 (d)(2), (d)(4) (if an anti-infective drug), (d)(5), (d)(6), and (f) for the listed drug on which the applicant relies shall be satisfied by reference to the listed drug under paragraph (a)(1)(iii) of this section.

(4) The applicant shall submit a field copy of the application that contains the technical section described in 314.50(d)(1), a copy of the information required under 314.50(a) and (c), and certification that the field copy is a true copy of the technical section described in 314.50(d)(1) contained in the archival and review copies of the application.

(b) An application may not be submitted under this section for a drug product whose only difference from the reference listed drug is that:

(1) The extent to which its active ingredient(s) is absorbed or otherwise made available to the site of action is less than that of the reference listed drug; or

(2) The rate at which its active ingredient(s) is absorbed or otherwise made available to the site of action is unintentionally less than that of the reference listed drug.

[57 FR 17982, Apr. 28, 1992; 57 FR 61612, Dec. 28, 1992, as amended at 58 FR 47351, Sept. 8, 1993; 59 FR 50364, Oct. 3, 1994]

Sec. 314.55 Pediatric use information.

(a) Required assessment. Except as provided in paragraphs (b), (c), and (d) of this section, each application for a new active ingredient, new indication, new dosage form, new dosing regimen, or new route of administration shall contain data that are adequate to assess the safety and effectiveness of the drug product for the claimed indications in all relevant pediatric subpopulations, and to support dosing and administration for each pediatric subpopulation for which the drug is safe and effective. Where the course of the disease and the effects of the drug are sufficiently similar in adults and pediatric patients, FDA may conclude that pediatric effectiveness can be extrapolated from adequate and well-controlled studies in adults usually supplemented with other information obtained in pediatric patients, such as pharmacokinetic studies. Studies may not be needed in each pediatric age group, if data from one age group can be extrapolated to another. Assessments of safety and effectiveness required under this section for a drug product that represents a meaningful therapeutic benefit over existing treatments for pediatric patients must be carried out using appropriate formulations for each age group(s) for which the assessment is required.

(b) Deferred submission.

(1) FDA may, on its own initiative or at the request of an applicant, defer submission of some or all assessments of safety and effectiveness described in paragraph (a) of this section until after approval of the drug product for use in adults. Deferral may be granted if, among other reasons, the drug is ready for approval in adults before studies in pediatric patients are complete, or pediatric studies should be delayed until additional safety or effectiveness data have been

collected. If an applicant requests deferred submission, the request must provide a certification from the applicant of the grounds for delaying pediatric studies, a description of the planned or ongoing studies, and evidence that the studies are being or will be conducted with due diligence and at the earliest possible time.

(2) If FDA determines that there is an adequate justification for temporarily delaying the submission of assessments of pediatric safety and effectiveness, the drug product may be approved for use in adults subject to the requirement that the applicant submit the required assessments within a specified time.

(c) Waivers –

(1) General. FDA may grant a full or partial waiver of the requirements of paragraph (a) of this section on its own initiative or at the request of an applicant. A request for a waiver must provide an adequate justification.

(2) Full waiver. An applicant may request a waiver of the requirements of paragraph (a) of this section if the applicant certifies that:

(i) The drug product does not represent a meaningful therapeutic benefit over existing treatments for pediatric patients and is not likely to be used in a substantial number of pediatric patients;

(ii) Necessary studies are impossible or highly impractical because, e.g., the number of such patients is so small or geographically dispersed; or

(iii) There is evidence strongly suggesting that the drug product would be ineffective or unsafe in all pediatric age groups.

(3) Partial waiver. An applicant may request a waiver of the requirements of paragraph (a) of this section with respect to a specified pediatric age group, if the applicant certifies that:

(i) The drug product does not represent a meaningful therapeutic benefit over existing treatments for pediatric patients in that age group, and is not likely to be used in a substantial number of patients in that age group;

Part 314

(ii) Necessary studies are impossible or highly impractical because, e.g., the number of patients in that age group is so small or geographically dispersed;

(iii) There is evidence strongly suggesting that the drug product would be ineffective or unsafe in that age group; or

(iv) The applicant can demonstrate that reasonable attempts to produce a pediatric formulation necessary for that age group have failed.

(4) FDA action on waiver. FDA shall grant a full or partial waiver, as appropriate, if the agency finds that there is a reasonable basis on which to conclude that one or more of the grounds for waiver specified in paragraphs (c)(2) or (c)(3) of this section have been met. If a waiver is granted on the ground that it is not possible to develop a pediatric formulation, the waiver will cover only those pediatric age groups requiring that formulation. If a waiver is granted because there is evidence that the product would be ineffective or unsafe in pediatric populations, this information will be included in the product's labeling.

(5) Definition of "meaningful therapeutic benefit." For purposes of this section and 201.23 of this chapter, a drug will be considered to offer a meaningful therapeutic benefit over existing therapies if FDA estimates that:

(i) If approved, the drug would represent a significant improvement in the treatment, diagnosis, or prevention of a disease, compared to marketed products adequately labeled for that use in the relevant pediatric population. Examples of how improvement might be demonstrated include, for example, evidence of increased effectiveness in treatment, prevention, or diagnosis of disease, elimination or substantial reduction of a treatment-limiting drug reaction, documented enhancement of compliance, or evidence of safety and effectiveness in a new subpopulation; or

(ii) The drug is in a class of drugs or for an indication for which there is a need for additional therapeutic options.

(d) Exemption for orphan drugs. This section does not apply to any drug for an indication or indications for which orphan designation has been granted under part 316, subpart C, of this chapter.

[63 FR 66670, Dec. 2, 1998]

Sec. 314.60 Amendments to an unapproved application, supplement, or resubmission.

(a) FDA generally assumes that when an original application, supplement to an approved application, or resubmission of an application or supplement is submitted to the agency for review, the applicant believes that the agency can approve the application, supplement, or resubmission as submitted. However, the applicant may submit an amendment to an application that has been filed under 314.101 but is not yet approved.

(b)(1) Submission of a major amendment to an original application, efficacy supplement, or resubmission of an application or efficacy supplement within 3 months of the end of the initial review cycle constitutes an agreement by the applicant under section 505(c) of the act to extend the initial review cycle by 3 months. (For references to a resubmission of an application or efficacy supplement in paragraph (b) of this section, the timeframe for reviewing the resubmission is the "review cycle" rather than the "initial review cycle.") FDA may instead defer review of the amendment until the subsequent review cycle. If the agency extends the initial review cycle for an original application, efficacy supplement, or resubmission under this paragraph, the division responsible for reviewing the application, supplement, or resubmission will notify the applicant of the extension. The initial review cycle for an original application, efficacy supplement, or resubmission of an application or efficacy supplement may be extended only once due to submission of a major amendment. FDA may, at its discretion, review any subsequent major amendment during the initial review cycle (as extended) or defer review until the subsequent review cycle.

(2) Submission of a major amendment to an original application, efficacy supplement, or resubmission of an application or efficacy supplement more than 3 months before the end of the initial review cycle will not extend the cycle. FDA may, at its discretion, review such an amendment during the initial review cycle or defer review until the subsequent review cycle.

(3) Submission of an amendment to an original application, efficacy supplement, or resubmission of an application or efficacy supplement that is not a major amendment will not

extend the initial review cycle. FDA may, at its discretion, review such an amendment during the initial review cycle or defer review until the subsequent review cycle.

(4) Submission of a major amendment to a manufacturing supplement within 2 months of the end of the initial review cycle constitutes an agreement by the applicant under section 505(c) of the act to extend the initial review cycle by 2 months. FDA may instead defer review of the amendment until the subsequent review cycle. If the agency extends the initial review cycle for a manufacturing supplement under this paragraph, the division responsible for reviewing the supplement will notify the applicant of the extension. The initial review cycle for a manufacturing supplement may be extended only once due to submission of a major amendment. FDA may, at its discretion, review any subsequent major amendment during the initial review cycle (as extended) or defer review until the subsequent review cycle.

(5) Submission of an amendment to a supplement other than an efficacy or manufacturing supplement will not extend the initial review cycle. FDA may, at its discretion, review such an amendment during the initial review cycle or defer review until the subsequent review cycle.

(6) A major amendment may not include data to support an indication or claim that was not included in the original application, supplement, or resubmission, but it may include data to support a minor modification of an indication or claim that was included in the original application, supplement, or resubmission.

(7) When FDA defers review of an amendment until the subsequent review cycle, the agency will notify the applicant of the deferral in the complete response letter sent to the applicant under 314.110 of this part.

(c)(1) An unapproved application may not be amended if all of the following conditions apply:

(i) The unapproved application is for a drug for which a previous application has been approved and granted a period of exclusivity in accordance with section 505(c)(3)(D)(ii) of the act that has not expired;

(ii) The applicant seeks to amend the unapproved application to include a published report of an investigation that was conducted or sponsored by the applicant entitled to exclusivity for the drug;

(iii) The applicant has not obtained a right of reference to the investigation described in paragraph (c)(1)(ii) of this section; and

(iv) The report of the investigation described in paragraph (c)(1)(ii) of this section would be essential to the approval of the unapproved application.

(2) The submission of an amendment described in paragraph (c)(1) of this section will cause the unapproved application to be deemed to be withdrawn by the applicant under 314.65 on the date of receipt by FDA of the amendment. The amendment will be considered a resubmission of the application, which may not be accepted except as provided in accordance with section 505(c)(3)(D)(ii) of the act.

(d) The applicant shall submit a field copy of each amendment to 314.50(d)(1). The applicant shall include in its submission of each such amendment to FDA a statement certifying that a field copy of the amendment has been sent to the applicant's home FDA district office.

[50 FR 7493, Feb. 22, 1985, as amended at 57 FR 17983, Apr. 28, 1992; 58 FR 47352, Sept. 8, 1993; 63 FR 5252, Feb. 2, 1998; 69 FR 18764, Apr. 8, 2004; 73 FR 39608, July 10, 2008]

Sec. 314.65 Withdrawal by the applicant of an unapproved application.

An applicant may at any time withdraw an application that is not yet approved by notifying the Food and Drug Administration in writing. If, by the time it receives such notice, the agency has identified any deficiencies in the application, we will list such deficiencies in the letter we send the applicant acknowledging the withdrawal. A decision to withdraw the application is without prejudice to refiling. The agency will retain the application and will provide a copy to the applicant on request under the fee schedule in 20.45 of FDA's public information regulations.

[50 FR 7493, Feb. 22, 1985, as amended at 68 FR 25287, May 12, 2003; 73 FR 39609, July 10, 2008]

Sec. 314.70 Supplements and other changes to an approved application.

    (a) Changes to an approved application.

        (1)(i) Except as provided in paragraph (a)(1)(ii) of this section, the applicant must notify FDA about each change in each condition established in an approved application beyond the variations already provided for in the application. The notice is required to describe the change fully. Depending on the type of change, the applicant must notify FDA about the change in a supplement under paragraph (b) or (c) of this section or by inclusion of the information in the annual report to the application under paragraph (d) of this section.

        (ii) The submission and grant of a written request for an exception or alternative under 201.26 of this chapter satisfies the applicable requirements in paragraphs (a) through (c) of this section. However, any grant of a request for an exception or alternative under 201.26 of this chapter must be reported as part of the annual report to the application under paragraph (d) of this section.

        (2) The holder of an approved application under section 505 of the act must assess the effects of the change before distributing a drug product made with a manufacturing change.

        (3) Notwithstanding the requirements of paragraphs (b) and (c) of this section, an applicant must make a change provided for in those paragraphs in accordance with a regulation or guidance that provides for a less burdensome notification of the change (for example, by submission of a supplement that does not require approval prior to distribution of the product or in an annual report).

        (4) The applicant must promptly revise all promotional labeling and advertising to make it consistent with any labeling change implemented in accordance with paragraphs (b) and (c) of this section.

        (5) Except for a supplement providing for a change in the labeling, the applicant must include in each supplement and amendment to a supplement providing for a change under paragraph (b) or (c) of this section a statement certifying that

a field copy has been provided in accordance with 314.440(a)(4).

(6) A supplement or annual report must include a list of all changes contained in the supplement or annual report. For supplements, this list must be provided in the cover letter.

(b) Changes requiring supplement submission and approval prior to distribution of the product made using the change (major changes).

(1) A supplement must be submitted for any change in the drug substance, drug product, production process, quality controls, equipment, or facilities that has a substantial potential to have an adverse effect on the identity, strength, quality, purity, or potency of the drug product as these factors may relate to the safety or effectiveness of the drug product.

(2) These changes include, but are not limited to:

(i) Except those described in paragraphs (c) and (d) of this section, changes in the qualitative or quantitative formulation of the drug product, including inactive ingredients, or in the specifications provided in the approved application;

(ii) Changes requiring completion of studies in accordance with part 320 of this chapter to demonstrate the equivalence of the drug product to the drug product as manufactured without the change or to the reference listed drug;

(iii) Changes that may affect drug substance or drug product sterility assurance, such as changes in drug substance, drug product, or component sterilization method(s) or an addition, deletion, or substitution of steps in an aseptic processing operation;

(iv) Changes in the synthesis or manufacture of the drug substance that may affect the impurity profile and/or the physical, chemical, or biological properties of the drug substance;

(v) The following labeling changes:

(A) Changes in labeling, except those described in paragraphs (c)(6)(iii), (d)(2)(ix), or (d)(2)(x) of this section;

Part 314

(B) If applicable, any change to a Medication Guide required under part 208 of this chapter, except for changes in the information specified in 208.20(b)(8)(iii) and (b)(8)(iv) of this chapter; and

(C) Any change to the information required by 201.57(a) of this chapter, with the following exceptions that may be reported in an annual report under paragraph (d)(2)(x) of this section:

(1) Removal of a listed section(s) specified in 201.57(a)(5) of this chapter; and

(2) Changes to the most recent revision date of the labeling as specified in 201.57(a)(15) of this chapter.

(vi) Changes in a drug product container closure system that controls the drug product delivered to a patient or changes in the type (e.g., glass to high density polyethylene (HDPE), HDPE to polyvinyl chloride, vial to syringe) or composition (e.g., one HDPE resin to another HDPE resin) of a packaging component that may affect the impurity profile of the drug product.

(vii) Changes solely affecting a natural product, a recombinant DNA-derived protein/polypeptide, or a complex or conjugate of a drug substance with a monoclonal antibody for the following:

(A) Changes in the virus or adventitious agent removal or inactivation method(s);

(B) Changes in the source material or cell line; and

(C) Establishment of a new master cell bank or seed.

(viii) Changes to a drug product under an application that is subject to a validity assessment because of significant questions regarding the integrity of the data supporting that application.

(3) The applicant must obtain approval of a supplement from FDA prior to distribution of a drug product made using a change under paragraph (b) of this section. Except for submissions under paragraph (e) of this section, the following information must be contained in the supplement:

(i) A detailed description of the proposed change;

(ii) The drug product(s) involved;

(iii) The manufacturing site(s) or area(s) affected;

(iv) A description of the methods used and studies performed to assess the effects of the change;

(v) The data derived from such studies;

(vi) For a natural product, a recombinant DNA-derived protein/polypeptide, or a complex or conjugate of a drug substance with a monoclonal antibody, relevant validation protocols and a list of relevant standard operating procedures must be provided in addition to the requirements in paragraphs (b)(3)(iv) and (b)(3)(v) of this section; and

(vii) For sterilization process and test methodologies related to sterilization process validation, relevant validation protocols and a list of relevant standard operating procedures must be provided in addition to the requirements in paragraphs (b)(3)(iv) and (b)(3)(v) of this section.

(4) An applicant may ask FDA to expedite its review of a supplement for public health reasons or if a delay in making the change described in it would impose an extraordinary hardship on the applicant. Such a supplement and its mailing cover should be plainly marked: "Prior Approval Supplement-Expedited Review Requested."

(c) Changes requiring supplement submission at least 30 days prior to distribution of the drug product made using the change (moderate changes).

(1) A supplement must be submitted for any change in the drug substance, drug product, production process, quality controls, equipment, or facilities that has a moderate potential to have an adverse effect on the identity, strength, quality, purity, or potency of the drug product as these factors may relate to the safety or effectiveness of the drug product. If the supplement provides for a labeling change under paragraph (c)(6)(iii) of this section, 12 copies of the final printed labeling must be included.

(2) These changes include, but are not limited to:

Part 314

    (i) A change in the container closure system that does not affect the quality of the drug product, except those described in paragraphs (b) and (d) of this section; and

    (ii) Changes solely affecting a natural protein, a recombinant DNA-derived protein/polypeptide or a complex or conjugate of a drug substance with a monoclonal antibody, including:

        (A) An increase or decrease in production scale during finishing steps that involves different equipment; and

        (B) Replacement of equipment with that of a different design that does not affect the process methodology or process operating parameters.

    (iii) Relaxation of an acceptance criterion or deletion of a test to comply with an official compendium that is consistent with FDA statutory and regulatory requirements.

(3) A supplement submitted under paragraph (c)(1) of this section is required to give a full explanation of the basis for the change and identify the date on which the change is to be made. The supplement must be labeled "Supplement--Changes Being Effected in 30 Days" or, if applicable under paragraph (c)(6) of this section, "Supplement--Changes Being Effected."

(4) Pending approval of the supplement by FDA, except as provided in paragraph (c)(6) of this section, distribution of the drug product made using the change may begin not less than 30 days after receipt of the supplement by FDA. The information listed in paragraphs (b)(3)(i) through (b)(3)(vii) of this section must be contained in the supplement.

(5) The applicant must not distribute the drug product made using the change if within 30 days following FDA's receipt of the supplement, FDA informs the applicant that either:

    (i) The change requires approval prior to distribution of the drug product in accordance with paragraph (b) of this section; or

    (ii) Any of the information required under paragraph (c)(4) of this section is missing; the applicant must not distribute the drug product made using the change until the supplement has been amended to provide the missing information.

(6) The agency may designate a category of changes for the purpose of providing that, in the case of a change in such category, the holder of an approved application may commence distribution of the drug product involved upon receipt by the agency of a supplement for the change. These changes include, but are not limited to:

(i) Addition to a specification or changes in the methods or controls to provide increased assurance that the drug substance or drug product will have the characteristics of identity, strength, quality, purity, or potency that it purports or is represented to possess;

(ii) A change in the size and/or shape of a container for a nonsterile drug product, except for solid dosage forms, without a change in the labeled amount of drug product or from one container closure system to another;

(iii) Changes in the labeling to reflect newly acquired information, except for changes to the information required in 201.57(a) of this chapter (which must be made under paragraph (b)(2)(v)(C) of this section), to accomplish any of the following:

(A) To add or strengthen a contraindication, warning, precaution, or adverse reaction for which the evidence of a causal association satisfies the standard for inclusion in the labeling under 201.57(c) of this chapter;

(B) To add or strengthen a statement about drug abuse, dependence, psychological effect, or overdosage;

(C) To add or strengthen an instruction about dosage and administration that is intended to increase the safe use of the drug product;

(D) To delete false, misleading, or unsupported indications for use or claims for effectiveness; or

(E) Any labeling change normally requiring a supplement submission and approval prior to distribution of the drug product that FDA specifically requests be submitted under this provision.

(7) If the agency disapproves the supplemental application, it may order the manufacturer to cease distribution of the drug product(s) made with the manufacturing change.

(d) Changes to be described in an annual report (minor changes).

(1) Changes in the drug substance, drug product, production process, quality controls, equipment, or facilities that have a minimal potential to have an adverse effect on the identity, strength, quality, purity, or potency of the drug product as these factors may relate to the safety or effectiveness of the drug product must be documented by the applicant in the next annual report in accordance with 314.81(b)(2).

(2) These changes include, but are not limited to:

(i) Any change made to comply with a change to an official compendium, except a change described in paragraph (c)(2)(iii) of this section, that is consistent with FDA statutory and regulatory requirements.

(ii) The deletion or reduction of an ingredient intended to affect only the color of the drug product;

(iii) Replacement of equipment with that of the same design and operating principles except those equipment changes described in paragraph (c) of this section;

(iv) A change in the size and/or shape of a container containing the same number of dosage units for a nonsterile solid dosage form drug product, without a change from one container closure system to another;

(v) A change within the container closure system for a nonsterile drug product, based upon a showing of equivalency to the approved system under a protocol approved in the application or published in an official compendium;

(vi) An extension of an expiration dating period based upon full shelf life data on production batches obtained from a protocol approved in the application;

(vii) The addition or revision of an alternative analytical procedure that provides the same or increased assurance of the identity, strength, quality, purity, or potency of the material being tested as the analytical procedure described in the approved application, or deletion of an alternative analytical procedure;

(viii) The addition by embossing, debossing, or engraving of a code imprint to a solid oral dosage form drug product other than a modified release dosage form, or a minor change in an existing code imprint;

(ix) A change in the labeling concerning the description of the drug product or in the information about how the drug product is supplied, that does not involve a change in the dosage strength or dosage form; and

(x) An editorial or similar minor change in labeling, including a change to the information allowed by paragraphs (b)(2)(v)(C)(1) and (2) of this section.

(3) For changes under this category, the applicant is required to submit in the annual report:

(i) A statement by the holder of the approved application that the effects of the change have been assessed;

(ii) A full description of the manufacturing and controls changes, including the manufacturing site(s) or area(s) involved;

(iii) The date each change was implemented;

(iv) Data from studies and tests performed to assess the effects of the change; and,

(v) For a natural product, recombinant DNA-derived protein/polypeptide, complex or conjugate of a drug substance with a monoclonal antibody, sterilization process or test methodology related to sterilization process validation, a cross-reference to relevant validation protocols and/or standard operating procedures.

(e) Protocols. An applicant may submit one or more protocols describing the specific tests and studies and acceptance criteria to be achieved to demonstrate the lack of adverse effect for specified types of manufacturing changes on the identity, strength, quality, purity, and potency of the drug product as these factors may relate to the safety or effectiveness of the drug product. Any such protocols, if not included in the approved application, or changes to an approved protocol, must be submitted as a supplement requiring approval from FDA prior to distribution of a drug product produced with the manufacturing change. The

Part 314

supplement, if approved, may subsequently justify a reduced reporting category for the particular change because the use of the protocol for that type of change reduces the potential risk of an adverse effect.

(f) Patent information. The applicant must comply with the patent information requirements under section 505(c)(2) of the act.

(g) Claimed exclusivity. If an applicant claims exclusivity under 314.108 upon approval of a supplement for change to its previously approved drug product, the applicant must include with its supplement the information required under 314.50(j).

[69 FR 18764, Apr. 8, 2004, as amended at 71 FR 3997, Jan. 24, 2006; 72 FR 73600, Dec. 28, 2007; 73 FR 49609, Aug. 22, 2008]

Sec. 314.71 Procedures for submission of a supplement to an approved application.

(a) Only the applicant may submit a supplement to an application.

(b) All procedures and actions that apply to an application under 314.50 also apply to supplements, except that the information required in the supplement is limited to that needed to support the change. A supplement is required to contain an archival copy and a review copy that include an application form and appropriate technical sections, samples, and labeling; except that a supplement for a change other than a change in labeling is required also to contain a field copy.

(c) All procedures and actions that apply to applications under this part, including actions by applicants and the Food and Drug Administration, also apply to supplements except as specified otherwise in this part.

[50 FR 7493, Feb. 22, 1985, as amended at 50 FR 21238, May 23, 1985; 58 FR 47352, Sept. 8, 1993; 67 FR 9586, Mar. 4, 2002; 73 FR 39609, July 10, 2008]

Sec. 314.72 Change in ownership of an application.

(a) An applicant may transfer ownership of its application. At the time of transfer the new and former owners are required to submit information to the Food and Drug Administration as follows:

(1) The former owner shall submit a letter or other document that states that all rights to the application have been transferred to the new owner.

(2) The new owner shall submit an application form signed by the new owner and a letter or other document containing the following:

  (i) The new owner's commitment to agreements, promises, and conditions made by the former owner and contained in the application;

  (ii) The date that the change in ownership is effective; and

  (iii) Either a statement that the new owner has a complete copy of the approved application, including supplements and records that are required to be kept under 314.81, or a request for a copy of the application from FDA's files. FDA will provide a copy of the application to the new owner under the fee schedule in 20.45 of FDA's public information regulations.

(b) The new owner shall advise FDA about any change in the conditions in the approved application under 314.70, except the new owner may advise FDA in the next annual report about a change in the drug product's label or labeling to change the product's brand or the name of its manufacturer, packer, or distributor.

[50 FR 7493, Feb. 22, 1985; 50 FR 14212, Apr. 11, 1985, as amended at 50 FR 21238, May 23, 1985; 67 FR 9586, Mar. 4, 2002; 68 FR 25287, May 12, 2003]

Sec. 314.80 Postmarketing reporting of adverse drug experiences.

(a) Definitions. The following definitions of terms apply to this section:

Adverse drug experience. Any adverse event associated with the use of a drug in humans, whether or not considered drug related, including the following: An adverse event occurring in the course of the use of a drug product in professional practice; an adverse event occurring from drug overdose whether accidental or intentional; an adverse event occurring from drug abuse; an adverse event occurring from drug

Part 314

withdrawal; and any failure of expected pharmacological action.

Disability. A substantial disruption of a person's ability to conduct normal life functions.

Life-threatening adverse drug experience. Any adverse drug experience that places the patient, in the view of the initial reporter, atimmediate risk of death from the adverse drug experience as it occurred,i.e. , it does not include an adverse drug experience that, had it occurred in a more severe form, might have caused death.

Serious adverse drug experience. Any adverse drug experience occurring at any dose that results in any of the following outcomes: Death, a life-threatening adverse drug experience, inpatient hospitalization or prolongation of existing hospitalization, a persistent or significant disability/incapacity, or a congenital anomaly/birth defect. Important medical events that may not result in death, be life-threatening, or require hospitalization may be considered a serious adverse drug experience when, based upon appropriate medical judgment, they may jeopardize the patient or subject and may require medical or surgical intervention to prevent one of the outcomes listed in this definition. Examples of such medical events include allergic bronchospasm requiring intensive treatment in an emergency room or at home, blood dyscrasias or convulsions that do not result in inpatient hospitalization, or the development of drug dependency or drug abuse.

Unexpected adverse drug experience. Any adverse drug experience that is not listed in the current labeling for the drug product. This includes events that may be symptomatically and pathophysiologically related to an event listed in the labeling, but differ from the event because of greater severity or specificity. For example, under this definition, hepatic necrosis would be unexpected (by virtue of greater severity) if the labeling only referred to elevated hepatic enzymes or hepatitis. Similarly, cerebral thromboembolism and cerebral vasculitis would be unexpected (by virtue of greater specificity) if the labeling only listed cerebral vascular accidents. "Unexpected," as used in this definition, refers to an adverse drug experience that has not been previously observed (i.e. , included in the labeling) rather than from the perspective of such experience not being anticipated from the pharmacological properties of the pharmaceutical product.

(b) Review of adverse drug experiences. Each applicant having an approved application under 314.50 or, in the case of a 505(b)(2) application, an effective approved application, shall promptly review all adverse drug experience information obtained or otherwise received by the applicant from any source, foreign or domestic, including information derived from commercial marketing experience, postmarketing clinical investigations, postmarketing epidemiological/surveillance studies, reports in the scientific literature, and unpublished scientific papers. Applicants are not required to resubmit to FDA adverse drug experience reports forwarded to the applicant by FDA; however, applicants must submit all followup information on such reports to FDA. Any person subject to the reporting requirements under paragraph (c) of this section shall also develop written procedures for the surveillance, receipt, evaluation, and reporting of postmarketing adverse drug experiences to FDA.

(c) Reporting requirements. The applicant shall report to FDA adverse drug experience information, as described in this section. The applicant shall submit two copies of each report described in this section to the Central Document Room, 5901-B Ammendale Rd., Beltsville, MD 20705-1266. FDA may waive the requirement for the second copy in appropriate instances.

(1)(i) Postmarketing 15-day "Alert reports". The applicant shall report each adverse drug experience that is both serious and unexpected, whether foreign or domestic, as soon as possible but in no case later than 15 calendar days of initial receipt of the information by the applicant.

(ii) Postmarketing 15-day "Alert reports"--followup. The applicant shall promptly investigate all adverse drug experiences that are the subject of these postmarketing 15-day Alert reports and shall submit followup reports within 15 calendar days of receipt of new information or as requested by FDA. If additional information is not obtainable, records should be maintained of the unsuccessful steps taken to seek additional information. Postmarketing 15-day Alert reports and followups to them shall be submitted under separate cover.

(iii) Submission of reports. The requirements of paragraphs (c)(1)(i) and (c)(1)(ii) of this section, concerning the submission of postmarketing 15-day Alert reports, shall also apply to any person other than the applicant (nonapplicant) whose name appears on the label of an approved drug product as a manufacturer, packer, or distributor. To avoid unnecessary duplication in the submission to FDA of reports required by paragraphs (c)(1)(i) and (c)(1)(ii) of this section, obligations of a nonapplicant may be met by submission of all reports of serious adverse drug experiences to the applicant. If a nonapplicant elects to submit adverse drug experience reports to the applicant rather than to FDA, the nonapplicant shall submit each report to the applicant within 5 calendar days of receipt of the report by the nonapplicant, and the applicant shall then comply with the requirements of this section. Under this circumstance, the nonapplicant shall maintain a record of this action which shall include:

(A) A copy of each adverse drug experience report;

(B) The date the report was received by the nonapplicant;

(C) The date the report was submitted to the applicant; and

(D) The name and address of the applicant.

(iv) Report identification. Each report submitted under this paragraph shall bear prominent identification as to its contents,i.e. , "15-day Alert report," or "15-day Alert report-followup."

(2) Periodic adverse drug experience reports.

(i) The applicant shall report each adverse drug experience not reported under paragraph (c)(1)(i) of this section at quarterly intervals, for 3 years from the date of approval of the application, and then at annual intervals. The applicant shall submit each quarterly report within 30 days of the close of the quarter (the first quarter beginning on the date of approval of the application) and each annual report within 60 days of the anniversary date of approval of the application. Upon written notice, FDA may extend or reestablish the requirement that an applicant submit quarterly reports, or require that the applicant submit reports under this section at different times than those stated. For example, the agency may reestablish a quarterly reporting requirement following the approval of a major supplement. Followup information to adverse drug experiences submitted in a periodic report may be submitted in the next periodic report.

(ii) Each periodic report is required to contain: (a) a narrative summary and analysis of the information in the report and an analysis of the 15-day Alert reports submitted during the reporting interval (all 15-day Alert reports being appropriately referenced by the applicant's patient identification number, adverse reaction term(s), and date of submission to FDA); (b) a FDA Form 3500A (Adverse Reaction Report) for each adverse drug experience not reported under paragraph (c)(1)(i) of this section (with an index consisting of a line listing of the applicant's patient identification number and adverse reaction term(s)); and (c) a history of actions taken since the last report because of adverse drug experiences (for example, labeling changes or studies initiated).

(iii) Periodic reporting, except for information regarding 15-day Alert reports, does not apply to adverse drug experience information obtained from postmarketing studies (whether or not conducted under an investigational new drug application), from reports in the scientific literature, and from foreign marketing experience.

(d) Scientific literature.

(1) A 15-day Alert report based on information from the scientific literature is required to be accompanied by a copy of the published article. The 15-day reporting requirements in paragraph (c)(1)(i) of this section (i.e. , serious, unexpected adverse drug experiences) apply only to reports found in scientific and medical journals either as case reports or as the result of a formal clinical trial.

(2) As with all reports submitted under paragraph (c)(1)(i) of this section, reports based on the scientific literature shall be submitted on FDA Form 3500A or comparable format as prescribed by paragraph (f) of this section. In cases where the

Part 314

applicant believes that preparing the FDA Form 3500A constitutes an undue hardship, the applicant may arrange with the Office of Surveillance and Epidemiology for an acceptable alternative reporting format.

(e) Postmarketing studies.

(1) An applicant is not required to submit a 15-day Alert report under paragraph (c) of this section for an adverse drug experience obtained from a postmarketing study (whether or not conducted under an investigational new drug application) unless the applicant concludes that there is a reasonable possibility that the drug caused the adverse experience.

(2) The applicant shall separate and clearly mark reports of adverse drug experiences that occur during a postmarketing study as being distinct from those experiences that are being reported spontaneously to the applicant.

(f) Reporting FDA Form 3500A.

(1) Except as provided in paragraph (f)(3) of this section, the applicant shall complete FDA Form 3500A for each report of an adverse drug experience (foreign events may be submitted either on an FDA Form 3500A or, if preferred, on a CIOMS I form).

(2) Each completed FDA Form 3500A should refer only to an individual patient or a single attached publication.

(3) Instead of using FDA Form 3500A, an applicant may use a computer-generated FDA Form 3500A or other alternative format (e.g., a computer-generated tape or tabular listing) provided that:

(i) The content of the alternative format is equivalent in all elements of information to those specified in FDA Form 3500A; and

(ii) The format is agreed to in advance by the Office of Surveillance and Epidemiology.

(4) FDA Form 3500A and instructions for completing the form are available on the Internet athttp://www.fda.gov/medwatch/index.html.

(g) Multiple reports. An applicant should not include in reports under this section any adverse drug experiences that occurred in clinical trials if they were previously submitted as part of the approved application. If a report applies to a drug for which an applicant holds more than one approved application, the applicant should submit the report to the application that was first approved. If a report refers to more than one drug marketed by an applicant, the applicant should submit the report to the application for the drug listed first in the report.

(h) Patient privacy. An applicant should not include in reports under this section the names and addresses of individual patients; instead, the applicant should assign a unique code number to each report, preferably not more than eight characters in length. The applicant should include the name of the reporter from whom the information was received. Names of patients, health care professionals, hospitals, and geographical identifiers in adverse drug experience reports are not releasable to the public under FDA's public information regulations in part 20.

(i) Recordkeeping. The applicant shall maintain for a period of 10 years records of all adverse drug experiences known to the applicant, including raw data and any correspondence relating to adverse drug experiences.

(j) Withdrawal of approval. If an applicant fails to establish and maintain records and make reports required under this section, FDA may withdraw approval of the application and, thus, prohibit continued marketing of the drug product that is the subject of the application.

(k) Disclaimer. A report or information submitted by an applicant under this section (and any release by FDA of that report or information) does not necessarily reflect a conclusion by the applicant or FDA that the report or information constitutes an admission that the drug caused or contributed to an adverse effect. An applicant need not admit, and may deny, that the report or information submitted under this section constitutes an admission that the drug caused or contributed to an adverse effect. For purposes of this provision, the term "applicant" also includes any person reporting under paragraph (c)(1)(iii) of this section.

[50 FR 7493, Feb. 22, 1985; 50 FR 14212, Apr. 11, 1985, as amended at 50 FR 21238, May 23, 1985; 51 FR 24481, July 3, 1986; 52 FR 37936, Oct. 13, 1987; 55 FR 11580, Mar. 29, 1990; 57 FR 17983, Apr. 28, 1992; 62 FR 34168, June 25, 1997; 62 FR 52251, Oct. 7, 1997; 63 FR 14611, Mar. 26, 1998; 67 FR 9586, Mar. 4, 2002; 69 FR 13473, Mar. 23, 2004; 74 FR 13113, Mar. 26, 2009]

Part 314

Sec. 314.81 Other postmarketing reports.

(a) Applicability. Each applicant shall make the reports for each of its approved applications and abbreviated applications required under this section and section 505(k) of the act.

(b) Reporting requirements. The applicant shall submit to the Food and Drug Administration at the specified times two copies of the following reports:

    (1) NDA--Field alert report. The applicant shall submit information of the following kinds about distributed drug products and articles to the FDA district office that is responsible for the facility involved within 3 working days of receipt by the applicant. The information may be provided by telephone or other rapid communication means, with prompt written followup. The report and its mailing cover should be plainly marked: "NDA--Field Alert Report."

        (i) Information concerning any incident that causes the drug product or its labeling to be mistaken for, or applied to, another article.

        (ii) Information concerning any bacteriological contamination, or any significant chemical, physical, or other change or deterioration in the distributed drug product, or any failure of one or more distributed batches of the drug product to meet the specification established for it in the application.

    (2) Annual report. The applicant shall submit each year within 60 days of the anniversary date of U.S. approval of the application, two copies of the report to the FDA division responsible for reviewing the application. Each annual report is required to be accompanied by a completed transmittal Form FDA 2252 (Transmittal of Periodic Reports for Drugs for Human Use), and must include all the information required under this section that the applicant received or otherwise obtained during the annual reporting interval that ends on the U.S. anniversary date. The report is required to contain in the order listed:

        (i) Summary. A brief summary of significant new information from the previous year that might affect the safety, effectiveness, or labeling of the drug product. The report is also required to contain a brief description of actions the applicant has taken or intends to take as a result of this new information, for example, submit a labeling supplement, add a warning to the labeling, or initiate a new study. The summary shall briefly state whether labeling supplements for pediatric use have been submitted and whether new studies in the pediatric population to support appropriate labeling for the pediatric population have been initiated. Where possible, an estimate of patient exposure to the drug product, with special reference to the pediatric population (neonates, infants, children, and adolescents) shall be provided, including dosage form.

(ii)(a) Distribution data. Information about the quantity of the drug product distributed under the approved application, including that distributed to distributors. The information is required to include the National Drug Code (NDC) number, the total number of dosage units of each strength or potency distributed (e.g., 100,000/5 milligram tablets, 50,000/10 milliliter vials), and the quantities distributed for domestic use and the quantities distributed for foreign use. Disclosure of financial or pricing data is not required.

(b) Authorized generic drugs. If applicable, the date each authorized generic drug (as defined in 314.3) entered the market, the date each authorized generic drug ceased being distributed, and the corresponding trade or brand name. Each dosage form and/or strength is a different authorized generic drug and should be listed separately. The first annual report submitted on or after January 25, 2010 must include the information listed in this paragraph for any authorized generic drug that was marketed during the time period covered by an annual report submitted after January 1, 1999. If information is included in the annual report with respect to any authorized generic drug, a copy of that portion of the annual report must be sent to the Food and Drug Administration, Center for Drug Evaluation and Research, Office of New Drug Quality Assessment, Bldg. 21, rm. 2562, 10903 New Hampshire Ave., Silver Spring, MD 20993-0002, and marked "Authorized Generic Submission" or, by e-mail, to the Authorized Generics electronic mailbox

Part 314

atAuthorizedGenerics@fda.hhs.gov with
"Authorized Generic Submission" indicated in the
subject line. However, at such time that FDA has
required that annual reports be submitted in an
electronic format, the information required by this
paragraph must be submitted as part of the annual
report, in the electronic format specified for
submission of annual reports at that time, and not as
a separate submission under the preceding sentence
in this paragraph.

(iii) Labeling.

(a) Currently used professional labeling, patient
     brochures or package inserts (if any), and a
     representative sample of the package labels.

(b) The content of labeling required under 201.100(d)(3)
     of this chapter (i.e. , the package insert or
     professional labeling), including all text, tables, and
     figures, must be submitted in electronic format.
     Electronic format submissions must be in a form
     that FDA can process, review, and archive. FDA will
     periodically issue guidance on how to provide the
     electronic submission (e.g., method of transmission,
     media, file formats, preparation and organization of
     files). Submissions under this paragraph must be
     made in accordance with part 11 of this chapter,
     except for the requirements of 11.10(a), (c) through
     (h), and (k), and the corresponding requirements of
     11.30.

(c) A summary of any changes in labeling that have
     been made since the last report listed by date in the
     order in which they were implemented, or if no
     changes, a statement of that fact.

(iv) Chemistry, manufacturing, and controls changes.

(a) Reports of experiences, investigations, studies, or
     tests involving chemical or physical properties, or
     any other properties of the drug (such as the drug's
     behavior or properties in relation to microorganisms,
     including both the effects of the drug on
     microorganisms and the effects of microorganisms
     on the drug). These reports are only required for
     new information that may affect FDA's previous

conclusions about the safety or effectiveness of the drug product.

(b) A full description of the manufacturing and controls changes not requiring a supplemental application under 314.70 (b) and (c), listed by date in the order in which they were implemented.

(v) Nonclinical laboratory studies. Copies of unpublished reports and summaries of published reports of new toxicological findings in animal studies and in vitro studies (e.g., mutagenicity) conducted by, or otherwise obtained by, the applicant concerning the ingredients in the drug product. The applicant shall submit a copy of a published report if requested by FDA.

(vi) Clinical data.

(a) Published clinical trials of the drug (or abstracts of them), including clinical trials on safety and effectiveness; clinical trials on new uses; biopharmaceutic, pharmacokinetic, and clinical pharmacology studies; and reports of clinical experience pertinent to safety (for example, epidemiologic studies or analyses of experience in a monitored series of patients) conducted by or otherwise obtained by the applicant. Review articles, papers describing the use of the drug product in medical practice, papers and abstracts in which the drug is used as a research tool, promotional articles, press clippings, and papers that do not contain tabulations or summaries of original data should not be reported.

(b) Summaries of completed unpublished clinical trials, or prepublication manuscripts if available, conducted by, or otherwise obtained by, the applicant. Supporting information should not be reported. (A study is considered completed 1 year after it is concluded.)

(c) Analysis of available safety and efficacy data in the pediatric population and changes proposed in the labeling based on this information. An assessment of data needed to ensure appropriate labeling for the pediatric population shall be included.

(vii) Status reports of postmarketing study commitments. A status report of each postmarketing study of the drug product concerning clinical safety, clinical efficacy, clinical pharmacology, and nonclinical toxicology that is required by FDA (e.g., accelerated approval clinical benefit studies, pediatric studies) or that the applicant has committed, in writing, to conduct either at the time of approval of an application for the drug product or a supplement to an application, or after approval of the application or a supplement. For pediatric studies, the status report shall include a statement indicating whether postmarketing clinical studies in pediatric populations were required by FDA under 201.23 of this chapter. The status of these postmarketing studies shall be reported annually until FDA notifies the applicant, in writing, that the agency concurs with the applicant's determination that the study commitment has been fulfilled or that the study is either no longer feasible or would no longer provide useful information.

(a) Content of status report. The following information must be provided for each postmarketing study reported under this paragraph:

(1) Applicant's name.

(2) Product name. Include the approved drug product's established name and proprietary name, if any.

(3) NDA, ANDA, and supplement number.

(4) Date of U.S. approval of NDA or ANDA.

(5) Date of postmarketing study commitment.

(6) Description of postmarketing study commitment. The description must include sufficient information to uniquely describe the study. This information may include the purpose of the study, the type of study, the patient population addressed by the study and the indication(s) and dosage(s) that are to be studied.

(7) Schedule for completion and reporting of the postmarketing study commitment. The schedule should include the actual or projected dates for

submission of the study protocol to FDA, completion of patient accrual or initiation of an animal study, completion of the study, submission of the final study report to FDA, and any additional milestones or submissions for which projected dates were specified as part of the commitment. In addition, it should include a revised schedule, as appropriate. If the schedule has been previously revised, provide both the original schedule and the most recent, previously submitted revision.

(8) Current status of the postmarketing study commitment. The status of each postmarketing study should be categorized using one of the following terms that describes the study's status on the anniversary date of U.S. approval of the application or other agreed upon date:

(i) Pending. The study has not been initiated, but does not meet the criterion for delayed.

(ii) Ongoing. The study is proceeding according to or ahead of the original schedule described under paragraph (b)(2)(vii)(a)(7) of this section.

(iii) Delayed. The study is behind the original schedule described under paragraph (b)(2)(vii)(a)(7) of this section.

(iv) Terminated. The study was ended before completion but a final study report has not been submitted to FDA.

(v) Submitted. The study has been completed or terminated and a final study report has been submitted to FDA.

(9) Explanation of the study's status. Provide a brief description of the status of the study, including the patient accrual rate (expressed by providing the number of patients or subjects enrolled to date, and the total planned enrollment), and an explanation of the study's status identified under paragraph (b)(2)(vii)(a)(8) of this section. If the study has been completed, include the date the

study was completed and the date the final study report was submitted to FDA, as applicable. Provide a revised schedule, as well as the reason(s) for the revision, if the schedule under paragraph (b)(2)(vii)(a)(7) of this section has changed since the last report.

(b) Public disclosure of information. Except for the information described in this paragraph, FDA may publicly disclose any information described in paragraph (b)(2)(vii) of this section, concerning a postmarketing study, if the agency determines that the information is necessary to identify the applicant or to establish the status of the study, including the reasons, if any, for failure to conduct, complete, and report the study. Under this section, FDA will not publicly disclose trade secrets, as defined in 20.61 of this chapter, or information, described in 20.63 of this chapter, the disclosure of which would constitute an unwarranted invasion of personal privacy.

(viii) Status of other postmarketing studies. A status report of any postmarketing study not included under paragraph (b)(2)(vii) of this section that is being performed by, or on behalf of, the applicant. A status report is to be included for any chemistry, manufacturing, and controls studies that the applicant has agreed to perform and for all product stability studies.

(ix) Log of outstanding regulatory business. To facilitate communications between FDA and the applicant, the report may, at the applicant's discretion, also contain a list of any open regulatory business with FDA concerning the drug product subject to the application (e.g., a list of the applicant's unanswered correspondence with the agency, a list of the agency's unanswered correspondence with the applicant).

(3) Other reporting –

(i) Advertisements and promotional labeling. The applicant shall submit specimens of mailing pieces and any other labeling or advertising devised for promotion of the drug product at the time of initial dissemination of the labeling and at the time of initial publication of the advertisement for a prescription drug product. Mailing pieces and labeling that are designed to contain samples of a drug product are required to be complete, except the sample of the drug product may be omitted. Each submission is required to be accompanied by a completed transmittal Form FDA-2253 (Transmittal of Advertisements and Promotional Labeling for Drugs for Human Use) and is required to include a copy of the product's current professional labeling. Form FDA-2253 is available on the Internet at http://www.fda.gov/opacom/morechoices/fdaforms/cder.html.

(ii) Special reports. Upon written request the agency may require that the applicant submit the reports under this section at different times than those stated.

(iii) Notification of discontinuance.

    (a) An applicant who is the sole manufacturer of an approved drug product must notify FDA in writing at least 6 months prior to discontinuing manufacture of the drug product if:

        (1) The drug product is life supporting, life sustaining, or intended for use in the prevention of a serious disease or condition; and

        (2) The drug product was not originally derived from human tissue and replaced by a recombinant product.

    (b) For drugs regulated by the Center for Drug Evaluation and Research (CDER) or the Center for Biologics Evaluation and Research (CBER), one copy of the notification required by paragraph (b)(3)(iii)(a) of this section must be sent to the CDER Drug Shortage Coordinator, at the address of the Director of CDER; one copy to the CDER Drug Registration and Listing Team, Division of Compliance Risk Management and Surveillance; and one copy to either the director of the review division in CDER that is responsible for reviewing the application, or the director of the office in CBER that is responsible for reviewing the application.

    (c) FDA will publicly disclose a list of all drug products to be discontinued under paragraph (b)(3)(iii)(a) of

Part 314

this section. If the notification period is reduced under 314.91, the list will state the reason(s) for such reduction and the anticipated date that manufacturing will cease.

(iv) Withdrawal of approved drug product from sale.

    (a) The applicant shall submit on Form FDA 2657 (Drug Product Listing), within 15 working days of the withdrawal from sale of a drug product, the following information:

        (1) The National Drug Code (NDC) number.

        (2) The identity of the drug product by established name and by proprietary name.

        (3) The new drug application or abbreviated application number.

        (4) The date of withdrawal from sale. It is requested but not required that the reason for withdrawal of the drug product from sale be included with the information.

    (b) The applicant shall submit each Form FDA-2657 to the Records Repository Team (HFD-143), Center for Drug Evaluation and Research, Food and Drug Administration, 5600 Fishers Lane, Rockville, MD 20857.

    (c) Reporting under paragraph (b)(3)(iv) of this section constitutes compliance with the requirements under 207.30(a) of this chapter to report "at the discretion of the registrant when the change occurs."

(c) General requirements –

    (1) Multiple applications. For all reports required by this section, the applicant shall submit the information common to more than one application only to the application first approved, and shall not report separately on each application. The submission is required to identify all the applications to which the report applies.

    (2) Patient identification. Applicants should not include in reports under this section the names and addresses of individual patients; instead, the applicant should code the patient names whenever possible and retain the code in the

applicant's files. The applicant shall maintain sufficient patient identification information to permit FDA, by using that information alone or along with records maintained by the investigator of a study, to identify the name and address of individual patients; this will ordinarily occur only when the agency needs to investigate the reports further or when there is reason to believe that the reports do not represent actual results obtained.

(d) Withdrawal of approval. If an applicant fails to make reports required under this section, FDA may withdraw approval of the application and, thus, prohibit continued marketing of the drug product that is the subject of the application.

[50 FR 7493, Feb. 22, 1985; 50 FR 14212, Apr. 11, 1985, as amended at 50 FR 21238, May 23, 1985; 55 FR 11580, Mar. 29, 1990; 57 FR 17983, Apr. 28, 1992; 63 FR 66670, Dec. 2, 1998; 64 FR 401, Jan. 5, 1999; 65 FR 64617, Oct. 30, 2000; 66 FR 10815, Feb. 20, 2001; 68 FR 69019, Dec. 11, 2003; 69 FR 18766, Apr. 8, 2004; 69 FR 48775, Aug. 11, 2004; 72 FR 58999, Oct. 18, 2007; 74 FR 13113, Mar. 26, 2009; 74 FR 37167, July 28, 2009]

Sec. 314.90 Waivers.

(a) An applicant may ask the Food and Drug Administration to waive under this section any requirement that applies to the applicant under 314.50 through 314.81. An applicant may ask FDA to waive under 314.126(c) any criteria of an adequate and well-controlled study described in 314.126(b). A waiver request under this section is required to be submitted with supporting documentation in an application, or in an amendment or supplement to an application. The waiver request is required to contain one of the following:

(1) An explanation why the applicant's compliance with the requirement is unnecessary or cannot be achieved;

(2) A description of an alternative submission that satisfies the purpose of the requirement; or

(3) Other information justifying a waiver.

(b) FDA may grant a waiver if it finds one of the following:

(1) The applicant's compliance with the requirement is unnecessary for the agency to evaluate the application or compliance cannot be achieved;

Part 314

(2) The applicant's alternative submission satisfies the requirement; or

(3) The applicant's submission otherwise justifies a waiver.

[50 FR 7493, Feb. 22, 1985, as amended at 50 FR 21238, May 23, 1985; 67 FR 9586, Mar. 4, 2002]

Sec. 314.91 Obtaining a reduction in the discontinuance notification period.

(a) What is the discontinuance notification period? The discontinuance notification period is the 6-month period required under 314.81(b)(3)(iii)(a). The discontinuance notification period begins when an applicant who is the sole manufacturer of certain products notifies FDA that it will discontinue manufacturing the product. The discontinuance notification period ends when manufacturing ceases.

(b) When can FDA reduce the discontinuance notification period? FDA can reduce the 6-month discontinuance notification period when it finds good cause exists for the reduction. FDA may find good cause exists based on information certified by an applicant in a request for a reduction of the discontinuance notification period. In limited circumstances, FDA may find good cause exists based on information already known to the agency. These circumstances can include the withdrawal of the drug from the market based upon formal FDA regulatory action (e.g., under the procedures described in 314.150 for the publication of a notice of opportunity for a hearing describing the basis for the proposed withdrawal of a drug from the market) or resulting from the applicant's consultations with the agency.

(c) How can an applicant request a reduction in the discontinuance notification period?

(1) The applicant must certify in a written request that, in its opinion and to the best of its knowledge, good cause exists for the reduction. The applicant must submit the following certification:

The undersigned certifies that good cause exists for a reduction in the 6-month notification period required in 314.81(b)(3)(iii)(a) for discontinuing the manufacture of (name of the drug product). The following circumstances establish good cause (one or more of the circumstances in paragraph (d) of this section).

(2) The certification must be signed by the applicant or the applicant's attorney, agent (representative), or other authorized official. If the person signing the certification does not reside or have a place of business within the United States, the certification must contain the name and address of, and must also be signed by, an attorney, agent, or other authorized official who resides or maintains a place of business within the United States.

(3) For drugs regulated by the Center for Drug Evaluation and Research (CDER) or the Center for Biologics Evaluation and Research (CBER), one copy of the certification must be submitted to the Drug Shortage Coordinator at the address of the Director of CDER, one copy to the CDER Drug Registration and Listing Team, Division of Compliance Risk Management and Surveillance in CDER, and one copy to either the director of the review division in CDER responsible for reviewing the application, or the director of the office in CBER responsible for reviewing the application.

(d) What circumstances and information can establish good cause for a reduction in the discontinuance notification period?

(1) A public health problem may result from continuation of manufacturing for the 6-month period. This certification must include a detailed description of the potential threat to the public health.

(2) A biomaterials shortage prevents the continuation of the manufacturing for the 6-month period. This certification must include a detailed description of the steps taken by the applicant in an attempt to secure an adequate supply of biomaterials to enable manufacturing to continue for the 6-month period and an explanation of why the biomaterials could not be secured.

(3) A liability problem may exist for the manufacturer if the manufacturing is continued for the 6-month period. This certification must include a detailed description of the potential liability problem.

(4) Continuation of the manufacturing for the 6-month period may cause substantial economic hardship for the manufacturer. This certification must include a detailed

Part 314

description of the financial impact of continuing to manufacture the drug product over the 6-month period.

(5) The manufacturer has filed for bankruptcy under chapter 7 or 11 of title 11, United States Code (11 U.S.C. 701et seq. and 1101et seq.). This certification must be accompanied by documentation of the filing or proof that the filing occurred.

(6) The manufacturer can continue distribution of the drug product to satisfy existing market need for 6 months. This certification must include a detailed description of the manufacturer's processes to ensure such distribution for the 6-month period.

(7) Other good cause exists for the reduction. This certification must include a detailed description of the need for a reduction.

[72 FR 58999, Oct. 18, 2007]

Subpart C--Abbreviated Applications

Sec. 314.92 Drug products for which abbreviated applications may be submitted.

(a) Abbreviated applications are suitable for the following drug products within the limits set forth under 314.93:

(1) Drug products that are the same as a listed drug. A "listed drug" is defined in 314.3. For determining the suitability of an abbreviated new drug application, the term "same as" means identical in active ingredient(s), dosage form, strength, route of administration, and conditions of use, except that conditions of use for which approval cannot be granted because of exclusivity or an existing patent may be omitted. If a listed drug has been voluntarily withdrawn from or not offered for sale by its manufacturer, a person who wishes to submit an abbreviated new drug application for the drug shall comply with 314.122.

(2) [Reserved]

(3) Drug products that have been declared suitable for an abbreviated new drug application submission by FDA through the petition procedures set forth under 10.30 of this chapter and 314.93.

(b) FDA will publish in the list listed drugs for which abbreviated applications may be submitted. The list is available from the Superintendent of Documents, U.S. Government Printing Office, Washington, DC 20402, 202-783-3238.

[57 FR 17983, Apr. 28, 1992, as amended at 64 FR 401, Jan. 5, 1999]

Sec. 314.93 Petition to request a change from a listed drug.

(a) The only changes from a listed drug for which the agency will accept a petition under this section are those changes described in paragraph (b) of this section. Petitions to submit abbreviated new drug applications for other changes from a listed drug will not be approved.

(b) A person who wants to submit an abbreviated new drug application for a drug product which is not identical to a listed drug in route of administration, dosage form, and strength, or in which one active ingredient is substituted for one of the active ingredients in a listed combination drug, must first obtain permission from FDA to submit such an abbreviated application.

(c) To obtain permission to submit an abbreviated new drug application for a change described in paragraph (b) of this section, a person must submit and obtain approval of a petition requesting the change. A person seeking permission to request such a change from a reference listed drug shall submit a petition in accordance with 10.20 of this chapter and in the format specified in 10.30 of this chapter. The petition shall contain the information specified in 10.30 of this chapter and any additional information required by this section. If any provision of 10.20 or 10.30 of this chapter is inconsistent with any provision of this section, the provisions of this section apply.

(d) The petitioner shall identify a listed drug and include a copy of the proposed labeling for the drug product that is the subject of the petition and a copy of the approved labeling for the listed drug. The petitioner may, under limited circumstances, identify more than one listed drug, for example, when the proposed drug product is a combination product that differs from the combination reference listed drug with regard to an active ingredient, and the different active ingredient is an active ingredient of a listed drug. The petitioner shall also include information to show that:

Part 314

(1) The active ingredients of the proposed drug product are of the same pharmacological or therapeutic class as those of the reference listed drug.

(2) The drug product can be expected to have the same therapeutic effect as the reference listed drug when administered to patients for each condition of use in the reference listed drug's labeling for which the applicant seeks approval.

(3) If the proposed drug product is a combination product with one different active ingredient, including a different ester or salt, from the reference listed drug, that the different active ingredient has previously been approved in a listed drug or is a drug that does not meet the definition of "new drug" in section 201(b) of the act.

(e) No later than 90 days after the date a petition that is permitted under paragraph (a) of this section is submitted, FDA will approve or disapprove the petition.

(1) FDA will approve a petition properly submitted under this section unless it finds that:

(i) Investigations must be conducted to show the safety and effectiveness of the drug product or of any of its active ingredients, its route of administration, dosage form, or strength which differs from the reference listed drug; or

(ii) For a petition that seeks to change an active ingredient, the drug product that is the subject of the petition is not a combination drug; or

(iii) For a combination drug product that is the subject of the petition and has an active ingredient different from the reference listed drug:

(A) The drug product may not be adequately evaluated for approval as safe and effective on the basis of the information required to be submitted under 314.94; or

(B) The petition does not contain information to show that the different active ingredient of the drug product is of the same pharmacological or therapeutic class as the ingredient of the reference listed drug that is to be changed and that the drug product can be expected to have the same therapeutic effect as the reference listed drug when administered to patients for each condition of use in the listed drug's labeling for which the applicant seeks approval; or

(C) The different active ingredient is not an active ingredient in a listed drug or a drug that meets the requirements of section 201(p) of the act; or

(D) The remaining active ingredients are not identical to those of the listed combination drug; or

(iv) Any of the proposed changes from the listed drug would jeopardize the safe or effective use of the product so as to necessitate significant labeling changes to address the newly introduced safety or effectiveness problem; or

(v) FDA has determined that the reference listed drug has been withdrawn from sale for safety or effectiveness reasons under 314.161, or the reference listed drug has been voluntarily withdrawn from sale and the agency has not determined whether the withdrawal is for safety or effectiveness reasons.

(2) For purposes of this paragraph, "investigations must be conducted" means that information derived from animal or clinical studies is necessary to show that the drug product is safe or effective. Such information may be contained in published or unpublished reports.

(3) If FDA approves a petition submitted under this section, the agency's response may describe what additional information, if any, will be required to support an abbreviated new drug application for the drug product. FDA may, at any time during the course of its review of an abbreviated new drug application, request additional information required to evaluate the change approved under the petition.

(f) FDA may withdraw approval of a petition if the agency receives any information demonstrating that the petition no longer satisfies the conditions under paragraph (e) of this section.

Sec. 314.94 Content and format of an abbreviated application.

Abbreviated applications are required to be submitted in the form and contain the information required under this section. Three copies of the application are required, an archival copy, a review copy, and a field copy. FDA will maintain guidance documents on the format and content of applications to assist applicants in their preparation.

(a) Abbreviated new drug applications. Except as provided in paragraph (b) of this section, the applicant shall submit a complete archival copy of the abbreviated new drug application that includes the following:

(1) Application form. The applicant shall submit a completed and signed application form that contains the information described under 314.50(a)(1), (a)(3), (a)(4), and (a)(5). The applicant shall state whether the submission is an abbreviated application under this section or a supplement to an abbreviated application under 314.97.

(2) Table of contents. the archival copy of the abbreviated new drug application is required to contain a table of contents that shows the volume number and page number of the contents of the submission.

(3) Basis for abbreviated new drug application submission. An abbreviated new drug application must refer to a listed drug. Ordinarily, that listed drug will be the drug product selected by the agency as the reference standard for conducting bioequivalence testing. The application shall contain:

(i) The name of the reference listed drug, including its dosage form and strength. For an abbreviated new drug application based on an approverd petition under 10.30 of this chapter or 314.93, the reference listed drug must be the same as the listed drug approved in the petition.

(ii) A statement as to whether, according to the information published in the list, the reference listed drug is entitled to a period of marketing exclusivity under section 505(j)(4)(D) of the act.

(iii) For an abbreviated new drug application based on an approved petition under 10.30 of this chapter or 314.93, a reference to FDA-assigned docket number for the petition and a copy of FDA's correspondence approving the petition.

(4) Conditions of use.

(i) A statement that the conditions of use prescribed, recommended, or suggested in the labeling proposed for the drug product have been previously approved for the reference listed drug.

(ii) A reference to the applicant's annotated proposed labeling and to the currently approved labeling for the reference listed drug provided under paragraph (a)(8) of this section.

(5) Active ingredients.

(i) For a single-active-ingredient drug product, information to show that the active ingredient is the same as that of the reference single-active-ingredient listed drug, as follows:

(A) A statement that the active ingredient of the proposed drug product is the same as that of the reference listed drug.

(B) A reference to the applicant's annotated proposed labeling and to the currently approved labeling for the reference listed drug provided under paragraph (a)(8) of this section.

(ii) For a combination drug product, information to show that the active ingredients are the same as those of the reference listed drug except for any different active ingredient that has been the subject of an approved petition, as follows:

(A) A statement that the active ingredients of the proposed drug product are the same as those of the reference listed drug, or if one of the active ingredients differs from one of the active ingredients of the reference listed drug and the abbreviated application is submitted under the approval of a petition under 314.93 to vary such active ingredient, information to show that the other active ingredients of the drug product are the same as the other active ingredients of the reference listed drug, information to show that the different active ingredient is an active ingredient of another listed drug or of a drug that does not meet the definition of "new drug" in section 201(p) of the act, and such other information about the different active ingredient that FDA may require.

   (B) A reference to the applicant's annotated proposed labeling and to the currently approved labeling for the reference listed drug provided under paragraph (a)(8) of this section.

 (6) Route of administration, dosage form, and strength.

  (i) Information to show that the route of administration, dosage form, and strength of the drug product are the same as those of the reference listed drug except for any differences that have been the subject of an approved petition, as follows:

   (A) A statement that the route of administration, dosage form, and strength of the proposed drug product are the same as those of the reference listed drug.

   (B) A reference to the applicant's annotated proposed labeling and to the currently approved labeling for the reference listed drug provided under paragraph (a)(8) of this section.

  (ii) If the route of administration, dosage form, or strength of the drug product differs from the reference listed drug and the abbreviated application is submitted under an approved petition under 314.93, such information about the different route of administration, dosage form, or strength that FDA may require.

 (7) Bioequivalence.

  (i) Information that shows that the drug product is bioequivalent to the reference listed drug upon which the applicant relies. A complete study report must be submitted for the bioequivalence study upon which the applicant relies for approval. For all other bioequivalence studies conducted on the same drug product formulation as defined in 320.1(g) of this chapter, the applicant must submit either a complete or summary report. If a summary report of a bioequivalence study is submitted and FDA determines that there may be bioequivalence issues or concerns with the product, FDA may require that the applicant submit a complete report of the bioequivalence study to FDA; or

  (ii) If the abbreviated new drug application is submitted under a petition approved under 314.93, the results of any bioavailability of bioequivalence testing required by the agency, or any other information required by the agency to show that the active ingredients of the proposed drug product are of the same pharmacological or therapeutic class as those in the reference listed drug and that the proposed drug product can be expected to have the same therapeutic effect as the reference listed drug. If the proposed drug product contains a different active ingredient than the reference listed drug, FDA will consider the proposed drug product to have the same therapeutic effect as the reference listed drug if the applicant provides information demonstrating that:

(A) There is an adequate scientific basis for determining that substitution of the specific proposed dose of the different active ingredient for the dose of the member of the same pharmacological or therapeutic class in the reference listed drug will yield a resulting drug product whose safety and effectiveness have not been adversely affected.

(B) The unchanged active ingredients in the proposed drug product are bioequivalent to those in the reference listed drug.

(C) The different active ingredient in the proposed drug product is bioequivalent to an approved dosage form containing that ingredient and approved for the same indication as the proposed drug product or is bioequivalent to a drug product offered for that indication which does not meet the definition of "new drug" under section 201(p) of the act.

(iii) For each in vivo bioequivalence study contained in the abbreviated new drug application, a description of the analytical and statistical methods used in each study and a statement with respect to each study that it either was conducted in compliance with the institutional review board regulations in part 56 of this chapter, or was not subject to the regulations under 56.104 or 56.105 of this chapter and that each study was conducted in compliance with the informed consent regulations in part 50 of this chapter.

(8) Labeling –

(i) Listed drug labeling. A copy of the currently approved labeling (including, if applicable, any Medication Guide

required under part 208 of this chapter) for the listed
drug referred to in the abbreviated new drug application,
if the abbreviated new drug application relies on a
reference listed drug.

(ii) Copies of proposed labeling. Copies of the label and all
labeling for the drug product including, if applicable, any
Medication Guide required under part 208 of this chapter
(4 copies of draft labeling or 12 copies of final printed
labeling).

(iii) Statement on proposed labeling. A statement that the
applicant's proposed labeling including, if applicable, any
Medication Guide required under part 208 of this chapter
is the same as the labeling of the reference listed drug
except for differences annotated and explained under
paragraph (a)(8)(iv) of this section.

(iv) Comparison of approved and proposed labeling. A side-
by-side comparison of the applicant's proposed labeling
including, if applicable, any Medication Guide required
under part 208 of this chapter with the approved labeling
for the reference listed drug with all differences annotated
and explained. Labeling (including the container label,
package insert, and, if applicable, Medication Guide)
proposed for the drug product must be the same as the
labeling approved for the reference listed drug, except for
changes required because of differences approved under
a petition filed under 314.93 or because the drug product
and the reference listed drug are produced or distributed
by different manufacturers. Such differences between the
applicant's proposed labeling and labeling approved for
the reference listed drug may include differences in
expiration date, formulation, bioavailability, or
pharmacokinetics, labeling revisions made to comply with
current FDA labeling guidelines or other guidance, or
omission of an indication or other aspect of labeling
protected by patent or accorded exclusivity under section
505(j)(4)(D) of the act.

(9) Chemistry, manufacturing, and controls.

(i) The information required under 314.50(d)(1), except that
314.50(d)(1)(ii)(c) shall contain the proposed or actual
master production record, including a description of the

equipment, to be used for the manufacture of a commercial lot of the drug product.

(ii) Inactive ingredients. Unless otherwise stated in paragraphs (a)(9)(iii) through (a)(9)(v) of this section, an applicant shall identify and characterize the inactive ingredients in the proposed drug product and provide information demonstrating that such inactive ingredients do not affect the safety or efficacy of the proposed drug product.

(iii) Inactive ingredient changes permitted in drug products intended for parenteral use. Generally, a drug product intended for parenteral use shall contain the same inactive ingredients and in the same concentration as the reference listed drug identified by the applicant under paragraph (a)(3) of this section. However, an applicant may seek approval of a drug product that differs from the reference listed drug in preservative, buffer, or antioxidant provided that the applicant identifies and characterizes the differences and provides information demonstrating that the differences do not affect the safety or efficacy of the proposed drug product.

(iv) Inactive ingredient changes permitted in drug products intended for ophthalmic or otic use. Generally, a drug product intended for ophthalmic or otic use shall contain the same inactive ingredients and in the same concentration as the reference listed drug identified by the applicant under paragraph (a)(3) of this section. However, an applicant may seek approval of a drug product that differs from the reference listed drug in preservative, buffer, substance to adjust tonicity, or thickening agent provided that the applicant identifies and characterizes the differences and provides information demonstrating that the differences do not affect the safety or efficacy of the proposed drug product, except that, in a product intended for ophthalmic use, an applicant may not change a buffer or substance to adjust tonicity for the purpose of claiming a therapeutic advantage over or difference from the listed drug, e.g., by using a balanced salt solution as a diluent as opposed to an isotonic saline solution, or by making a significant change in the pH or other change that may raise questions of irritability.

(v) Inactive ingredient changes permitted in drug products intended for topical use. Generally, a drug product intended for topical use, solutions for aerosolization or nebulization, and nasal solutions shall contain the same inactive ingredients as the reference listed drug identified by the applicant under paragraph (a)(3) of this section. However, an abbreviated application may include different inactive ingredients provided that the applicant identifies and characterizes the differences and provides information demonstrating that the differences do not affect the safety or efficacy of the proposed drug product.

(10) Samples. The information required under 314.50(e)(1) and (e)(2)(i). Samples need not be submitted until requested by FDA.

(11) Other. The information required under 314.50(g).

(12) Patent certification –

(i) Patents claiming drug, drug product, or method of use.

(A) Except as provided in paragraph (a)(12)(iv) of this section, a certification with respect to each patent issued by the United States Patent and Trademark Office that, in the opinion of the applicant and to the best of its knowledge, claims the reference listed drug or that claims a use of such listed drug for which the applicant is seeking approval under section 505(j) of the act and for which information is required to be filed under section 505(b) and (c) of the act and 314.53. For each such patent, the applicant shall provide the patent number and certify, in its opinion and to the best of its knowledge, one of the following circumstances:

(1) That the patent information has not been submitted to FDA. The applicant shall entitle such a certification "Paragraph I Certification";

(2) That the patent has expired. The applicant shall entitle such a certification "Paragraph II Certification";

(3) The date on which the patent will expire. The applicant shall entitle such a certification "Paragraph III Certification"; or

(4) That the patent is invalid, unenforceable, or will not be infringed by the manufacture, use, or sale of the drug product for which the abbreviated application is submitted. The applicant shall entitle such a certification "Paragraph IV Certification". This certification shall be submitted in the following form:

I, (name of applicant), certify that Patent No. _____ (is invalid, unenforceable, or will not be infringed by the manufacture, use, or sale of) (name of proposed drug product) for which this application is submitted.

The certification shall be accompanied by a statement that the applicant will comply with the requirements under 314.95(a) with respect to providing a notice to each owner of the patent or their representatives and to the holder of the approved application for the listed drug, and with the requirements under 314.95(c) with respect to the content of the notice.

(B) If the abbreviated new drug application refers to a listed drug that is itself a licensed generic product of a patented drug first approved under section 505(b) of the act, the appropriate patent certification under paragraph (a)(12)(i) of this section with respect to each patent that claims the first-approved patented drug or that claims a use for such drug.

(ii) No relevant patents. If, in the opinion of the applicant and to the best of its knowledge, there are no patents described in paragraph (a)(12)(i) of this section, a certification in the following form:

In the opinion and to the best knowledge of (name of applicant), there are no patents that claim the listed drug referred to in this application or that claim a use of the listed drug.

(iii) Method of use patent.

(A) If patent information is submitted under section 505(b) or (c) of the act and 314.53 for a patent claiming a method of using the listed drug, and the labeling for the drug product for which the applicant

Part 314

is seeking approval does not include any indications that are covered by the use patent, a statement explaining that the method of use patent does not claim any of the proposed indications.

(B) If the labeling of the drug product for which the applicant is seeking approval includes an indication that, according to the patent information submitted under section 505(b) or (c) of the act and 314.53 or in the opinion of the applicant, is claimed by a use patent, an applicable certification under paragraph (a)(12)(i) of this section.

(iv) Method of manufacturing patent. An applicant is not required to make a certification with respect to any patent that claims only a method of manufacturing the listed drug.

(v) Licensing agreements. If the abbreviated new drug application is for a drug or method of using a drug claimed by a patent and the applicant has a licensing agreement with the patent owner, a certification under paragraph (a)(12)(i)(A)(4) of this section ("Paragraph IV Certification") as to that patent and a statement that it has been granted a patent license.

(vi) Late submission of patent information. If a patent on the listed drug is issued and the holder of the approved application for the listed drug does not submit the required information on the patent within 30 days of issuance of the patent, an applicant who submitted an abbreviated new drug application for that drug that contained an appropriate patent certification before the submission of the patent information is not required to submit an amended certification. An applicant whose abbreviated new drug application is submitted after a late submission of patent information, or whose pending abbreviated application was previously submitted but did not contain an appropriate patent certification at the time of the patent submission, shall submit a certification under paragraph (a)(12)(i) of this section or a statement under paragraph (a)(12)(iii) of this section as to that patent.

(vii) Disputed patent information. If an applicant disputes the accuracy or relevance of patent information submitted to

FDA, the applicant may seek a confirmation of the correctness of the patent information in accordance with the procedures under 314.53(f). Unless the patent information is withdrawn or changed, the applicant shall submit an appropriate certification for each relevant patent.

(viii) Amended certifications. A certification submitted under paragraphs (a)(12)(i) through (a)(12)(iii) of this section may be amended at any time before the effective date of the approval of the application. However, an applicant who has submitted a paragraph IV patent certification may not change it to a paragraph III certification if a patent infringement suit has been filed against another paragraph IV applicant unless the agency has determined that no applicant is entitled to 180-day exclusivity or the patent expires before the lawsuit is resolved or expires after the suit is resolved but before the end of the 180-day exclusivity period. If an applicant with a pending application voluntarily makes a patent certification for an untimely filed patent, the applicant may withdraw the patent certification for the untimely filed patent. An applicant shall submit an amended certification by letter or as an amendment to a pending application or by letter to an approved application. Once an amendment or letter is submitted, the application will no longer be considered to contain the prior certification.

(A) After finding of infringement. An applicant who has submitted a certification under paragraph (a)(12)(i)(A)(4) of this section and is sued for patent infringement within 45 days of the receipt of notice sent under 314.95 shall amend the certification if a final judgment in the action against the applicant is entered finding the patent to be infringed. In the amended certification, the applicant shall certify under paragraph (a)(12)(i)(A)(3) of this section that the patent will expire on a specific date. Once an amendment or letter for the change has been submitted, the application will no longer be considered to be one containing a certification under paragraph (a)(12)(i)(A)(4) of this section. If a final judgment finds the patent to be invalid and infringed, an amended certification is not required.

(B) After removal of a patent from the list. If a patent is removed from the list, any applicant with a pending application (including a tentatively approved application with a delayed effective date) who has made a certification with respect to such patent shall amend its certification. The applicant shall certify under paragraph (a)(12)(ii) of this section that no patents described in paragraph (a)(12)(i) of this section claim the drug or, if other relevant patents claim the drug, shall amend the certification to refer only to those relevant patents. In the amendment, the applicant shall state the reason for the change in certification (that the patent is or has been removed from the list). A patent that is the subject of a lawsuit under 314.107(c) shall not be removed from the list until FDA determines either that no delay in effective dates of approval is required under that section as a result of the lawsuit, that the patent has expired, or that any such period of delay in effective dates of approval is ended. An applicant shall submit an amended certification. Once an amendment or letter for the change has been submitted, the application will no longer be considered to be one containing a certification under paragraph (a)(12)(i)(A)(4) of this section.

(C) Other amendments.

(1) Except as provided in paragraphs (a)(12)(vi) and (a)(12)(viii)(C)(2) of this section, an applicant shall amend a submitted certification if, at any time before the effective date of the approval of the application, the applicant learns that the submitted certification is no longer accurate.

(2) An applicant is not required to amend a submitted certification when information on a patent on the listed drug is submitted after the effective date of approval of the abbreviated application.

(13) Financial certification or disclosure statement. An abbreviated application shall contain a financial certification or disclosure statement as required by part 54 of this chapter.

(b) Drug products subject to the Drug Efficacy Study Implementation (DESI) review. If the abbreviated new drug application is for a duplicate of a drug product that is subject to FDA's DESI review (a review of drug products approved as safe between 1938 and 1962) or other DESI-like review and the drug product evaluated in the review is a listed drug, the applicant shall comply with the provisions of paragraph (a) of this section.

(c) [Reserved]

(d) Format of an abbreviated application.

   (1) The applicant must submit a complete archival copy of the abbreviated application as required under paragraphs (a) and (c) of this section. FDA will maintain the archival copy during the review of the application to permit individual reviewers to refer to information that is not contained in their particular technical sections of the application, to give other agency personnel access to the application for official business, and to maintain in one place a complete copy of the application.

     (i) Format of submission. An applicant may submit portions of the archival copy of the abbreviated application in any form that the applicant and FDA agree is acceptable, except as provided in paragraph (d)(1)(ii) of this section.

     (ii) Labeling. The content of labeling required under 201.100(d)(3) of this chapter (commonly referred to as the package insert or professional labeling), including all text, tables, and figures, must be submitted to the agency in electronic format as described in paragraph (d)(1)(iii) of this section. This requirement applies to the content of labeling for the proposed drug product only and is in addition to the requirements of paragraph (a)(8)(ii) of this section that copies of the formatted label and all proposed labeling be submitted. Submissions under this paragraph must be made in accordance with part 11 of this chapter, except for the requirements of 11.10(a), (c) through (h), and (k), and the corresponding requirements of 11.30.

     (iii) Electronic format submissions. Electronic format submissions must be in a form that FDA can process, review, and archive. FDA will periodically issue guidance on how to provide the electronic submission (e.g.,

method of transmission, media, file formats, preparation
and organization of files).

(2) For abbreviated new drug applications, the applicant shall
submit a review copy of the abbreviated application that
contains two separate sections. One section shall contain the
information described under paragraphs (a)(2) through (a)(6),
(a)(8), and (a)(9) of this section 505(j)(2)(A)(vii) of the act and
one copy of the analytical procedures and descriptive
information needed by FDA's laboratories to perform tests
on samples of the proposed drug product and to validate the
applicant's analytical procedures. The other section shall
contain the information described under paragraphs (a)(3),
(a)(7), and (a)(8) of this section. Each of the sections in the
review copy is required to contain a copy of the application
form described under 314.50(a).

(3) [Reserved]

(4) The applicant may obtain from FDA sufficient folders to
bind the archival, the review, and the field copies of the
abbreviated application.

(5) The applicant shall submit a field copy of the abbreviated
application that contains the technical section described in
paragraph (a)(9) of this section, a copy of the application
form required under paragraph (a)(1) of this section, and a
certification that the field copy is a true copy of the technical
section described in paragraph (a)(9) of this section contained
in the archival and review copies of the abbreviated
application.

[57 FR 17983, Apr. 28, 1992; 57 FR 29353, July 1, 1992, as amended at 58 FR
47352, Sept. 8, 1993; 59 FR 50364, Oct. 3, 1994; 63 FR 5252, Feb. 2, 1998; 63
FR 66399, Dec. 1, 1998; 64 FR 401, Jan. 5, 1999; 65 FR 56479, Sept. 19, 2000;
67 FR 77672, Dec. 19, 2002; 68 FR 69019, Dec. 11, 2003; 69 FR 18766, Apr. 8,
2004; 74 FR 2861, Jan. 16, 2009]

Sec. 314.95 Notice of certification of invalidity or noninfringement of a patent.

(a) Notice of certification. For each patent that claims the listed drug
or that claims a use for such listed drug for which the applicant is
seeking approval and that the applicant certifies under
314.94(a)(12) is invalid, unenforceable, or will not be infringed, the
applicant shall send notice of such certification by registered or

certified mail, return receipt requested to each of the following persons:

(1) Each owner of the patent which is the subject of the certification or the representative designated by the owner to receive the notice. The name and address of the patent owner or its representative may be obtained from the United States Patent and Trademark Office; and

(2) The holder of the approved application under section 505(b) of the act for the listed drug that is claimed by the patent and for which the applicant is seeking approval, or, if the application holder does not reside or maintain a place of business within the United States, the application holder's attorney, agent, or other authorized official. The name and address of the application holder or its attorney, agent, or authorized official may be obtained from the Orange Book Staff, Office of Generic Drugs, 7500 Standish Pl., Rockville, MD 20855.

(3) This paragraph does not apply to a use patent that claims no uses for which the applicant is seeking approval.

(b) Sending the notice. The applicant shall send the notice required by paragraph (a) of this section when it receives from FDA an acknowledgment letter stating that its abbreviated new drug application is sufficiently complete to permit a substantive review. At the same time, the applicant shall amend its abbreviated new drug application to include a statement certifying that the notice has been provided to each person identified under paragraph (a) of this section and that the notice met the content requirements under paragraph (c) of this section.

(c) Contents of a notice. In the notice, the applicant shall cite section 505(j)(2)(B)(ii) of the act and shall include, but not be limited to, the following information:

(1) A statement that FDA has received an abbreviated new drug application submitted by the applicant containing any required bioavailability or bioequivalence data or information.

(2) The abbreviated application number.

(3) The established name, if any, as defined in section 502(e)(3) of the act, of the proposed drug product.

(4) The active ingredient, strength, and dosage form of the proposed drug product.

(5) The patent number and expiration date, as submitted to the agency or as known to the applicant, of each patent alleged to be invalid, unenforceable, or not infringed.

(6) A detailed statement of the factual and legal basis of the applicant's opinion that the patent is not valid, unenforceable, or will not be infringed. The applicant shall include in the detailed statement:

    (i) For each claim of a patent alleged not to be infringed, a full and detailed explanation of why the claim is not infringed.

    (ii) For each claim of a patent alleged to be invalid or unenforceable, a full and detailed explanation of the grounds supporting the allegation.

(7) If the applicant does not reside or have a place of business in the United States, the name and address of an agent in the United States authorized to accept service of process for the applicant.

(d) Amendment to an abbreviated application. If an abbreviated application is amended to include the certification described in 314.94(a)(12)(i)(A)(4), the applicant shall send the notice required by paragraph (a) of this section at the same time that the amendment to the abbreviated application is submitted to FDA.

(e) Documentation of receipt of notice. The applicant shall amend its abbreviated application to document receipt of the notice required under paragraph (a) of this section by each person provided the notice. The applicant shall include a copy of the return receipt or other similar evidence of the date the notification was received. FDA will accept as adequate documentation of the date of receipt a return receipt or a letter acknowledging receipt by the person provided the notice. An applicant may rely on another form of documentation only if FDA has agreed to such documentation in advance. A copy of the notice itself need not be submitted to the agency.

(f) Approval. If the requirements of this section are met, FDA will presume the notice to be complete and sufficient, and it will count the day following the date of receipt of the notice by the patent owner or its representative and by the approved application holder as the first day of the 45-day period provided for in section 505(j)(4)(B)(iii) of the act. FDA may, if the applicant provides a written statement to FDA that a later date should be used, count from such later date.

[59 FR 50366, Oct. 3, 1994, as amended at 68 FR 36705, June 18, 2003; 69 FR 11310, Mar. 10, 2004; 74 FR 9766, Mar. 6, 2009; 74 FR 36605, July 24, 2009]

Sec. 314.96 Amendments to an unapproved abbreviated application.

(a) Abbreviated new drug application.

(1) An applicant may amend an abbreviated new drug application that is submitted under 314.94, but not yet approved, to revise existing information or provide additional information. Amendments containing bioequivalence studies must contain reports of all bioequivalence studies conducted by the applicant on the same drug product formulation, unless the information has previously been submitted to FDA in the abbreviated new drug application. A complete study report must be submitted for any bioequivalence study upon which the applicant relies for approval. For all other bioequivalence studies conducted on the same drug product formulation as defined in 320.1(g) of this chapter, the applicant must submit either a complete or summary report. If a summary report of a bioequivalence study is submitted and FDA determines that there may be bioequivalence issues or concerns with the product, FDA may require that the applicant submit a complete report of the bioequivalence study to FDA.

(2) Submission of an amendment containing significant data or information before the end of the initial review cycle constitutes an agreement between FDA and the applicant to extend the initial review cycle only for the time necessary to review the significant data or information and for no more than 180 days.

(b) The applicant shall submit a field copy of each amendment to 314.94(a)(9). The applicant, other than a foreign applicant, shall include in its submission of each such amendment to FDA a statement certifying that a field copy of the amendment has been sent to the applicant's home FDA district office.

Part 314

[57 FR 17983, Apr. 28, 1992, as amended at 58 FR 47352, Sept. 8, 1993; 64 FR 401, Jan. 5, 1999; 73 FR 39609, July 10, 2008; 74 FR 2861, Jan. 16, 2009]

Sec. 314.97 Supplements and other changes to an approved abbreviated application.

The applicant shall comply with the requirements of 314.70 and 314.71 regarding the submission of supplemental applications and other changes to an approved abbreviated application.

Sec. 314.98 Postmarketing reports.

(a) Except as provided in paragraph (b) of this section, each applicant having an approved abbreviated new drug application under 314.94 that is effective shall comply with the requirements of 314.80 regarding the reporting and recordkeeping of adverse drug experiences.

(b) Each applicant shall submit one copy of each report required under 314.80 to the Central Document Room, Center for Drug Evaluation and Research, Food and Drug Administration, 5901-B Ammendale Rd., Beltsville, MD 20705-1266.

(c) Each applicant shall make the reports required under 314.81 and section 505(k) of the act for each of its approved abbreviated applications.

[57 FR 17983, Apr. 28, 1992, as amended at 64 FR 401, Jan. 5, 1999; 74 FR 13113, Mar. 26, 2009]

Sec. 314.99 Other responsibilities of an applicant of an abbreviated application.

(a) An applicant shall comply with the requirements of 314.65 regarding withdrawal by the applicant of an unapproved abbreviated application and 314.72 regarding a change in ownership of an abbreviated application.

(b) An applicant may ask FDA to waive under this section any requirement that applies to the applicant under 314.92 through 314.99. The applicant shall comply with the requirements for a waiver under 314.90.

Subpart D--FDA Action on Applications and Abbreviated Applications

Sec. 314.100 Timeframes for reviewing applications and abbreviated applications.

(a) Except as provided in paragraph (c) of this section, within 180 days of receipt of an application for a new drug under section 505(b) of the act or an abbreviated application for a new drug under section 505(j) of the act, FDA will review it and send the applicant either an approval letter under 314.105 or a complete response letter under 314.110. This 180-day period is called the "initial review cycle."

(b) At any time before approval, an applicant may withdraw an application under 314.65 or an abbreviated application under 314.99 and later submit it again for consideration.

(c) The initial review cycle may be adjusted by mutual agreement between FDA and an applicant or as provided in 314.60 and 314.96, as the result of a major amendment.

[73 FR 39609, July 10, 2008]

Sec. 314.101 Filing an application and receiving an abbreviated new drug application.

(a)(1) Within 60 days after FDA receives an application, the agency will determine whether the application may be filed. The filing of an application means that FDA has made a threshold determination that the application is sufficiently complete to permit a substantive review.

(2) If FDA finds that none of the reasons in paragraphs (d) and (e) of this section for refusing to file the application apply, the agency will file the application and notify the applicant in writing. The date of filing will be the date 60 days after the date FDA received the application. The date of filing begins the 180-day period described in section 505(c) of the act. This 180-day period is called the "filing clock."

(3) If FDA refuses to file the application, the agency will notify the applicant in writing and state the reason under paragraph (d) or (e) of this section for the refusal. If FDA refuses to file

the application under paragraph (d) of this section, the applicant may request in writing within 30 days of the date of the agency's notification an informal conference with the agency about whether the agency should file the application. If, following the informal conference, the applicant requests that FDA file the application (with or without amendments to correct the deficiencies), the agency will file the application over protest under paragraph (a)(2) of this section, notify the applicant in writing, and review it as filed. If the application is filed over protest, the date of filing will be the date 60 days after the date the applicant requested the informal conference. The applicant need not resubmit a copy of an application that is filed over protest. If FDA refuses to file the application under paragraph (e) of this section, the applicant may amend the application and resubmit it, and the agency will make a determination under this section whether it may be filed.

(b)(1) An abbreviated new drug application will be reviewed after it is submitted to determine whether the abbreviated application may be received. Receipt of an abbreviated new drug application means that FDA has made a threshold determination that the abbreviated application is sufficiently complete to permit a substantive review.

(2) If FDA finds that none of the reasons in paragraphs (d) and (e) of this section for considering the abbreviated new drug application not to have been received applies, the agency will receive the abbreviated new drug application and notify the applicant in writing.

(3) If FDA considers the abbreviated new drug application not to have been received under paragraph (d) or (e) of this section, FDA will notify the applicant, ordinarily by telephone. The applicant may then:

(i) Withdraw the abbreviated new drug application under 314.99; or

(ii) Amend the abbreviated new drug application to correct the deficiencies; or

(iii) Take no action, in which case FDA will refuse to receive the abbreviated new drug application.

(c) [Reserved]

(d) FDA may refuse to file an application or may not consider an abbreviated new drug application to be received if any of the following applies:

(1) The application does not contain a completed application form.

(2) The application is not submitted in the form required under 314.50 or 314.94.

(3) The application or abbreviated application is incomplete because it does not on its face contain information required under section 505(b), section 505(j), or section 507 of the act and 314.50 or 314.94.

(4) The applicant fails to submit a complete environmental assessment, which addresses each of the items specified in the applicable format under 25.40 of this chapter or fails to provide sufficient information to establish that the requested action is subject to categorical exclusion under 25.30 or 25.31 of this chapter.

(5) The application or abbreviated application does not contain an accurate and complete English translation of each part of the application that is not in English.

(6) The application does not contain a statement for each nonclinical laboratory study that it was conducted in compliance with the requirements set forth in part 58 of this chapter, or, for each study not conducted in compliance with part 58 of this chapter, a brief statement of the reason for the noncompliance.

(7) The application does not contain a statement for each clinical study that it was conducted in compliance with the institutional review board regulations in part 56 of this chapter, or was not subject to those regulations, and that it was conducted in compliance with the informed consent regulations in part 50 of this chapter, or, if the study was subject to but was not conducted in compliance with those regulations, the application does not contain a brief statement of the reason for the noncompliance.

(8) The drug product that is the subject of the submission is already covered by an approved application or abbreviated application and the applicant of the submission:

(i) Has an approved application or abbreviated application for the same drug product; or

(ii) Is merely a distributor and/or repackager of the already approved drug product.

(9) The application is submitted as a 505(b)(2) application for a drug that is a duplicate of a listed drug and is eligible for approval under section 505(j) of the act.

(e) The agency will refuse to file an application or will consider an abbreviated new drug application not to have been received if any of the following applies:

(1) The drug product is subject to licensing by FDA under the Public Health Service Act (42 U.S.C. 201et seq.) and subchapter F of this chapter.

(2) In the case of a 505(b)(2) application or an abbreviated new drug application, the drug product contains the same active moiety as a drug that:

(i) Was approved after September 24, 1984, in an application under section 505(b) of the act, and

(ii) Is entitled to a 5-year period of exclusivity under section 505(c)(3)(D)(ii) and (j)(4)(D)(ii) of the act and 314.108(b)(2), unless the 5-year exclusivity period has elapsed or unless 4 years of the 5-year period have elapsed and the application or abbreviated application contains a certification of patent invalidity or noninfringement described in 314.50(i)(1)(i)(A)(4) or 314.94(a)(12)(i)(A)(4).

(f)(1) Within 180 days after the date of filing, plus the period of time the review period was extended (if any), FDA will either:

(i) Approve the application; or

(ii) Issue a notice of opportunity for a hearing if the applicant asked FDA to provide it an opportunity for a hearing on an application in response to a complete response letter.

(2) Within 180 days after the date of receipt, plus the period of time the review clock was extended (if any), FDA will either approve or disapprove the abbreviated new drug application. If FDA disapproves the abbreviated new drug application, FDA will issue a notice of opportunity for hearing if the

applicant asked FDA to provide it an opportunity for a hearing on an abbreviated new drug application in response to a complete response letter.

(3) This paragraph does not apply to applications or abbreviated applications that have been withdrawn from FDA review by the applicant.

[57 FR 17987, Apr. 28, 1992; 57 FR 29353, July 1, 1992, as amended at 59 FR 50366, Oct. 3, 1994; 62 FR 40599, July 29, 1997; 64 FR 402, Jan. 5, 1999; 73 FR 39609, July 10, 2008]

Sec. 314.102 Communications between FDA and applicants.

(a) General principles. During the course of reviewing an application or an abbreviated application, FDA shall communicate with applicants about scientific, medical, and procedural issues that arise during the review process. Such communication may take the form of telephone conversations, letters, or meetings, whichever is most appropriate to discuss the particular issue at hand. Communications shall be appropriately documented in the application in accordance with 10.65 of this chapter. Further details on the procedures for communication between FDA and applicants are contained in a staff manual guide that is publicly available.

(b) Notification of easily correctable deficiencies. FDA reviewers shall make every reasonable effort to communicate promptly to applicants easily correctable deficiencies found in an application or an abbreviated application when those deficiencies are discovered, particularly deficiencies concerning chemistry, manufacturing, and controls issues. The agency will also inform applicants promptly of its need for more data or information or for technical changes in the application or the abbreviated application needed to facilitate the agency's review. This early communication is intended to permit applicants to correct such readily identified deficiencies relatively early in the review process and to submit an amendment before the review period has elapsed. Such early communication would not ordinarily apply to major scientific issues, which require consideration of the entire pending application or abbreviated application by agency managers as well as reviewing staff. Instead, major scientific issues will ordinarily be addressed in a complete response letter.

(c) Ninety-day conference. Approximately 90 days after the agency receives the application, FDA will provide applicants with an opportunity to meet with agency reviewing officials. The purpose of the meeting will be to inform applicants of the general progress and status of their applications, and to advise applicants of deficiencies that have been identified by that time and that have not already been communicated. This meeting will be available on applications for all new chemical entities and major new indications of marketed drugs. Such meetings will be held at the applicant's option, and may be held by telephone if mutually agreed upon. Such meetings would not ordinarily be held on abbreviated applications because they are not submitted for new chemical entities or new indications.

(d) End-of-review conference. At the conclusion of FDA's review of an NDA as designated by the issuance of a complete response letter, FDA will provide the applicant with an opportunity to meet with agency reviewing officials. The purpose of the meeting will be to discuss what further steps need to be taken by the applicant before the application can be approved. Requests for such meetings must be directed to the director of the division responsible for reviewing the application.

(e) Other meetings. Other meetings between FDA and applicants may be held, with advance notice, to discuss scientific, medical, and other issues that arise during the review process. Requests for meetings shall be directed to the director of the division responsible for reviewing the application or abbreviated application. FDA will make every attempt to grant requests for meetings that involve important issues and that can be scheduled at mutually convenient times. However, "drop-in" visits (i.e. , an unannounced and unscheduled visit by a company representative) are discouraged except for urgent matters, such as to discuss an important new safety issue.

[57 FR 17988, Apr. 28, 1992; 57 FR 29353, July 1, 1992, as amended at 73 FR 39609, July 10, 2008]

Sec. 314.103 Dispute resolution.

(a) General. FDA is committed to resolving differences between applicants and FDA reviewing divisions with respect to technical requirements for applications or abbreviated applications as quickly and amicably as possible through the cooperative exchange of information and views.

(b) Administrative and procedural issues. When administrative or procedural disputes arise, the applicant should first attempt to resolve the matter with the division responsible for reviewing the application or abbreviated application, beginning with the consumer safety officer assigned to the application or abbreviated application. If resolution is not achieved, the applicant may raise the matter with the person designated as ombudsman, whose function shall be to investigate what has happened and to facilitate a timely and equitable resolution. Appropriate issues to raise with the ombudsman include resolving difficulties in scheduling meetings, obtaining timely replies to inquiries, and obtaining timely completion of pending reviews. Further details on this procedure are contained in a staff manual guide that is publicly available under FDA's public information regulations in part 20.

(c) Scientific and medical disputes.

(1) Because major scientific issues are ordinarily communicated to applicants in a complete response letter pursuant to 314.110, the "end-of-review conference" described in 314.102(d) will provide a timely forum for discussing and resolving, if possible, scientific and medical issues on which the applicant disagrees with the agency. In addition, the "ninety-day conference" described in 314.102(c) will provide a timely forum for discussing and resolving, if possible, issues identified by that date.

(2) When scientific or medical disputes arise at other times during the review process, applicants should discuss the matter directly with the responsible reviewing officials. If necessary, applicants may request a meeting with the appropriate reviewing officials and management representatives in order to seek a resolution. Ordinarily, such meetings would be held first with the Division Director, then with the Office Director, and finally with the Center Director if the matter is still unresolved. Requests for such meetings shall be directed to the director of the division responsible for reviewing the application or abrreviated application. FDA will make every attempt to grant requests for meetings that involve important issues and that can be scheduled at mutually convenient times.

Part 314

(3) In requesting a meeting designed to resolve a scientific or medical dispute, applicants may suggest that FDA seek the advice of outside experts, in which case FDA may, in its discretion, invite to the meeting one or more of its advisory committee members or other consultants, as designated by the agency. Applicants may also bring their own consultants. For major scientific and medical policy issues not resolved by informal meetings, FDA may refer the matter to one of its standing advisory committees for its consideration and recommendations.

[50 FR 7493, Feb. 22, 1985; 50 FR 14212, Apr. 11, 1985, as amended at 57 FR 17989, Apr. 28, 1992; 73 FR 39609, July 10, 2008]

Sec. 314.104 Drugs with potential for abuse.

The Food and Drug Administration will inform the Drug Enforcement Administration under section 201(f) of the Controlled Substances Act (21 U.S.C. 801) when an application or abbreviated application is submitted for a drug that appears to have an abuse potential.

[57 FR 17989, Apr. 28, 1992]

Sec. 314.105 Approval of an application and an abbreviated application.

(a) The Food and Drug Administration will approve an application and send the applicant an approval letter if none of the reasons in 314.125 for refusing to approve the application applies. An approval becomes effective on the date of the issuance of the approval letter, except with regard to an approval under section 505(b)(2) of the act with a delayed effective date. An approval with a delayed effective date is tentative and does not become final until the effective date. A new drug product or antibiotic approved under this paragraph may not be marketed until an approval is effective.

(b) FDA will approve an application and issue the applicant an approval letter on the basis of draft labeling if the only deficiencies in the application concern editorial or similar minor deficiencies in the draft labeling. Such approval will be conditioned upon the applicant incorporating the specified labeling changes exactly as directed, and upon the applicant submitting to FDA a copy of the final printed labeling prior to marketing.

(c) FDA will approve an application after it determines that the drug meets the statutory standards for safety and effectiveness, manufacturing and controls, and labeling, and an abbreviated application after it determines that the drug meets the statutory standards for manufacturing and controls, labeling, and, where applicable, bioequivalence. While the statutory standards apply to all drugs, the many kinds of drugs that are subject to the statutory standards and the wide range of uses for those drugs demand flexibility in applying the standards. Thus FDA is required to exercise its scientific judgment to determine the kind and quantity of data and information an applicant is required to provide for a particular drug to meet the statutory standards. FDA makes its views on drug products and classes of drugs available through guidance documents, recommendations, and other statements of policy.

(d) FDA will approve an abbreviated new drug application and send the applicant an approval letter if none of the reasons in 314.127 for refusing to approve the abbreviated new drug application applies. The approval becomes effective on the date of the issuance of the agency's approval letter unless the approval letter provides for a delayed effective date. An approval with a delayed effective date is tentative and does not become final until the effective date. A new drug product approved under this paragraph may not be introduced or delivered for introduction into interstate commerce until approval of the abbreviated new drug application is effective. Ordinarily, the effective date of approval will be stated in the approval letter.

[57 FR 17989, Apr. 28, 1992, as amended at 64 FR 402, Jan. 5, 1999; 65 FR 56479, Sept. 19, 2000; 73 FR 39609, July 10, 2008]

Sec. 314.106 Foreign data.

(a) General. The acceptance of foreign data in an application generally is governed by 312.120 of this chapter.

(b) As sole basis for marketing approval. An application based solely on foreign clinical data meeting U.S. criteria for marketing approval may be approved if: (1) The foreign data are applicable to the U.S. population and U.S. medical practice; (2) the studies have been performed by clinical investigators of recognized competence; and (3) the data may be considered valid without the need for an on-site inspection by FDA or, if FDA considers such an inspection to be necessary, FDA is able to validate the data through an on-site inspection or other appropriate means. Failure of an application to meet any of these criteria will result in the application not being approvable based on the foreign data alone. FDA will apply this policy in a flexible manner according to the nature of the drug and the data being considered.

(c) Consultation between FDA and applicants. Applicants are encouraged to meet with agency officials in a "presubmission" meeting when approval based solely on foreign data will be sought.

[50 FR 7493, Feb. 22, 1985, as amended at 55 FR 11580, Mar. 29, 1990]

Sec. 314.107 Effective date of approval of a 505(b)(2) application or abbreviated new drug application under section 505(j) of the act.

(a) General. A drug product may be introduced or delivered for introduction into interstate commerce when approval of the application or abbreviated application for the drug product becomes effective. Except as provided in this section, approval of an application or abbreviated application for a drug product becomes effective on the date FDA issues an approval letter under 314.105 for the application or abbreviated application.

(b) Effect of patent on the listed drug. If approval of an abbreviated new drug application submitted under section 505(j) of the act or of a 505(b)(2) application is granted, that approval will become effective in accordance with the following:

(1) Date of approval letter. Except as provided in paragraphs (b)(3), (b)(4), and (c) of this section, approval will become effective on the date FDA issues an approval letter under 314.105 if the applicant certifies under 314.50(i) or 314.94(a)(12) that:

(i) There are no relevant patents; or

(ii) The applicant is aware of a relevant patent but the patent information required under section 505 (b) or (c) of the act has not been submitted to FDA; or

(iii) The relevant patent has expired; or

(iv) The relevant patent is invalid, unenforceable, or will not be infringed.

(2) Patent expiration. If the applicant certifies under 314.50(i) or 314.94(a)(12) that the relevant patent will expire on a specified date, approval will become effective on the specified date.

(3) Disposition of patent litigation.

(i)(A) Except as provided in paragraphs (b)(3)(ii), (b)(3)(iii), and (b)(3)(iv) of this section, if the applicant certifies under 314.50(i) or 314.94(a)(12) that the relevant patent is invalid, unenforceable, or will not be infringed, and the patent owner or its representative or the exclusive patent licensee brings suit for patent infringement within 45 days of receipt by the patent owner of the notice of certification from the applicant under 314.52 or 314.95, approval may be made effective 30 months after the date of the receipt of the notice of certification by the patent owner or by the exclusive licensee (or their representatives) unless the court has extended or reduced the period because of a failure of either the plaintiff or defendant to cooperate reasonably in expediting the action; or

(B) If the patented drug product qualifies for 5 years of exclusive marketing under 314.108(b)(2) and the patent owner or its representative or the exclusive patent licensee brings suit for patent infringement during the 1-year period beginning 4 years after the date the patented drug was approved and within 45 days of receipt by the patent owner of the notice of certification, the approval may be made effective at the expiration of the 71/2years from the date of approval of the application for the patented drug product.

(ii) If before the expiration of the 30-month period, or 71/2years where applicable, the court issues a final order that the patent is invalid, unenforceable, or not infringed, approval may be made effective on the date the court enters judgment;

(iii) If before the expiration of the 30-month period, or 71/2years where applicable, the court issues a final order or judgment that the patent has been infringed, approval may be made effective on the date the court determines that the patent will expire or otherwise orders; or

(iv) If before the expiration of the 30-month period, or 71/2years where applicable, the court grants a preliminary injunction prohibiting the applicant from engaging in the commercial manufacture or sale of the drug product until the court decides the issues of patent validity and infringement, and if the court later decides that the patent is invalid, unenforceable, or not infringed, approval may be made effective on the date the court enters a final order or judgment that the patent is invalid, unenforceable, or not infringed.

(v) FDA will issue a tentative approval letter when tentative approval is appropriate in accordance with paragraph (b)(3) of this section. In order for an approval to be made effective under paragraph (b)(3) of this section, the applicant must receive an approval letter from the agency indicating that the application has received final approval. Tentative approval of an application does not constitute "approval" of an application and cannot, absent a final approval letter from the agency, result in an effective approval under paragraph (b)(3) of this section.

(4) Multiple certifications. If the applicant has submitted certifications under 314.50(i) or 314.94(a)(12) for more than one patent, the date of approval will be calculated for each certification, and the approval will become effective on the last applicable date.

(c) Subsequent abbreviated new drug application submission.

(1) If an abbreviated new drug application contains a certification that a relevant patent is invalid, unenforceable, or will not be infringed and the application is for a generic copy of the same listed drug for which one or more substantially complete abbreviated new drug applications were previously submitted containing a certification that the same patent was invalid, unenforceable, or would not be infringed, approval of the subsequent abbreviated new drug application will be made effective no sooner than 180 days from whichever of the following dates is earlier:

(i) The date the applicant submitting the first application first commences commercial marketing of its drug product; or

(ii) The date of a decision of the court holding the relevant patent invalid, unenforceable, or not infringed.

(2) For purposes of paragraph (c)(1) of this section, the "applicant submitting the first application" is the applicant that submits an application that is both substantially complete and contains a certification that the patent was invalid, unenforceable, or not infringed prior to the submission of any other application for the same listed drug that is both substantially complete and contains the same certification. A "substantially complete" application must contain the results of any required bioequivalence studies, or, if applicable, a request for a waiver of such studies.

(3) For purposes of paragraph (c)(1) of this section, if FDA concludes that the applicant submitting the first application is not actively pursuing approval of its abbreviated application, FDA will make the approval of subsequent abbreviated applications immediately effective if they are otherwise eligible for an immediately effective approval.

(4) For purposes of paragraph (c)(1)(i) of this section, the applicant submitting the first application shall notify FDA of the date that it commences commercial marketing of its drug product. Commercial marketing commences with the first date of introduction or delivery for introduction into interstate commerce outside the control of the manufacturer of a drug product, except for investigational use under part 312 of this chapter, but does not include transfer of the drug product for reasons other than sale within the control of the manufacturer or application holder. If an applicant does not promptly notify FDA of such date, the effective date of approval shall be deemed to be the date of the commencement of first commercial marketing.

(d) *Delay due to exclusivity.* The agency will also delay the effective date of the approval of an abbreviated new drug application under section 505(j) of the act or a 505(b)(2) application if delay is required by the exclusivity provisions in 314.108. When the effective date of an application is delayed under both this section and 314.108, the effective date will be the later of the 2 days specified under this section and 314.108.

Part 314

(e) Notification of court actions. The applicant shall submit a copy of the entry of the order or judgment to the Office of Generic Drugs (HFD-600), or to the appropriate division in the Office of New Drugs within 10 working days of a final judgment.

(f) Computation of 45-day time clock.

(1) The 45-day clock described in paragraph (b)(3) of this section begins on the day after the date of receipt of the applicant's notice of certification by the patent owner or its representative, and by the approved application holder. When the 45th day falls on Saturday, Sunday, or a Federal holiday, the 45th day will be the next day that is not a Saturday, Sunday, or a Federal holiday.

(2) The abbreviated new drug applicant or the 505(b)(2) applicant shall notify FDA immediately of the filing of any legal action filed within 45 days of receipt of the notice of certification. If the applicant submitting the abbreviated new drug application or the 505(b)(2) application or patent owner or its representative does not notify FDA in writing before the expiration of the 45-day time period or the completion of the agency's review of the application, whichever occurs later, that a legal action for patent infringement was filed within 45 days of receipt of the notice of certification, approval of the abbreviated new drug application or the 505(b)(2) application will be made effective immediately upon expiration of the 45 days or upon completion of the agency's review and approval of the application, whichever is later. The notification to FDA of the legal action shall include:

(i) The abbreviated new drug application or 505(b)(2) application number.

(ii) The name of the abbreviated new drug or 505(b)(2) application applicant.

(iii) The established name of the drug product or, if no established name exists, the name(s) of the active ingredient(s), the drug product's strength, and dosage form.

(iv) A certification that an action for patent infringement identified by number, has been filed in an appropriate court on a specified date.

The applicant of an abbreviated new drug application shall send the notification to FDA's Office of Generic Drugs (HFD-600). A 505(b)(2) applicant shall send the notification to the appropriate division in the Office of New Drugs reviewing the application. A patent owner or its representative may also notify FDA of the filing of any legal action for patent infringement. The notice should contain the information and be sent to the offices or divisions described in this paragraph.

(3) If the patent owner or approved application holder who is an exclusive patent licensee waives its opportunity to file a legal action for patent infringement within 45 days of a receipt of the notice of certification and the patent owner or approved application holder who is an exclusive patent licensee submits to FDA a valid waiver before the 45 days elapse, approval of the abbreviated new drug application or the 505(b)(2) application will be made effective upon completion of the agency's review and approval of the application. FDA will only accept a waiver in the following form:

(Name of patent owner or exclusive patent licensee) has received notice from (name of applicant) under (section 505(b)(3) or 505(j)(2)(B) of the act) and does not intend to file an action for patent infringement against (name of applicant) concerning the drug (name of drug) before (date on which 45 days elapses. (Name of patent owner or exclusive patent licensee) waives the opportunity provided by (section 505(c)(3)(C) or 505(j)(B)(iii) of the act) and does not object to FDA's approval of (name of applicant)'s (505(b)(2) or abbreviated new drug application) for (name of drug) with an immediate effective date on or after the date of this letter.

[59 FR 50367, Oct. 3, 1994, as amended at 63 FR 59712, Nov. 5, 1998; 65 FR 43235, July 13, 2000; 73 FR 39609, July 10, 2008; 74 FR 9766, Mar. 6, 2009]

Sec. 314.108 New drug product exclusivity.

(a) Definitions. The following definitions of terms apply to this section:

Active moiety means the molecule or ion, excluding those appended portions of the molecule that cause the drug to be an ester, salt (including a salt with hydrogen or coordination bonds), or other noncovalent derivative (such as a complex,

Part 314

chelate, or clathrate) of the molecule, responsible for the physiological or pharmacological action of the drug substance.

Approved under section 505(b) means an application submitted under section 505(b) and approved on or after October 10, 1962, or an application that was "deemed approved" under section 107(c)(2) of Pub. L. 87-781.

Clinical investigation means any experiment other than a bioavailability study in which a drug is administered or dispensed to, or used on, human subjects.

Conducted or sponsored by the applicant with regard to an investigation means that before or during the investigation, the applicant was named in Form FDA-1571 filed with FDA as the sponsor of the investigational new drug application under which the investigation was conducted, or the applicant or the applicant's predecessor in interest, provided substantial support for the investigation. To demonstrate "substantial support," an applicant must either provide a certified statement from a certified public accountant that the applicant provided 50 percent or more of the cost of conducting the study or provide an explanation why FDA should consider the applicant to have conducted or sponsored the study if the applicant's financial contribution to the study is less than 50 percent or the applicant did not sponsor the investigational new drug. A predecessor in interest is an entity, e.g., a corporation, that the applicant has taken over, merged with, or purchased, or from which the applicant has purchased all rights to the drug. Purchase of nonexclusive rights to a clinical investigation after it is completed is not sufficient to satisfy this definition.

Date of approval means the date on the letter from FDA stating that the new drug application is approved, whether or not final printed labeling or other materials must yet be submitted as long as approval of such labeling or materials is not expressly required. "Date of approval" refers only to a final approval and not to a tentative approval that may become effective at a later date.

Essential to approval means, with regard to an investigation, that there are no other data available that could support approval of the application.

FDA means the Food and Drug Administration.

New chemical entity means a drug that contains no active moiety that has been approved by FDA in any other application submitted under section 505(b) of the act.

New clinical investigation means an investigation in humans the results of which have not been relied on by FDA to demonstrate substantial evidence of effectiveness of a previously approved drug product for any indication or of safety for a new patient population and do not duplicate the results of another investigation that was relied on by the agency to demonstrate the effectiveness or safety in a new patient population of a previously approved drug product. For purposes of this section, data from a clinical investigation previously submitted for use in the comprehensive evaluation of the safety of a drug product but not to support the effectiveness of the drug product would be considered new.

(b) Submission of and effective date of approval of an abbreviated new drug application submitted under section 505(j) of the act or a 505(b)(2) application. (1) [Reserved]

   (2) If a drug product that contains a new chemical entity was approved after September 24, 1984, in an application submitted under section 505(b) of the act, no person may submit a 505(b)(2) application or abbreviated new drug application under section 505(j) of the act for a drug product that contains the same active moiety as in the new chemical entity for a period of 5 years from the date of approval of the first approved new drug application, except that the 505(b)(2) application or abbreviated application may be submitted after 4 years if it contains a certification of patent invalidity or noninfringement described in 314.50(i)(1)(i)(A)(4) or 314.94(a)(12)(i)(A)(4).

   (3) The approval of a 505(b)(2) application or abbreviated application described in paragraph (b)(2) of this section will become effective as provided in 314.107(b)(1) or (b)(2), unless the owner of a patent that claims the drug, the patent owner's representative, or exclusive licensee brings suit for patent infringement against the applicant during the 1-year period beginning 48 months after the date of approval of the new drug application for the new chemical entity and within 45 days after receipt of the notice described at 314.52 or 314.95, in which case, approval of the 505(b)(2) application or

Part 314

abbreviated application will be made effective as provided in
314.107(b)(3).

(4) If an application:

    (i) Was submitted under section 505(b) of the act;

    (ii) Was approved after September 24, 1984;

    (iii) Was for a drug product that contains an active moiety
that has been previously approved in another application
under section 505(b) of the act; and

    (iv) Contained reports of new clinical investigations (other
than bioavailability studies) conducted or sponsored by
the applicant that were essential to approval of the
application, the agency will not make effective for a
period of 3 years after the date of approval of the
application the approval of a 505(b)(2) application or an
abbreviated new drug application for the conditions of
approval of the original application, or an abbreviated
new drug application submitted pursuant to an approved
petition under section 505(j)(2)(C) of the act that relies on
the information supporting the conditions of approval of
an original new drug application.

(5) If a supplemental application:

    (i) Was approved after September 24, 1984; and

    (ii) Contained reports of new clinical investigations (other
than bioavailability studies) that were conducted or
sponsored by the applicant that were essential to approval
of the supplemental application, the agency will not make
effective for a period of 3 years after the date of approval
of the supplemental application the approval of a
505(b)(2) application or an abbreviated new drug
application for a change, or an abbreviated new drug
application submitted pursuant to an approved petition
under section 505(j)(2)(C) of the act that relies on the
information supporting a change approved in the
supplemental new drug application.

[59 FR 50368, Oct. 3, 1994]

Sec. 314.110 Complete response letter to the applicant.

(a) Complete response letter. FDA will send the applicant a complete response letter if the agency determines that we will not approve the application or abbreviated application in its present form for one or more of the reasons given in 314.125 or 314.127, respectively.

  (1) Description of specific deficiencies. A complete response letter will describe all of the specific deficiencies that the agency has identified in an application or abbreviated application, except as stated in paragraph (a)(3) of this section.

  (2) Complete review of data. A complete response letter reflects FDA's complete review of the data submitted in an original application or abbreviated application (or, where appropriate, a resubmission) and any amendments that the agency has reviewed. The complete response letter will identify any amendments that the agency has not yet reviewed.

  (3) Inadequate data. If FDA determines, after an application is filed or an abbreviated application is received, that the data submitted are inadequate to support approval, the agency might issue a complete response letter without first conducting required inspections and/or reviewing proposed product labeling.

  (4) Recommendation of actions for approval. When possible, a complete response letter will recommend actions that the applicant might take to place the application or abbreviated application in condition for approval.

(b) Applicant actions. After receiving a complete response letter, the applicant must take one of following actions:

  (1) Resubmission. Resubmit the application or abbreviated application, addressing all deficiencies identified in the complete response letter.

    (i) A resubmission of an application or efficacy supplement that FDA classifies as a Class 1 resubmission constitutes an agreement by the applicant to start a new 2-month review cycle beginning on the date FDA receives the resubmission.

Part 314

(ii) A resubmission of an application or efficacy supplement that FDA classifies as a Class 2 resubmission constitutes an agreement by the applicant to start a new 6-month review cycle beginning on the date FDA receives the resubmission.

(iii) A resubmission of an NDA supplement other than an efficacy supplement constitutes an agreement by the applicant to start a new review cycle the same length as the initial review cycle for the supplement (excluding any extension due to a major amendment of the initial supplement), beginning on the date FDA receives the resubmission.

(iv) A major resubmission of an abbreviated application constitutes an agreement by the applicant to start a new 6-month review cycle beginning on the date FDA receives the resubmission.

(v) A minor resubmission of an abbreviated application constitutes an agreement by the applicant to start a new review cycle beginning on the date FDA receives the resubmission.

(2) Withdrawal. Withdraw the application or abbreviated application. A decision to withdraw an application or abbreviated application is without prejudice to a subsequent submission.

(3) Request opportunity for hearing. Ask the agency to provide the applicant an opportunity for a hearing on the question of whether there are grounds for denying approval of the application or abbreviated application under section 505(d) or (j)(4) of the act, respectively. The applicant must submit the request to the Associate Director for Policy, Center for Drug Evaluation and Research, Food and Drug Administration, 10903 New Hampshire Ave., Silver Spring, MD 20993. Within 60 days of the date of the request for an opportunity for a hearing, or within a different time period to which FDA and the applicant agree, the agency will either approve the application or abbreviated application under 314.105, or refuse to approve the application under 314.125 or abbreviated application under 314.127 and give the applicant written notice of an opportunity for a hearing under 314.200 and section 505(c)(1)(B) or (j)(5)(c) of the act on the question of whether there are grounds for denying approval of the

application or abbreviated application under section 505(d) or (j)(4) of the act, respectively.

(c) Failure to take action.

(1) An applicant agrees to extend the review period under section 505(c)(1) or (j)(5)(A) of the act until it takes any of the actions listed in paragraph (b) of this section. For an application or abbreviated application, FDA may consider an applicant's failure to take any of such actions within 1 year after issuance of a complete response letter to be a request by the applicant to withdraw the application, unless the applicant has requested an extension of time in which to resubmit the application. FDA will grant any reasonable request for such an extension. FDA may consider an applicant's failure to resubmit the application within the extended time period or to request an additional extension to be a request by the applicant to withdraw the application.

(2) If FDA considers an applicant's failure to take action in accordance with paragraph (c)(1) of this section to be a request to withdraw the application, the agency will notify the applicant in writing. The applicant will have 30 days from the date of the notification to explain why the application should not be withdrawn and to request an extension of time in which to resubmit the application. FDA will grant any reasonable request for an extension. If the applicant does not respond to the notification within 30 days, the application will be deemed to be withdrawn.

[73 FR 39609, July 10, 2008]

Sec. 314.120 [Reserved]

Sec. 314.122 Submitting an abbreviated application for, or a 505(j)(2)(C) petition that relies on, a listed drug that is no longer marketed.

(a) An abbreviated new drug application that refers to, or a petition under section 505(j)(2)(C) of the act and 314.93 that relies on, a listed drug that has been voluntarily withdrawn from sale in the United States must be accompanied by a petition seeking a determination whether the listed drug was withdrawn for safety or effectiveness reasons. The petition must be submitted under 10.25(a) and 10.30 of this chapter and must contain all evidence

Part 314

available to the petitioner concerning the reasons for the withdrawal from sale.

(b) When a petition described in paragraph (a) of this section is submitted, the agency will consider the evidence in the petition and any other evidence before the agency, and determine whether the listed drug is withdrawn from sale for safety or effectiveness reasons, in accordance with the procedures in 314.161.

(c) An abbreviated new drug application described in paragraph (a) of this section will be disapproved, under 314.127(a)(11), and a 505(j)(2)(C) petition described in paragraph (a) of this section will be disapproved, under 314.93(e)(1)(iv), unless the agency determines that the withdrawal of the listed drug was not for safety or effectiveness reasons.

(d) Certain drug products approved for safety and effectiveness that were no longer marketed on September 24, 1984, are not included in the list. Any person who wishes to obtain marketing approval for such a drug product under an abbreviated new drug application must petition FDA for a determination whether the drug product was withdrawn from the market for safety or effectiveness reasons and request that the list be amended to include the drug product. A person seeking such a determination shall use the petition procedures established in 10.30 of this chapter. The petitioner shall include in the petition information to show that the drug product was approved for safety and effectiveness and all evidence available to the petitioner concerning the reason that marketing of the drug product ceased.

[57 FR 17990, Apr. 28, 1992; 57 FR 29353, July 1, 1992]

Sec. 314.125 Refusal to approve an application.

(a) The Food and Drug Administration will refuse to approve the application and for a new drug give the applicant written notice of an opportunity for a hearing under 314.200 on the question of whether there are grounds for denying approval of the application under section 505(d) of the act, if:

(1) FDA sends the applicant a complete response letter under 314.110;

(2) The applicant requests an opportunity for hearing for a new drug on the question of whether the application is approvable; and

(3) FDA finds that any of the reasons given in paragraph (b) of this section apply.

(b) FDA may refuse to approve an application for any of the following reasons:

(1) The methods to be used in, and the facilities and controls used for, the manufacture, processing, packing, or holding of the drug substance or the drug product are inadequate to preserve its identity, strength, quality, purity, stability, and bioavailability.

(2) The investigations required under section 505(b) of the act do not include adequate tests by all methods reasonably applicable to show whether or not the drug is safe for use under the conditions prescribed, recommended, or suggested in its proposed labeling.

(3) The results of the tests show that the drug is unsafe for use under the conditions prescribed, recommended, or suggested in its proposed labeling or the results do not show that the drug product is safe for use under those conditions.

(4) There is insufficient information about the drug to determine whether the product is safe for use under the conditions prescribed, recommended, or suggested in its proposed labeling.

(5) There is a lack of substantial evidence consisting of adequate and well-controlled investigations, as defined in 314.126, that the drug product will have the effect it purports or is represented to have under the conditions of use prescribed, recommended, or suggested in its proposed labeling.

(6) The proposed labeling is false or misleading in any particular.

(7) The application contains an untrue statement of a material fact.

(8) The drug product's proposed labeling does not comply with the requirements for labels and labeling in part 201.

(9) The application does not contain bioavailability or bioequivalence data required under part 320 of this chapter.

Part 314

(10) A reason given in a letter refusing to file the application under 314.101(d), if the deficiency is not corrected.

(11) The drug will be manufactured or processed in whole or in part in an establishment that is not registered and not exempt from registration under section 510 of the act and part 207.

(12) The applicant does not permit a properly authorized officer or employee of the Department of Health and Human Services an adequate opportunity to inspect the facilities, controls, and any records relevant to the application.

(13) The methods to be used in, and the facilities and controls used for, the manufacture, processing, packing, or holding of the drug substance or the drug product do not comply with the current good manufacturing practice regulations in parts 210 and 211.

(14) The application does not contain an explanation of the omission of a report of any investigation of the drug product sponsored by the applicant, or an explanation of the omission of other information about the drug pertinent to an evaluation of the application that is received or otherwise obtained by the applicant from any source.

(15) A nonclinical laboratory study that is described in the application and that is essential to show that the drug is safe for use under the conditions prescribed, recommended, or suggested in its proposed labeling was not conducted in compliance with the good laboratory practice regulations in part 58 of this chapter and no reason for the noncompliance is provided or, if it is, the differences between the practices used in conducting the study and the good laboratory practice regulations do not support the validity of the study.

(16) Any clinical investigation involving human subjects described in the application, subject to the institutional review board regulations in part 56 of this chapter or informed consent regulations in part 50 of this chapter, was not conducted in compliance with those regulations such that the rights or safety of human subjects were not adequately protected.

(17) The applicant or contract research organization that conducted a bioavailability or bioequivalence study described in 320.38 or 320.63 of this chapter that is contained in the application refuses to permit an inspection of facilities or records relevant to the study by a properly authorized officer

or employee of the Department of Health and Human Services or refuses to submit reserve samples of the drug products used in the study when requested by FDA.

(18) For a new drug, the application failed to contain the patent information required by section 505(b)(1) of the act.

(c) For drugs intended to treat life-threatening or severely-debilitating illnesses that are developed in accordance with 312.80 through 312.88 of this chapter, the criteria contained in paragraphs (b) (3), (4), and (5) of this section shall be applied according to the considerations contained in 312.84 of this chapter.

[50 FR 7493, Feb. 22, 1985, as amended at 53 FR 41524, Oct. 21, 1988; 57 FR 17991, Apr. 28, 1992; 58 FR 25926, Apr. 28, 1993; 64 FR 402, Jan. 5, 1999; 73 FR 39610, July 10, 2008; 74 FR 9766, Mar. 6, 2009]

Sec. 314.126 Adequate and well-controlled studies.

(a) The purpose of conducting clinical investigations of a drug is to distinguish the effect of a drug from other influences, such as spontaneous change in the course of the disease, placebo effect, or biased observation. The characteristics described in paragraph (b) of this section have been developed over a period of years and are recognized by the scientific community as the essentials of an adequate and well-controlled clinical investigation. The Food and Drug Administration considers these characteristics in determining whether an investigation is adequate and well-controlled for purposes of section 505 of the act. Reports of adequate and well-controlled investigations provide the primary basis for determining whether there is "substantial evidence" to support the claims of effectiveness for new drugs. Therefore, the study report should provide sufficient details of study design, conduct, and analysis to allow critical evaluation and a determination of whether the characteristics of an adequate and well-controlled study are present.

(b) An adequate and well-controlled study has the following characteristics:

(1) There is a clear statement of the objectives of the investigation and a summary of the proposed or actual methods of analysis in the protocol for the study and in the report of its results. In addition, the protocol should contain a description of the proposed methods of analysis, and the

study report should contain a description of the methods of analysis ultimately used. If the protocol does not contain a description of the proposed methods of analysis, the study report should describe how the methods used were selected.

(2) The study uses a design that permits a valid comparison with a control to provide a quantitative assessment of drug effect. The protocol for the study and report of results should describe the study design precisely; for example, duration of treatment periods, whether treatments are parallel, sequential, or crossover, and whether the sample size is predetermined or based upon some interim analysis. Generally, the following types of control are recognized:

(i) Placebo concurrent control. The test drug is compared with an inactive preparation designed to resemble the test drug as far as possible. A placebo-controlled study may include additional treatment groups, such as an active treatment control or a dose-comparison control, and usually includes randomization and blinding of patients or investigators, or both.

(ii) Dose-comparison concurrent control. At least two doses of the drug are compared. A dose-comparison study may include additional treatment groups, such as placebo control or active control. Dose-comparison trials usually include randomization and blinding of patients or investigators, or both.

(iii) No treatment concurrent control. Where objective measurements of effectiveness are available and placebo effect is negligible, the test drug is compared with no treatment. No treatment concurrent control trials usually include randomization.

(iv) Active treatment concurrent control. The test drug is compared with known effective therapy; for example, where the condition treated is such that administration of placebo or no treatment would be contrary to the interest of the patient. An active treatment study may include additional treatment groups, however, such as a placebo control or a dose-comparison control. Active treatment trials usually include randomization and blinding of patients or investigators, or both. If the intent of the trial is to show similarity of the test and control drugs, the report of the study should assess the ability of the study to have detected a difference between treatments. Similarity of test drug and active control can mean either that both drugs were effective or that neither was effective. The analysis of the study should explain why the drugs should be considered effective in the study, for example, by reference to results in previous placebo-controlled studies of the active control drug.

(v) Historical control. The results of treatment with the test drug are compared with experience historically derived from the adequately documented natural history of the disease or condition, or from the results of active treatment, in comparable patients or populations. Because historical control populations usually cannot be as well assessed with respect to pertinent variables as can concurrent control populations, historical control designs are usually reserved for special circumstances. Examples include studies of diseases with high and predictable mortality (for example, certain malignancies) and studies in which the effect of the drug is self-evident (general anesthetics, drug metabolism).

(3) The method of selection of subjects provides adequate assurance that they have the disease or condition being studied, or evidence of susceptibility and exposure to the condition against which prophylaxis is directed.

(4) The method of assigning patients to treatment and control groups minimizes bias and is intended to assure comparability of the groups with respect to pertinent variables such as age, sex, severity of disease, duration of disease, and use of drugs or therapy other than the test drug. The protocol for the study and the report of its results should describe how subjects were assigned to groups. Ordinarily, in a concurrently controlled study, assignment is by randomization, with or without stratification.

(5) Adequate measures are taken to minimize bias on the part of the subjects, observers, and analysts of the data. The protocol and report of the study should describe the procedures used to accomplish this, such as blinding.

(6) The methods of assessment of subjects' response are well-defined and reliable. The protocol for the study and the report of results should explain the variables measured, the methods of observation, and criteria used to assess response.

Part 314

(7) There is an analysis of the results of the study adequate to assess the effects of the drug. The report of the study should describe the results and the analytic methods used to evaluate them, including any appropriate statistical methods. The analysis should assess, among other things, the comparability of test and control groups with respect to pertinent variables, and the effects of any interim data analyses performed.

(c) The Director of the Center for Drug Evaluation and Research may, on the Director's own initiative or on the petition of an interested person, waive in whole or in part any of the criteria in paragraph (b) of this section with respect to a specific clinical investigation, either prior to the investigation or in the evaluation of a completed study. A petition for a waiver is required to set forth clearly and concisely the specific criteria from which waiver is sought, why the criteria are not reasonably applicable to the particular clinical investigation, what alternative procedures, if any, are to be, or have been employed, and what results have been obtained. The petition is also required to state why the clinical investigations so conducted will yield, or have yielded, substantial evidence of effectiveness, notwithstanding nonconformance with the criteria for which waiver is requested.

(d) For an investigation to be considered adequate for approval of a new drug, it is required that the test drug be standardized as to identity, strength, quality, purity, and dosage form to give significance to the results of the investigation.

(e) Uncontrolled studies or partially controlled studies are not acceptable as the sole basis for the approval of claims of effectiveness. Such studies carefully conducted and documented, may provide corroborative support of well-controlled studies regarding efficacy and may yield valuable data regarding safety of the test drug. Such studies will be considered on their merits in the light of the principles listed here, with the exception of the requirement for the comparison of the treated subjects with controls. Isolated case reports, random experience, and reports lacking the details which permit scientific evaluation will not be considered.

[50 FR 7493, Feb. 22, 1985, as amended at 50 FR 21238, May 23, 1985; 55 FR 11580, Mar. 29, 1990; 64 FR 402, Jan. 5, 1999; 67 FR 9586, Mar. 4, 2002]

Sec. 314.127 Refusal to approve an abbreviated new drug application.

(a) FDA will refuse to approve an abbreviated application for a new drug under section 505(j) of the act for any of the following reasons:

(1) The methods used in, or the facilities and controls used for, the manufacture, processing, and packing of the drug product are inadequate to ensure and preserve its identity, strength, quality, and purity.

(2) Information submitted with the abbreviated new drug application is insufficient to show that each of the proposed conditions of use has been previously approved for the listed drug referred to in the application.

(3)(i) If the reference listed drug has only one active ingredient, information submitted with the abbreviated new drug application is insufficient to show that the active ingredient is the same as that of the reference listed drug;

(ii) If the reference listed drug has more than one active ingredient, information submitted with the abbreviated new drug application is insufficient to show that the active ingredients are the same as the active ingredients of the reference listed drug; or

(iii) If the reference listed drug has more than one active ingredient and if the abbreviated new drug application is for a drug product that has an active ingredient different from the reference listed drug:

(A) Information submitted with the abbreviated new drug application is insufficient to show:

(1) That the other active ingredients are the same as the active ingredients of the reference listed drug; or

(2) That the different active ingredient is an active ingredient of a listed drug or a drug that does not meet the requirements of section 201(p) of the act; or

(B) No petition to submit an abbreviated application for the drug product with the different active ingredient was approved under 314.93.

(4)(i) If the abbreviated new drug application is for a drug product whose route of administration, dosage form, or strength purports to be the same as that of the listed drug referred to in the abbreviated new drug application, information submitted in the abbreviated new drug application is insufficient to show that the route of administration, dosage form, or strength is the same as that of the reference listed drug; or

(ii) If the abbreviated new drug application is for a drug product whose route of administration, dosage form, or strength is different from that of the listed drug referred to in the application, no petition to submit an abbreviated new drug application for the drug product with the different route of administration, dosage form, or strength was approved under 314.93.

(5) If the abbreviated new drug application was submitted under the approval of a petition under 314.93, the abbreviated new drug application did not contain the information required by FDA with respect to the active ingredient, route of administration, dosage form, or strength that is not the same as that of the reference listed drug.

(6)(i) Information submitted in the abbreviated new drug application is insufficient to show that the drug product is bioequivalent to the listed drug referred to in the abbreviated new drug application; or

(ii) If the abbreviated new drug application was submitted under a petition approved under 314.93, information submitted in the abbreviated new drug application is insufficient to show that the active ingredients of the drug product are of the same pharmacological or therapeutic class as those of the reference listed drug and that the drug product can be expected to have the same therapeutic effect as the reference listed drug when administered to patients for each condition of use approved for the reference listed drug.

(7) Information submitted in the abbreviated new drug application is insufficient to show that the labeling proposed for the drug is the same as the labeling approved for the listed drug referred to in the abbreviated new drug application except for changes required because of differences approved in a petition under 314.93 or because the drug product and

the reference listed drug are produced or distributed by different manufacturers or because aspects of the listed drug's labeling are protected by patent, or by exclusivity, and such differences do not render the proposed drug product less safe or effective than the listed drug for all remaining, nonprotected conditions of use.

(8)(i) Information submitted in the abbreviated new drug application of any other information available to FDA shows that:

(A) The inactive ingredients of the drug product are unsafe for use, as described in paragraph (a)(8)(ii) of this section, under the conditions prescribed, recommended, or suggested in the labeling proposed for the drug product; or

(B) The composition of the drug product is unsafe, as described in paragraph (a)(8)(ii) of this section, under the conditions prescribed, recommended, or suggested in the proposed labeling because of the type or quantity of inactive ingredients included or the manner in which the inactive ingredients are included.

(ii)(A) FDA will consider the inactive ingredients or composition of a drug product unsafe and refuse to approve an abbreviated new drug application under paragraph (a)(8)(i) of this section if, on the basis of information available to the agency, there is a reasonable basis to conclude that one or more of the inactive ingredients of the proposed drug or its composition raises serious questions of safety or efficacy. From its experience with reviewing inactive ingredients, and from other information available to it, FDA may identify changes in inactive ingredients or composition that may adversely affect a drug product's safety or efficacy. The inactive ingredients or composition of a proposed drug product will be considered to raise serious questions of safety or efficacy if the product incorporates one or more of these changes. Examples of the changes that may raise serious questions of safety or efficacy include, but are not limited to, the following:

(1) A change in an inactive ingredient so that the product does not comply with an official compendium.

(2) A change in composition to include an inactive ingredient that has not been previously approved in a drug product for human use by the same route of administration.

(3) A change in the composition of a parenteral drug product to include an inactive ingredient that has not been previously approved in a parenteral drug product.

(4) A change in composition of a drug product for ophthalmic use to include an inactive ingredient that has not been previously approved in a drug for ophthalmic use.

(5) The use of a delivery or a modified release mechanism never before approved for the drug.

(6) A change in composition to include a significantly greater content of one or more inactive ingredients than previously used in the drug product.

(7) If the drug product is intended for topical administration, a change in the properties of the vehicle or base that might increase absorption of certain potentially toxic active ingredients thereby affecting the safety of the drug product, or a change in the lipophilic properties of a vehicle or base, e.g., a change from an oleaginous to a water soluble vehicle or base.

(B) FDA will consider an inactive ingredient in, or the composition of, a drug product intended for parenteral use to be unsafe and will refuse to approve the abbreviated new drug application unless it contains the same inactive ingredients, other than preservatives, buffers, and antioxidants, in the same concentration as the listed drug, and, if it differs from the listed drug in a preservative, buffer, or antioxidant, the application contains sufficient information to demonstrate that the difference does not affect the safety or efficacy of the drug product.

(C) FDA will consider an inactive ingredient in, or the composition of, a drug product intended for ophthalmic or otic use unsafe and will refuse to approve the abbreviated new drug application unless it contains the same inactive ingredients, other than preservatives, buffers, substances to adjust tonicity, or thickening agents, in the same concentration as the listed drug, and if it differs from the listed drug in a preservative, buffer, substance to adjust tonicity, or thickening agent, the application contains sufficient information to demonstrate that the difference does not affect the safety or efficacy of the drug product and the labeling does not claim any therapeutic advantage over or difference from the listed drug.

(9) Approval of the listed drug referred to in the abbreviated new drug application has been withdrawn or suspended for grounds described in 314.150(a) or FDA has published a notice of opportunity for hearing to withdraw approval of the reference listed drug under 314.150(a).

(10) Approval of the listed drug referred to in the abbreviated new drug application has been withdrawn under 314.151 or FDA has proposed to withdraw approval of the reference listed drug under 314.151(a).

(11) FDA has determined that the reference listed drug has been withdrawn from sale for safety or effectiveness reasons under 314.161, or the reference listed drug has been voluntarily withdrawn from sale and the agency has not determined whether the withdrawal is for safety or effectiveness reasons, or approval of the reference listed drug has been suspended under 314.153, or the agency has issued an initial decision proposing to suspend the reference listed drug under 314.153(a)(1).

(12) The abbreviated new drug application does not meet any other requirement under section 505(j)(2)(A) of the act.

(13) The abbreviated new drug application contains an untrue statement of material fact.

(b) FDA may refuse to approve an abbreviated application for a new drug if the applicant or contract research organization that conducted a bioavailability or bioequivalence study described in 320.63 of this chapter that is contained in the abbreviated new drug application refuses to permit an inspection of facilities or records relevant to the study by a properly authorized officer of employee of the Department of Health and Human Services or refuses to submit reserve samples of the drug products used in the study when requested by FDA.

[57 FR 17991, Apr. 28, 1992; 57 FR 29353, July 1, 1992, as amended at 58 FR 25927, Apr. 28, 1993; 67 FR 77672, Dec. 19, 2002]

Sec. 314.150 Withdrawal of approval of an application or abbreviated application.

(a) The Food and Drug Administration will notify the applicant, and, if appropriate, all other persons who manufacture or distribute identical, related, or similar drug products as defined in 310.6 and 314.151(a) of this chapter and for a new drug afford an opportunity for a hearing on a proposal to withdraw approval of the application or abbreviated new drug application under section 505(e) of the act and under the procedure in 314.200, if any of the following apply:

(1) The Secretary of Health and Human Services has suspended the approval of the application or abbreviated application for a new drug on a finding that there is an imminent hazard to the public health. FDA will promptly afford the applicant an expedited hearing following summary suspension on a finding of imminent hazard to health.

(2) FDA finds:

(i) That clinical or other experience, tests, or other scientific data show that the drug is unsafe for use under the conditions of use upon the basis of which the application or abbreviated application was approved; or

(ii) That new evidence of clinical experience, not contained in the application or not available to FDA until after the application or abbreviated application was approved, or tests by new methods, or tests by methods not deemed reasonably applicable when the application or abbreviated application was approved, evaluated together with the evidence available when the application or abbreviated application was approved, reveal that the drug is not shown to be safe for use under the conditions of use upon the basis of which the application or abbreviated application was approved; or

(iii) Upon the basis of new information before FDA with respect to the drug, evaluated together with the evidence available when the application or abbreviated application was approved, that there is a lack of substantial evidence from adequate and well-controlled investigations as defined in 314.126, that the drug will have the effect it is purported or represented to have under the conditions of use prescribed, recommended, or suggested in its labeling; or

(iv) That the application or abbreviated application contains any untrue statement of a material fact; or

(v) That the patent information prescribed by section 505(c) of the act was not submitted within 30 days after the receipt of written notice from FDA specifying the failure to submit such information; or

(b) FDA may notify the applicant, and, if appropriate, all other persons who manufacture or distribute identical, related, or similar drug products as defined in 310.6, and for a new drug afford an opportunity for a hearing on a proposal to withdraw approval of the application or abbreviated new drug application under section 505(e) of the act and under the procedure in 314.200, if the agency finds:

(1) That the applicant has failed to establish a system for maintaining required records, or has repeatedly or deliberately failed to maintain required records or to make required reports under section 505(k) or 507(g) of the act and 314.80, 314.81, or 314.98, or that the applicant has refused to permit access to, or copying or verification of, its records.

(2) That on the basis of new information before FDA, evaluated together with the evidence available when the application or abbreviated application was approved, the methods used in, or the facilities and controls used for, the manufacture, processing, and packing of the drug are inadequate to ensure and preserve its identity, strength, quality, and purity and were not made adequate within a reasonable time after receipt of written notice from the agency.

(3) That on the basis of new information before FDA, evaluated together with the evidence available when the application or

Part 314

abbreviated application was approved, the labeling of the drug, based on a fair evaluation of all material facts, is false or misleading in any particular, and the labeling was not corrected by the applicant within a reasonable time after receipt of written notice from the agency.

(4) That the applicant has failed to comply with the notice requirements of section 510(j)(2) of the act.

(5) That the applicant has failed to submit bioavailability or bioequivalence data required under part 320 of this chapter.

(6) The application or abbreviated application does not contain an explanation of the omission of a report of any investigation of the drug product sponsored by the applicant, or an explanation of the omission of other information about the drug pertinent to an evaluation of the application or abbreviated application that is received or otherwise obtained by the applicant from any source.

(7) That any nonclinical laboratory study that is described in the application or abbreviated application and that is essential to show that the drug is safe for use under the conditions prescribed, recommended, or suggested in its labeling was not conducted in compliance with the good laboratory practice regulations in part 58 of this chapter and no reason for the noncompliance was provided or, if it was, the differences between the practices used in conducting the study and the good laboratory practice regulations do not support the validity of the study.

(8) Any clinical investigation involving human subjects described in the application or abbreviated application, subject to the institutional review board regulations in part 56 of this chapter or informed consent regulations in part 50 of this chapter, was not conducted in compliance with those regulations such that the rights or safety of human subjects were not adequately protected.

(9) That the applicant or contract research organization that conducted a bioavailability or bioequivalence study described in 320.38 or 320.63 of this chapter that is contained in the application or abbreviated application refuses to permit an inspection of facilities or records relevant to the study by a properly authorized officer or employee of the Department of Health and Human Services or refuses to submit reserve

samples of the drug products used in the study when requested by FDA.

(10) That the labeling for the drug product that is the subject of the abbreviated new drug application is no longer consistent with that for the listed drug referred to in the abbreviated new drug application, except for differences approved in the abbreviated new drug application or those differences resulting from:

    (i) A patent on the listed drug issued after approval of the abbreviated new drug application; or

    (ii) Exclusivity accorded to the listed drug after approval of the abbreviated new drug application that do not render the drug product less safe or effective than the listed drug for any remaining, nonprotected condition(s) of use.

(c) FDA will withdraw approval of an application or abbreviated application if the applicant requests its withdrawal because the drug subject to the application or abbreviated application is no longer being marketed, provided none of the conditions listed in paragraphs (a) and (b) of this section applies to the drug. FDA will consider a written request for a withdrawal under this paragraph to be a waiver of an opportunity for hearing otherwise provided for in this section. Withdrawal of approval of an application or abbreviated application under this paragraph is without prejudice to refiling.

(d) FDA may notify an applicant that it believes a potential problem associated with a drug is sufficiently serious that the drug should be removed from the market and may ask the applicant to waive the opportunity for hearing otherwise provided for under this section, to permit FDA to withdraw approval of the application or abbreviated application for the product, and to remove voluntarily the product from the market. If the applicant agrees, the agency will not make a finding under paragraph (b) of this section, but will withdraw approval of the application or abbreviated application in a notice published in theFederal Registerthat contains a brief summary of the agency's and the applicant's views of the reasons for withdrawal.

[57 FR 17993, Apr. 28, 1992, as amended at 58 FR 25927, Apr. 28, 1993; 64 FR 402, Jan. 5, 1999]

Part 314

Sec. 314.151 Withdrawal of approval of an abbreviated new drug application under section 505(j)(5) of the act.

(a) Approval of an abbreviated new drug application approved under 314.105(d) may be withdrawn when the agency withdraws approval, under 314.150(a) or under this section, of the approved drug referred to in the abbreviated new drug application. If the agency proposed to withdraw approval of a listed drug under 314.150(a), the holder of an approved application for the listed drug has a right to notice and opportunity for hearing. The published notice of opportunity for hearing will identify all drug products approved under 314.105(d) whose applications are subject to withdrawal under this section if the listed drug is withdrawn, and will propose to withdraw such drugs. Holders of approved applications for the identified drug products will be provided notice and an opportunity to respond to the proposed withdrawal of their applications as described in paragraphs (b) and (c) of this section.

(b)(1) The published notice of opportunity for hearing on the withdrawal of the listed drug will serve as notice to holders of identified abbreviated new drug applications of the grounds for the proposed withdrawal.

(2) Holders of applications for drug products identified in the notice of opportunity for hearing may submit written comments on the notice of opportunity for hearing issued on the proposed withdrawal of the listed drug. If an abbreviated new drug application holder submits comments on the notice of opportunity for hearing and a hearing is granted, the abbreviated new drug application holder may participate in the hearing as a nonparty participant as provided for in 12.89 of this chapter.

(3) Except as provided in paragraphs (c) and (d) of this section, the approval of an abbreviated new drug application for a drug product identified in the notice of opportunity for hearing on the withdrawal of a listed drug will be withdrawn when the agency has completed the withdrawal of approval of the listed drug.

(c)(1) If the holder of an application for a drug identified in the notice of opportunity for hearing has submitted timely comments but does not have an opportunity to participate in a hearing because a hearing is not requested or is settled, the submitted comments will be considered by the agency, which will issue an initial decision. The initial decision will respond to the comments, and contain the agency's decision whether there are grounds to withdraw approval of the listed drug and of the abbreviated new drug applications on which timely comments were submitted. The initial decision will be sent to each abbreviated new drug application holder that has submitted comments.

(2) Abbreviated new drug application holders to whom the initial decision was sent may, within 30 days of the issuance of the initial decision, submit written objections.

(3) The agency may, at its discretion, hold a limited oral hearing to resolve dispositive factual issues that cannot be resolved on the basis of written submissions.

(4) If there are no timely objections to the initial decision, it will become final at the expiration of 30 days.

(5) If timely objections are submitted, they will be reviewed and responded to in a final decision.

(6) The written comments received, the initial decision, the evidence relied on in the comments and in the initial decision, the objections to the initial decision, and, if a limited oral hearing has been held, the transcript of that hearing and any documents submitted therein, shall form the record upon which the agency shall make a final decision.

(7) Except as provided in paragraph (d) of this section, any abbreviated new drug application whose holder submitted comments on the notice of opportunity for hearing shall be withdrawn upon the issuance of a final decision concluding that the listed drug should be withdrawn for grounds as described in 314.150(a). The final decision shall be in writing and shall constitute final agency action, reviewable in a judicial proceeding.

(8) Documents in the record will be publicly available in accordance with 10.20(j) of this chapter. Documents available for examination or copying will be placed on public display in the Division of Dockets Management (HFA-305), Food and Drug Administration, room. 1-23, 12420 Parklawn Dr., Rockville, MD 20857, promptly upon receipt in that office.

(d) If the agency determines, based upon information submitted by the holder of an abbreviated new drug application, that the grounds for withdrawal of the listed drug are not applicable to a drug identified in the notice of opportunity for hearing, the final decision will state that the approval of the abbreviated new drug application for such drug is not withdrawn.

[57 FR 17994, Apr. 28, 1992]

Sec. 314.152 Notice of withdrawal of approval of an application or abbreviated application for a new drug.

If the Food and Drug Administration withdraws approval of an application or abbreviated application for a new drug, FDA will publish a notice in theFederal Registerannouncing the withdrawal of approval. If the application or abbreviated application was withdrawn for grounds described in 314.150(a) or 314.151, the notice will announce the removal of the drug from the list of approved drugs published under section 505(j)(6) of the act and shall satisfy the requirement of 314.162(b).

[57 FR 17994, Apr. 28, 1992]

Sec. 314.153 Suspension of approval of an abbreviated new drug application.

(a) Suspension of approval. The approval of an abbreviated new drug application approved under 314.105(d) shall be suspended for the period stated when:

(1) The Secretary of the Department of Health and Human Services, under the imminent hazard authority of section 505(e) of the act or the authority of this paragraph, suspends approval of a listed drug referred to in the abbreviated new drug application, for the period of the suspension;

(2) The agency, in the notice described in paragraph (b) of this section, or in any subsequent written notice given an abbreviated new drug application holder by the agency, concludes that the risk of continued marketing and use of the drug is inappropriate, pending completion of proceedings to withdraw or suspend approval under 314.151 or paragraph (b) of this section; or

(3) The agency, under the procedures set forth in paragraph (b) of this section, issues a final decision stating the determination that the abbreviated application is suspended

because the listed drug on which the approval of the abbreviated new drug application depends has been withdrawn from sale for reasons of safety or effectiveness or has been suspended under paragraph (b) of this section. The suspension will take effect on the date stated in the decision and will remain in effect until the agency determines that the marketing of the drug has resumed or that the withdrawal is not for safety or effectiveness reasons.

(b) Procedures for suspension of abbreviated new drug applications when a listed drug is voluntarily withdrawn for safety or effectiveness reasons.

(1) If a listed drug is voluntarily withdrawn from sale, and the agency determines that the withdrawal from sale was for reasons of safety or effectiveness, the agency will send each holder of an approved abbreviated new drug application that is subject to suspension as a result of this determination a copy of the agency's initial decision setting forth the reasons for the determination. The initial decision will also be placed on file with the Division of Dockets Management (HFA-305), Food and Drug Administration, room 1-23, 12420 Parklawn Dr., Rockville, MD 20857.

(2) Each abbreviated new drug application holder will have 30 days from the issuance of the initial decision to present, in writing, comments and information bearing on the initial decision. If no comments or information is received, the initial decision will become final at the expiration of 30 days.

(3) Comments and information received within 30 days of the issuance of the initial decision will be considered by the agency and responded to in a final decision.

(4) The agency may, in its discretion, hold a limited oral hearing to resolve dispositive factual issues that cannot be resolved on the basis of written submissions.

(5) If the final decision affirms the agency's initial decision that the listed drug was withdrawn for reasons of safety or effectiveness, the decision will be published in theFederal Registerin compliance with 314.152, and will, except as provided in paragraph (b)(6) of this section, suspend approval of all abbreviated new drug applications identified under paragraph (b)(1) of this section and remove from the list the listed drug and any drug whose approval was suspended

Part 314

under this paragraph. The notice will satisfy the requirement of 314.162(b). The agency's final decision and copies of materials on which it relies will also be filed with the Division of Dockets Management (address in paragraph (b)(1) of this section).

(6) If the agency determines in its final decision that the listed drug was withdrawn for reasons of safety or effectiveness but, based upon information submitted by the holder of an abbreviated new drug application, also determines that the reasons for the withdrawal of the listed drug are not relevant to the safety and effectiveness of the drug subject to such abbreviated new drug application, the final decision will state that the approval of such abbreviated new drug application is not suspended.

(7) Documents in the record will be publicly available in accordance with 10.20(j) of this chapter. Documents available for examination or copying will be placed on public display in the Division of Dockets Management (address in paragraph (b)(1) of this section) promptly upon receipt in that office.

[57 FR 17995, Apr. 28, 1992]

Sec. 314.160 Approval of an application or abbreviated application for which approval was previously refused, suspended, or withdrawn.

Upon the Food and Drug Administration's own initiative or upon request of an applicant, FDA may, on the basis of new data, approve an application or abbreviated application which it had previously refused, suspended, or withdrawn approval. FDA will publish a notice in theFederal Registerannouncing the approval.

[57 FR 17995, Apr. 28, 1992]

Sec. 314.161 Determination of reasons for voluntary withdrawal of a listed drug.

(a) A determination whether a listed drug that has been voluntarily withdrawn from sale was withdrawn for safety or effectiveness reasons may be made by the agency at any time after the drug has been voluntarily withdrawn from sale, but must be made:

(1) Prior to approving an abbreviated new drug application that refers to the listed drug;

(2) Whenever a listed drug is voluntarily withdrawn from sale and abbreviated new drug applications that referred to the listed drug have been approved; and

(3) When a person petitions for such a determination under 10.25(a) and 10.30 of this chapter.

(b) Any person may petition under 10.25(a) and 10.30 of this chapter for a determination whether a listed drug has been voluntarily withdrawn for safety or effectiveness reasons. Any such petition must contain all evidence available to the petitioner concerning the reason that the drug is withdrawn from sale.

(c) If the agency determines that a listed drug is withdrawn from sale for safety or effectiveness reasons, the agency will, except as provided in paragraph (d) of this section, publish a notice of the determination in theFederal Register.

(d) If the agency determines under paragraph (a) of this section that a listed drug is withdrawn from sale for safety and effectiveness reasons and there are approved abbreviated new drug applications that are subject to suspension under section 505(j)(5) of the act, FDA will initiate a proceeding in accordance with 314.153(b).

(e) A drug that the agency determines is withdrawn for safety or effectiveness reasons will be removed from the list, under 314.162. The drug may be relisted if the agency has evidence that marketing of the drug has resumed or that the withdrawal is not for safety or effectiveness reasons. A determination that the drug is not withdrawn for safety or effectiveness reasons may be made at any time after its removal from the list, upon the agency's initiative, or upon the submission of a petition under 10.25(a) and 10.30 of this chapter. If the agency determines that the drug is not withdrawn for safety or effectiveness reasons, the agency shall publish a notice of this determination in theFederal Register.The notice will also announce that the drug is relisted, under 314.162(c). The notice will also serve to reinstate approval of all suspended abbreviated new drug applications that referred to the listed drug.

[57 FR 17995, Apr. 28, 1992]

Sec. 314.162 Removal of a drug product from the list.

(a) FDA will remove a previously approved new drug product from the list for the period stated when:

(1) The agency withdraws or suspends approval of a new drug application or an abbreviated new drug application under 314.150(a) or 314.151 or under the imminent hazard authority of section 505(e) of the act, for the same period as the withdrawal or suspension of the application; or

(2) The agency, in accordance with the procedures in 314.153(b) or 314.161, issues a final decision stating that the listed drug was withdrawn from sale for safety or effectiveness reasons, or suspended under 314.153(b), until the agency determines that the withdrawal from the market has ceased or is not for safety or effectiveness reasons.

(b) FDA will publish in theFederal Registera notice announcing the removal of a drug from the list.

(c) At the end of the period specified in paragraph (a)(1) or (a)(2) of this section, FDA will relist a drug that has been removed from the list. The agency will publish in theFederal Registera notice announcing the relisting of the drug.

[57 FR 17996, Apr. 28, 1992]

Sec. 314.170 Adulteration and misbranding of an approved drug.

All drugs, including those the Food and Drug Administration approves under section 505 of the act and this part, are subject to the adulteration and misbranding provisions in sections 501, 502, and 503 of the act. FDA is authorized to regulate approved new drugs by regulations issued through informal rulemaking under sections 501, 502, and 503 of the act.

[50 FR 7493, Feb. 22, 1985. Redesignated at 57 FR 17983, Apr. 28, 1992, and amended at 64 FR 402, Jan. 5, 1999]

Subpart E--Hearing Procedures for New Drugs

Sec. 314.200 Notice of opportunity for hearing; notice of participation and request for hearing; grant or denial of hearing.

(a) Notice of opportunity for hearing. The Director of the Center for Drug Evaluation and Research, Food and Drug Administration, will give the applicant, and all other persons who manufacture or distribute identical, related, or similar drug products as defined in 310.6 of this chapter, notice and an opportunity for a hearing on the Center's proposal to refuse to approve an application or to withdraw the approval of an application or abbreviated application under section 505(e) of the act. The notice will state the reasons for the action and the proposed grounds for the order.

(1) The notice may be general (that is, simply summarizing in a general way the information resulting in the notice) or specific (that is, either referring to specific requirements in the statute and regulations with which there is a lack of compliance, or providing a detailed description and analysis of the specific facts resulting in the notice).

(2) FDA will publish the notice in theFederal Registerand will state that the applicant, and other persons subject to the notice under 310.6, who wishes to participate in a hearing, has 30 days after the date of publication of the notice to file a written notice of participation and request for hearing. The applicant, or other persons subject to the notice under 310.6, who fails to file a written notice of participation and request for hearing within 30 days, waives the opportunity for a hearing.

(3) It is the responsibility of every manufacturer and distributor of a drug product to review every notice of opportunity for a hearing published in theFederal Registerto determine whether it covers any drug product that person manufactures or distributes. Any person may request an opinion of the applicability of a notice to a specific product that may be identical, related, or similar to a product listed in a notice by writing to the Division of New Drugs and Labeling Compliance, Office of Compliance, Center for Drug Evaluation and Research, Food and Drug Administration, 10903 New Hampshire Ave., Silver Spring, MD 20993-0002. A person shall request an opinion within 30 days of the date of publication of the notice to be eligible for an opportunity for a hearing under the notice. If a person requests an opinion, that person's time for filing an appearance and request for a hearing and supporting studies and analyses begins on the date the person receives the opinion from FDA.

Part 314

(b) FDA will provide the notice of opportunity for a hearing to applicants and to other persons subject to the notice under 310.6, as follows:

(1) To any person who has submitted an application or abbreviated application, by delivering the notice in person or by sending it by registered or certified mail to the last address shown in the application or abbreviated application.

(2) To any person who has not submitted an application or abbreviated application but who is subject to the notice under 310.6 of this chapter, by publication of the notice in theFederal Register.

(c)(1) Notice of participation and request for a hearing, and submission of studies and comments. The applicant, or any other person subject to the notice under 310.6, who wishes to participate in a hearing, shall file with the Division of Dockets Management (HFA-305), Food and Drug Administration, 5630 Fishers Lane, rm. 1061, Rockville, MD 20852, (i) within 30 days after the date of the publication of the notice (or of the date of receipt of an opinion requested under paragraph (a)(3) of this section) a written notice of participation and request for a hearing and (ii) within 60 days after the date of publication of the notice, unless a different period of time is specified in the notice of opportunity for a hearing, the studies on which the person relies to justify a hearing as specified in paragraph (d) of this section. The applicant, or other person, may incorporate by reference the raw data underlying a study if the data were previously submitted to FDA as part of an application, abbreviated application, or other report.

(2) FDA will not consider data or analyses submitted after 60 days in determining whether a hearing is warranted unless they are derived from well-controlled studies begun before the date of the notice of opportunity for hearing and the results of the studies were not available within 60 days after the date of publication of the notice. Nevertheless, FDA may consider other studies on the basis of a showing by the person requesting a hearing of inadvertent omission and hardship. The person requesting a hearing shall list in the request for hearing all studies in progress, the results of which the person intends later to submit in support of the request for a hearing. The person shall submit under paragraph

(c)(1)(ii) of this section a copy of the complete protocol, a list of the participating investigators, and a brief status report of the studies.

(3) Any other interested person who is not subject to the notice of opportunity for a hearing may also submit comments on the proposal to withdraw approval of the application or abbreviated application. The comments are requested to be submitted within the time and under the conditions specified in this section.

(d) The person requesting a hearing is required to submit under paragraph (c)(1)(ii) of this section the studies (including all protocols and underlying raw data) on which the person relies to justify a hearing with respect to the drug product. Except, a person who requests a hearing on the refusal to approve an application is not required to submit additional studies and analyses if the studies upon which the person relies have been submitted in the application and in the format and containing the summaries required under 314.50.

(1) If the grounds for FDA's proposed action concern the effectiveness of the drug, each request for hearing is required to be supported only by adequate and well-controlled clinical studies meeting all of the precise requirements of 314.126 and, for combination drug products, 300.50, or by other studies not meeting those requirements for which a waiver has been previously granted by FDA under 314.126. Each person requesting a hearing shall submit all adequate and well-controlled clinical studies on the drug product, including any unfavorable analyses, views, or judgments with respect to the studies. No other data, information, or studies may be submitted.

(2) The submission is required to include a factual analysis of all the studies submitted. If the grounds for FDA's proposed action concern the effectiveness of the drug, the analysis is required to specify how each study accords, on a point-by-point basis, with each criterion required for an adequate well-controlled clinical investigation established under 314.126 and, if the product is a combination drug product, with each of the requirements for a combination drug established in 300.50, or the study is required to be accompanied by an appropriate waiver previously granted by FDA. If a study concerns a drug or dosage form or condition of use or mode

of administration other than the one in question, that fact is required to be clearly stated. Any study conducted on the final marketed form of the drug product is required to be clearly identified.

(3) Each person requesting a hearing shall submit an analysis of the data upon which the person relies, except that the required information relating either to safety or to effectiveness may be omitted if the notice of opportunity for hearing does not raise any issue with respect to that aspect of the drug; information on compliance with 300.50 may be omitted if the drug product is not a combination drug product. A financial certification or disclosure statement or both as required by part 54 of this chapter must accompany all clinical data submitted. FDA can most efficiently consider submissions made in the following format.

I.   Safety data.

    A.   Animal safety data.

        1.   Individual active components.

            a.   Controlled studies.

            b.   Partially controlled or uncontrolled studies.

        2.   Combinations of the individual active components.

            a.   Controlled studies.

            b.   Partially controlled or uncontrolled studies.

    B.   Human safety data.

        1.   Individual active components.

            a.   Controlled studies.

            b.   Partially controlled or uncontrolled studies.

            c.   Documented case reports.

            d.   Pertinent marketing experiences that may influence a determination about the safety of each individual active component.

        2.   Combinations of the individual active components.

            a.   Controlled studies.

b. Partially controlled or uncontrolled studies.

c. Documented case reports.

d. Pertinent marketing experiences that may influence a determination about the safety of each individual active component.

II. Effectiveness data.

A. Individual active components: Controlled studies, with an analysis showing clearly how each study satisfies, on a point-by-point basis, each of the criteria required by 314.126.

B. Combinations of individual active components.

1. Controlled studies with an analysis showing clearly how each study satisfies on a point-by-point basis, each of the criteria required by 314.126.

2. An analysis showing clearly how each requirement of 300.50 has been satisfied.

III. A summary of the data and views setting forth the medical rationale and purpose for the drug and its ingredients and the scientific basis for the conclusion that the drug and its ingredients have been proven safe and/or effective for the intended use. If there is an absence of controlled studies in the material submitted or the requirements of any element of 300.50 or 314.126 have not been fully met, that fact is required to be stated clearly and a waiver obtained under 314.126 is required to be submitted.

IV. A statement signed by the person responsible for such submission that it includes in full (or incorporates by reference as permitted in 314.200(c)(2)) all studies and information specified in 314.200(d).

(Warning: A willfully false statement is a criminal offense, 18 U.S.C. 1001.)

(e) Contentions that a drug product is not subject to the new drug requirements. A notice of opportunity for a hearing encompasses all issues relating to the legal status of each drug product subject to it, including identical, related, and similar drug products as defined in 310.6. A notice of appearance and request for a hearing under paragraph (c)(1)(i) of this section is required to contain any contention that the product is not a new drug because it is generally recognized as safe and effective within the meaning of section 201(p) of the act, or because it is exempt from part or all of the new drug provisions of the act under the exemption for products marketed before June 25, 1938, contained in section 201(p) of the act or under section 107(c) of the Drug Amendments of 1962, or for any other reason. Each contention is required to be supported by a submission under paragraph (c)(1)(ii) of this section and the Commissioner of Food and Drugs will make an administrative determination on each contention. The failure of any person subject to a notice of opportunity for a hearing, including any person who manufactures or distributes an identical, related, or similar drug product as defined in 310.6, to submit a notice of participation and request for hearing or to raise all such contentions constitutes a waiver of any contentions not raised.

(1) A contention that a drug product is generally recognized as safe and effective within the meaning of section 201(p) of the act is required to be supported by submission of the same quantity and quality of scientific evidence that is required to obtain approval of an application for the product, unless FDA has waived a requirement for effectiveness (under 314.126) or safety, or both. The submission should be in the format and with the analyses required under paragraph (d) of this section. A person who fails to submit the required scientific evidence required under paragraph (d) waives the contention. General recognition of safety and effectiveness shall ordinarily be based upon published studies which may be corroborated by unpublished studies and other data and information.

(2) A contention that a drug product is exempt from part or all of the new drug provisions of the act under the exemption for products marketed before June 25, 1938, contained in section 201(p) of the act, or under section 107(c) of the Drug Amendments of 1962, is required to be supported by evidence of past and present quantitative formulas, labeling, and evidence of marketing. A person who makes such a contention should submit the formulas, labeling, and evidence of marketing in the following format.

I. Formulation.

   A. A copy of each pertinent document or record to establish the exact quantitative formulation of the drug (both active and inactive ingredients) on the date of initial marketing of the drug.

   B. A statement whether such formulation has at any subsequent time been changed in any manner. If any such change has been made, the exact date, nature, and rationale for each change in formulation, including any deletion or change in the concentration of any active ingredient and/or inactive ingredient, should be stated, together with a copy of each pertinent document or record to establish the date and nature of each such change, including, but not limited to, the formula which resulted from each such change. If no such change has been made, a copy of representative documents or records showing the formula at representative points in time should be submitted to support the statement.

II. Labeling.

   A. A copy of each pertinent document or record to establish the identity of each item of written, printed, or graphic matter used as labeling on the date the drug was initially marketed.

   B. A statement whether such labeling has at any subsequent time been discontinued or changed in any manner. If such discontinuance or change has been made, the exact date, nature, and rationale for each discontinuance or change and a copy of each pertinent document or record to establish each such discontinuance or change should be submitted, including, but not limited to, the labeling which resulted from each such discontinuance or change. If no such discontinuance or change has been made, a copy of representative documents or records showing labeling at representative points in time should be submitted to support the statement.

Part 314

III. Marketing.

    A. A copy of each pertinent document or record to establish the exact date the drug was initially marketed.

    B. A statement whether such marketing has at any subsequent time been discontinued. If such marketing has been discontinued, the exact date of each such discontinuance should be submitted, together with a copy of each pertinent document or record to establish each such date.

IV. Verification.

A statement signed by the person responsible for such submission, that all appropriate records have been searched and to the best of that person's knowledge and belief it includes a true and accurate presentation of the facts.

(Warning: A willfully false statement is a criminal offense, 18 U.S.C. 1001.)

(3) The Food and Drug Administration will not find a drug product, including any active ingredient, which is identical, related, or similar, as described in 310.6, to a drug product, including any active ingredient for which an application is or at any time has been effective or deemed approved, or approved under section 505 of the act, to be exempt from part or all of the new drug provisions of the act.

(4) A contention that a drug product is not a new drug for any other reason is required to be supported by submission of the factual records, data, and information that are necessary and appropriate to support the contention.

(5) It is the responsibility of every person who manufactures or distributes a drug product in reliance upon a "grandfather" provision of the act to maintain files that contain the data and information necessary fully to document and support that status.

(f) Separation of functions. Separation of functions commences upon receipt of a request for hearing. The Director of the Center for Drug Evaluation and Research, Food and Drug Administration, will prepare an analysis of the request and a proposed order ruling on the matter. The analysis and proposed order, the request for hearing, and any proposed order denying a hearing and response under paragraph (g) (2) or (3) of this section will be submitted to the Office of the Commissioner of Food and Drugs for review and decision. When the Center for Drug Evaluation and Research recommends denial of a hearing on all issues on which a hearing is requested, no representative of the Center will participate or advise in the review and decision by the Commissioner. When the Center for Drug Evaluation and Research recommends that a hearing be granted on one or more issues on which a hearing is requested, separation of functions terminates as to those issues, and representatives of the Center may participate or advise in the review and decision by the Commissioner on those issues. The Commissioner may modify the text of the issues, but may not deny a hearing on those issues. Separation of functions continues with respect to issues on which the Center for Drug Evaluation and Research has recommended denial of a hearing. The Commissioner will neither evaluate nor rule on the Center's recommendation on such issues and such issues will not be included in the notice of hearing. Participants in the hearing may make a motion to the presiding officer for the inclusion of any such issue in the hearing. The ruling on such a motion is subject to review in accordance with 12.35(b). Failure to so move constitutes a waiver of the right to a hearing on such an issue. Separation of functions on all issues resumes upon issuance of a notice of hearing. The Office of the General Counsel, Department of Health and Human Services, will observe the same separation of functions.

(g) Summary judgment. A person who requests a hearing may not rely upon allegations or denials but is required to set forth specific facts showing that there is a genuine and substantial issue of fact that requires a hearing with respect to a particular drug product specified in the request for hearing.

  (1) Where a specific notice of opportunity for hearing (as defined in paragraph (a)(1) of this section) is used, the Commissioner will enter summary judgment against a person who requests a hearing, making findings and conclusions, denying a hearing, if it conclusively appears from the face of the data, information, and factual analyses in the request for the hearing that there is no genuine and substantial issue of fact which precludes the refusal to approve the application or abbreviated application or the withdrawal of approval of the application or abbreviated application; for example, no

adequate and well-controlled clinical investigations meeting each of the precise elements of 314.126 and, for a combination drug product, 300.50 of this chapter, showing effectiveness have been identified. Any order entering summary judgment is required to set forth the Commissioner's findings and conclusions in detail and is required to specify why each study submitted fails to meet the requirements of the statute and regulations or why the request for hearing does not raise a genuine and substantial issue of fact.

(2) When following a general notice of opportunity for a hearing (as defined in paragraph (a)(1) of this section) the Director of the Center for Drug Evaluation and Research concludes that summary judgment against a person requesting a hearing should be considered, the Director will serve upon the person requesting a hearing by registered mail a proposed order denying a hearing. This person has 60 days after receipt of the proposed order to respond with sufficient data, information, and analyses to demonstrate that there is a genuine and substantial issue of fact which justifies a hearing.

(3) When following a general or specific notice of opportunity for a hearing a person requesting a hearing submits data or information of a type required by the statute and regulations, and the Director of the Center for Drug Evaluation and Research concludes that summary judgment against the person should be considered, the Director will serve upon the person by registered mail a proposed order denying a hearing. The person has 60 days after receipt of the proposed order to respond with sufficient data, information, and analyses to demonstrate that there is a genuine and substantial issue of fact which justifies a hearing.

(4) If review of the data, information, and analyses submitted show that the grounds cited in the notice are not valid, for example, that substantial evidence of effectiveness exists, the Commissioner will enter summary judgment for the person requesting the hearing, and rescind the notice of opportunity for hearing.

(5) If the Commissioner grants a hearing, it will begin within 90 days after the expiration of the time for requesting the hearing unless the parties otherwise agree in the case of denial of approval, and as soon as practicable in the case of withdrawal of approval.

(6) The Commissioner will grant a hearing if there exists a genuine and substantial issue of fact or if the Commissioner concludes that a hearing would otherwise be in the public interest.

(7) If the manufacturer or distributor of an identical, related, or similar drug product requests and is granted a hearing, the hearing may consider whether the product is in fact identical, related, or similar to the drug product named in the notice of opportunity for a hearing.

(8) A request for a hearing, and any subsequent grant or denial of a hearing, applies only to the drug products named in such documents.

(h) FDA will issue a notice withdrawing approval and declaring all products unlawful for drug products subject to a notice of opportunity for a hearing, including any identical, related, or similar drug product under 310.6, for which an opportunity for a hearing is waived or for which a hearing is denied. The Commissioner may defer or stay the action pending a ruling on any related request for a hearing or pending any related hearing or other administrative or judicial proceeding.

[50 FR 7493, Feb. 22, 1985; 50 FR 14212, Apr. 11, 1985, as amended at 50 FR 21238, May 23, 1985; 55 FR 11580, Mar. 29, 1990; 57 FR 17996, Apr. 28, 1992; 59 FR 14364, Mar. 28, 1994; 63 FR 5252, Feb. 2, 1998; 67 FR 9586, Mar. 4, 2002; 68 FR 24879, May 9, 2003; 69 FR 48775, Aug. 11, 2004; 74 FR 13113, Mar. 26, 2009]

Sec. 314.201 Procedure for hearings.

Parts 10 through 16 apply to hearings relating to new drugs under section 505 (d) and (e) of the act.

Sec. 314.235 Judicial review.

(a) The Commissioner of Food and Drugs will certify the transcript and record. In any case in which the Commissioner enters an order without a hearing under 314.200(g), the record certified by the Commissioner is required to include the requests for hearing together with the data and information submitted and the Commissioner's findings and conclusion.

(b) A manufacturer or distributor of an identical, related, or similar drug product under 310.6 may seek judicial review of an order withdrawing approval of a new drug application, whether or not a hearing has been held, in a United States court of appeals under section 505(h) of the act.

Subpart F [Reserved]

Subpart G--Miscellaneous Provisions

Sec. 314.410 Imports and exports of new drugs.

(a) Imports.

    (1) A new drug may be imported into the United States if: (i) It is the subject of an approved application under this part; or (ii) it complies with the regulations pertaining to investigational new drugs under part 312; and it complies with the general regulations pertaining to imports under subpart E of part 1.

    (2) A drug substance intended for use in the manufacture, processing, or repacking of a new drug may be imported into the United States if it complies with the labeling exemption in 201.122 pertaining to shipments of drug substances in domestic commerce.

(b) Exports.

    (1) A new drug may be exported if it is the subject of an approved application under this part or it complies with the regulations pertaining to investigational new drugs under part 312.

    (2) A new drug substance that is covered by an application approved under this part for use in the manufacture of an approved drug product may be exported by the applicant or any person listed as a supplier in the approved application, provided the drug substance intended for export meets the specification of, and is shipped with a copy of the labeling required for, the approved drug product.

    (3) Insulin or an antibiotic drug may be exported without regard to the requirements in section 802 of the act if the insulin or antibiotic drug meets the requirements of section 801(e)(1) of the act.

[50 FR 7493, Feb. 22, 1985, unless otherwise noted. Redesignated at 57 FR 17983, Apr. 28, 1992, and amended at 64 FR 402, Jan. 5, 1999; 69 FR 18766, Apr. 8, 2004]

Sec. 314.420 Drug master files.

(a) A drug master file is a submission of information to the Food and Drug Administration by a person (the drug master file holder) who intends it to be used for one of the following purposes: To permit the holder to incorporate the information by reference when the holder submits an investigational new drug application under part 312 or submits an application or an abbreviated application or an amendment or supplement to them under this part, or to permit the holder to authorize other persons to rely on the information to support a submission to FDA without the holder having to disclose the information to the person. FDA ordinarily neither independently reviews drug master files nor approves or disapproves submissions to a drug master file. Instead, the agency customarily reviews the information only in the context of an application under part 312 or this part. A drug master file may contain information of the kind required for any submission to the agency, including information about the following:

(1) [Reserved]

(2) Drug substance, drug substance intermediate, and materials used in their preparation, or drug product;

(3) Packaging materials;

(4) Excipient, colorant, flavor, essence, or materials used in their preparation;

(5) FDA-accepted reference information. (A person wishing to submit information and supporting data in a drug master file (DMF) that is not covered by Types II through IV DMF's must first submit a letter of intent to the Drug Master File Staff, Food and Drug Administration, 5901-B Ammendale Rd., Beltsville, MD 20705-1266.) FDA will then contact the person to discuss the proposed submission.

(b) An investigational new drug application or an application, abbreviated application, amendment, or supplement may incorporate by reference all or part of the contents of any drug master file in support of the submission if the holder authorizes the incorporation in writing. Each incorporation by reference is required to describe the incorporated material by name, reference number, volume, and page number of the drug master file.

(c) A drug master file is required to be submitted in two copies. The agency has prepared guidance that provides information about how to prepare a well-organized drug master file. If the drug master file holder adds, changes, or deletes any information in the file, the holder shall notify in writing, each person authorized to reference that information. Any addition, change, or deletion of information in a drug master file (except the list required under paragraph (d) of this section) is required to be submitted in two copies and to describe by name, reference number, volume, and page number the information affected in the drug master file.

(d) The drug master file is required to contain a complete list of each person currently authorized to incorporate by reference any information in the file, identifying by name, reference number, volume, and page number the information that each person is authorized to incorporate. If the holder restricts the authorization to particular drug products, the list is required to include the name of each drug product and the application number, if known, to which the authorization applies.

(e) The public availability of data and information in a drug master file, including the availability of data and information in the file to a person authorized to reference the file, is determined under part 20 and 314.430.

[50 FR 7493, Feb. 22, 1985, as amended at 50 FR 21238, May 23, 1985; 53 FR 33122, Aug. 30, 1988; 55 FR 28380, July 11, 1990; 65 FR 1780, Jan. 12, 2000; 65 FR 56479, Sept. 19, 2000; 67 FR 9586, Mar. 4, 2002; 69 FR 13473, Mar. 23, 2004]

Sec. 314.430 Availability for public disclosure of data and information in an application or abbreviated application.

(a) The Food and Drug Administration will determine the public availability of any part of an application or abbreviated application under this section and part 20 of this chapter. For purposes of this section, the application or abbreviated application includes all data and information submitted with or incorporated by reference in the application or abbreviated application, including investigational new drug applications, drug master files under 314.420, supplements submitted under 314.70 or 314.97, reports under 314.80 or 314.98, and other submissions. For purposes of this section, safety and effectiveness data include all studies and tests of a drug on animals and humans and all studies and tests of the drug for identity, stability, purity, potency, and bioavailability.

(b) FDA will not publicly disclose the existence of an application or abbreviated application before an approval letter is sent to the applicant under 314.105 or tentative approval letter is sent to the applicant under 314.107, unless the existence of the application or abbreviated application has been previously publicly disclosed or acknowledged.

(c) If the existence of an unapproved application or abbreviated application has not been publicly disclosed or acknowledged, no data or information in the application or abbreviated application is available for public disclosure.

(d)(1) If the existence of an application or abbreviated application has been publicly disclosed or acknowledged before the agency sends an approval letter to the applicant, no data or information contained in the application or abbreviated application is available for public disclosure before the agency sends an approval letter, but the Commissioner may, in his or her discretion, disclose a summary of selected portions of the safety and effectiveness data that are appropriate for public consideration of a specific pending issue; for example, for consideration of an open session of an FDA advisory committee.

(2) Notwithstanding paragraph (d)(1) of this section, FDA will make available to the public upon request the information in the investigational new drug application that was required to be filed in Docket Number 95S-0158 in the Division of Dockets Management (HFA-305), Food and Drug Administration, 5630 Fishers Lane, rm. 1061, Rockville, MD 20852, for investigations involving an exception from informed consent under 50.24 of this chapter. Persons wishing to request this information shall submit a request under the Freedom of Information Act.

(e) After FDA sends an approval letter to the applicant, the following data and information in the application or abbreviated application are immediately available for public disclosure, unless the applicant shows that extraordinary circumstances exist. A list of approved applications and abbreviated applications, entitled "Approved Drug Products with Therapeutic Equivalence

Part 314

Evaluations," is available from the Government Printing Office, Washington, DC 20402. This list is updated monthly.

(1) [Reserved]

(2) If the application applies to a new drug, all safety and effectiveness data previously disclosed to the public as set forth in 20.81 and a summary or summaries of the safety and effectiveness data and information submitted with or incorporated by reference in the application. The summaries do not constitute the full reports of investigations under section 505(b)(1) of the act (21 U.S.C. 355(b)(1)) on which the safety or effectiveness of the drug may be approved. The summaries consist of the following:

(i) For an application approved before July 1, 1975, internal agency records that describe safety and effectiveness data and information, for example, a summary of the basis for approval or internal reviews of the data and information, after deletion of the following:

(a) Names and any information that would identify patients or test subjects or investigators.

(b) Any inappropriate gratuitous comments unnecessary to an objective analysis of the data and information.

(ii) For an application approved on or after July 1, 1975, a Summary Basis of Approval (SBA) document that contains a summary of the safety and effectiveness data and information evaluated by FDA during the drug approval process. The SBA is prepared in one of the following ways:

(a) Before approval of the application, the applicant may prepare a draft SBA which the Center for Drug Evaluation and Research will review and may revise. The draft may be submitted with the application or as an amendment.

(b) The Center for Drug Evaluation and Research may prepare the SBA.

(3) A protocol for a test or study, unless it is shown to fall within the exemption established for trade secrets and confidential commercial information in 20.61.

(4) Adverse reaction reports, product experience reports, consumer complaints, and other similar data and information after deletion of the following:

   (i) Names and any information that would identify the person using the product.

   (ii) Names and any information that would identify any third party involved with the report, such as a physician or hospital or other institution.

(5) A list of all active ingredients and any inactive ingredients previously disclosed to the public as set forth in 20.81.

(6) An assay procedure or other analytical procedure, unless it serves no regulatory or compliance purpose and is shown to fall within the exemption established for trade secrets and confidential commercial information in 20.61.

(7) All correspondence and written summaries of oral discussions between FDA and the applicant relating to the application, under the provisions of part 20.

(f) All safety and effectiveness data and information which have been submitted in an application and which have not previously been disclosed to the public are available to the public, upon request, at the time any one of the following events occurs unless extraordinary circumstances are shown:

(1) No work is being or will be undertaken to have the application approved.

(2) A final determination is made that the application is not approvable and all legal appeals have been exhausted.

(3) Approval of the application is withdrawn and all legal appeals have been exhausted.

(4) A final determination has been made that the drug is not a new drug.

(5) For applications submitted under section 505(b) of the act, the effective date of the approval of the first abbreviated application submitted under section 505(j) of the act which refers to such drug, or the date on which the approval of an abbreviated application under section 505(j) of the act which refers to such drug could be made effective if such an abbreviated application had been submitted.

(6) For abbreviated applications submitted under section 505(j) of the act, when FDA sends an approval letter to the applicant.

(g) The following data and information in an application or abbreviated application are not available for public disclosure unless they have been previously disclosed to the public as set forth in 20.81 of this chapter or they relate to a product or ingredient that has been abandoned and they do not represent a trade secret or confidential commercial or financial information under 20.61 of this chapter:

(1) Manufacturing methods or processes, including quality control procedures.

(2) Production, sales distribution, and similar data and information, except that any compilation of that data and information aggregated and prepared in a way that does not reveal data or information which is not available for public disclosure under this provision is available for public disclosure.

(3) Quantitative or semiquantitative formulas.

(h) The compilations of information specified in 20.117 are available for public disclosure.

[50 FR 7493, Feb. 22, 1985, as amended at 50 FR 21238, May 23, 1985; 55 FR 11580, Mar. 29, 1990; 57 FR 17996, Apr. 28, 1992; 61 FR 51530, Oct. 2, 1996; 64 FR 26698, May 13, 1998; 64 FR 402, Jan. 5, 1999; 66 FR 1832, Jan. 10, 2001; 68 FR 24879, May 9, 2003; 69 FR 18766, Apr. 8, 2004; 73 FR 39610, July 10, 2008]

Sec. 314.440 Addresses for applications and abbreviated applications.

(a) Applicants shall send applications, abbreviated applications, and other correspondence relating to matters covered by this part, except for products listed in paragraph (b) of this section, to the appropriate office identified below:

(1) Except as provided in paragraph (a)(4) of this section, an application under 314.50 or 314.54 submitted for filing should be directed to the Central Document Room, 5901-B Ammendale Rd., Beltsville, MD 20705-1266. Applicants may obtain information about folders for binding applications on the Internet athttp://www.fda.gov/cder/ddms/binders.htm.

After FDA has filed the application, the agency will inform the applicant which division is responsible for the application. Amendments, supplements, resubmissions, requests for waivers, and other correspondence about an application that has been filed should be addressed to 5901-B Ammendale Rd., Beltsville, MD 20705-1266, to the attention of the appropriate division.

(2) Except as provided in paragraph (a)(4) of this section, an abbreviated application under 314.94, and amendments, supplements, and resubmissions should be directed to the Office of Generic Drugs (HFD-600), Center for Drug Evaluation and Research, Food and Drug Administration, Metro Park North VII, 7620 Standish Pl., Rockville, MD 20855. This includes items sent by parcel post or overnight courier service. Correspondence not associated with an abbreviated application should be addressed specifically to the intended office or division and to the person as follows: Office of Generic Drugs, Center for Drug Evaluation and Research, Food and Drug Administration, Attn: [insert name of person], Metro Park North II, HFD-[insert mail code of office or division], 7500 Standish Place, rm. 150, Rockville, MD 20855. The mail code for the Office of Generic Drugs is HFD-600, the mail codes for the Divisions of Chemistry I, II, and III are HFD-620, HFD-640, and HFD-630, respectively, and the mail code for the Division of Bioequivalence is HFD-650.

(3) A request for an opportunity for a hearing under 314.110 on the question of whether there are grounds for denying approval of an application, except an application under paragraph (b) of this section, should be directed to the Associate Director for Policy (HFD-5).

(4) The field copy of an application, an abbreviated application, amendments, supplements, resubmissions, requests for waivers, and other correspondence about an application and an abbreviated application shall be sent to the applicant's home FDA district office, except that a foreign applicant shall send the field copy to the appropriate address identified in paragraphs (a)(1) and (a)(2) of this section.

(b) Applicants shall send applications and other correspondence relating to matters covered by this part for the drug products listed below to the Document Control Center (HFM-99), Center for Biologics Evaluation and Research, 1401 Rockville Pike, suite

Part 314

200N, Rockville, MD 20852-1448, except applicants shall send a request for an opportunity for a hearing under 314.110 on the question of whether there are grounds for denying approval of an application to the Director, Center for Biologics Evaluation and Research (HFM-1), at the same address.

(1) Ingredients packaged together with containers intended for the collection, processing, or storage of blood and blood components;

(2) Plasma volume expanders and hydroxyethyl starch for leukapheresis;

(3) Blood component processing solutions and shelf life extenders; and

(4) Oxygen carriers.

[50 FR 7493, Feb. 22, 1985, as amended at 50 FR 21238, May 23, 1985; 55 FR 11581, Mar. 29, 1990; 57 FR 17997, Apr. 28, 1992; 58 FR 47352, Sept. 8, 1993; 62 FR 43639, Aug. 15, 1997; 69 FR 13473, Mar. 23, 2004; 70 FR 14981, Mar. 24, 2005; 73 FR 39610, July 10, 2008; 74 FR 13113, Mar. 26, 2009; 75 FR 37295, June 29, 2010]

Sec. 314.445 Guidance documents.

(a) FDA has made available guidance documents under 10.115 of this chapter to help you to comply with certain requirements of this part.

(b) The Center for Drug Evaluation and Research (CDER) maintains a list of guidance documents that apply to CDER's regulations. The list is maintained on the Internet and is published annually in theFederal Register.A request for a copy of the CDER list should be directed to the Office of Training and Communications, Division of Drug Information, Center for Drug Evaluation and Research, Food and Drug Administration, 10903 New Hampshire Ave., Silver Spring, MD 20993-0002.

[65 FR 56480, Sept. 19, 2000, as amended at 74 FR 13113, Mar. 26, 2009]

Subpart H--Accelerated Approval of New Drugs for Serious or Life-Threatening Illnesses

Sec. 314.500 Scope.

This subpart applies to certain new drug products that have been studied for their safety and effectiveness in treating serious or life-threatening illnesses and that provide meaningful therapeutic benefit to patients over existing treatments (e.g., ability to treat patients unresponsive to, or intolerant of, available therapy, or improved patient response over available therapy).

[57 FR 58958, Dec. 11, 1992, as amended at 64 FR 402, Jan. 5, 1999]

Sec. 314.510 Approval based on a surrogate endpoint or on an effect on a clinical endpoint other than survival or irreversible morbidity.

FDA may grant marketing approval for a new drug product on the basis of adequate and well-controlled clinical trials establishing that the drug product has an effect on a surrogate endpoint that is reasonably likely, based on epidemiologic, therapeutic, pathophysiologic, or other evidence, to predict clinical benefit or on the basis of an effect on a clinical endpoint other than survival or irreversible morbidity. Approval under this section will be subject to the requirement that the applicant study the drug further, to verify and describe its clinical benefit, where there is uncertainty as to the relation of the surrogate endpoint to clinical benefit, or of the observed clinical benefit to ultimate outcome. Postmarketing studies would usually be studies already underway. When required to be conducted, such studies must also be adequate and well-controlled. The applicant shall carry out any such studies with due diligence.

Sec. 314.520 Approval with restrictions to assure safe use.

(a) If FDA concludes that a drug product shown to be effective can be safely used only if distribution or use is restricted, FDA will require such postmarketing restrictions as are needed to assure safe use of the drug product, such as:

(1) Distribution restricted to certain facilities or physicians with special training or experience; or

(2) Distribution conditioned on the performance of specified medical procedures.

(b) The limitations imposed will be commensurate with the specific safety concerns presented by the drug product.

Sec. 314.530 Withdrawal procedures.

(a) For new drugs approved under 314.510 and 314.520, FDA may withdraw approval, following a hearing as provided in part 15 of this chapter, as modified by this section, if:

    (1) A postmarketing clinical study fails to verify clinical benefit;

    (2) The applicant fails to perform the required postmarketing study with due diligence;

    (3) Use after marketing demonstrates that postmarketing restrictions are inadequate to assure safe use of the drug product;

    (4) The applicant fails to adhere to the postmarketing restrictions agreed upon;

    (5) The promotional materials are false or misleading; or

    (6) Other evidence demonstrates that the drug product is not shown to be safe or effective under its conditions of use.

(b) Notice of opportunity for a hearing. The Director of the Center for Drug Evaluation and Research will give the applicant notice of an opportunity for a hearing on the Center's proposal to withdraw the approval of an application approved under 314.510 or 314.520. The notice, which will ordinarily be a letter, will state generally the reasons for the action and the proposed grounds for the order.

(c) Submission of data and information.

    (1) If the applicant fails to file a written request for a hearing within 15 days of receipt of the notice, the applicant waives the opportunity for a hearing.

    (2) If the applicant files a timely request for a hearing, the agency will publish a notice of hearing in theFederal Registerin accordance with 12.32(e) and 15.20 of this chapter.

    (3) An applicant who requests a hearing under this section must, within 30 days of receipt of the notice of opportunity for a hearing, submit the data and information upon which the applicant intends to rely at the hearing.

(d) Separation of functions. Separation of functions (as specified in 10.55 of this chapter) will not apply at any point in withdrawal proceedings under this section.

(e) Procedures for hearings. Hearings held under this section will be conducted in accordance with the provisions of part 15 of this chapter, with the following modifications:

(1) An advisory committee duly constituted under part 14 of this chapter will be present at the hearing. The committee will be asked to review the issues involved and to provide advice and recommendations to the Commissioner of Food and Drugs.

(2) The presiding officer, the advisory committee members, up to three representatives of the applicant, and up to three representatives of the Center may question any person during or at the conclusion of the person's presentation. No other person attending the hearing may question a person making a presentation. The presiding officer may, as a matter of discretion, permit questions to be submitted to the presiding officer for response by a person making a presentation.

(f) Judicial review. The Commissioner's decision constitutes final agency action from which the applicant may petition for judicial review. Before requesting an order from a court for a stay of action pending review, an applicant must first submit a petition for a stay of action under 10.35 of this chapter.

[57 FR 58958, Dec. 11, 1992, as amended at 64 FR 402, Jan. 5, 1999]

Sec. 314.540 Postmarketing safety reporting.

Drug products approved under this program are subject to the postmarketing recordkeeping and safety reporting applicable to all approved drug products, as provided in 314.80 and 314.81.

Sec. 314.550 Promotional materials.

For drug products being considered for approval under this subpart, unless otherwise informed by the agency, applicants must submit to the agency for consideration during the preapproval review period copies of all promotional materials, including promotional labeling as well as advertisements, intended for dissemination or publication within 120 days following marketing approval. After 120 days following marketing approval, unless otherwise informed by the

Part 314

agency, the applicant must submit promotional materials at least 30 days prior to the intended time of initial dissemination of the labeling or initial publication of the advertisement.

Sec. 314.560 Termination of requirements.

If FDA determines after approval that the requirements established in 314.520, 314.530, or 314.550 are no longer necessary for the safe and effective use of a drug product, it will so notify the applicant. Ordinarily, for drug products approved under 314.510, these requirements will no longer apply when FDA determines that the required postmarketing study verifies and describes the drug product's clinical benefit and the drug product would be appropriate for approval under traditional procedures. For drug products approved under 314.520, the restrictions would no longer apply when FDA determines that safe use of the drug product can be assured through appropriate labeling. FDA also retains the discretion to remove specific postapproval requirements upon review of a petition submitted by the sponsor in accordance with 10.30.

Subpart I--Approval of New Drugs When Human Efficacy Studies Are Not Ethical or Feasible

Sec. 314.600 Scope.

This subpart applies to certain new drug products that have been studied for their safety and efficacy in ameliorating or preventing serious or life-threatening conditions caused by exposure to lethal or permanently disabling toxic biological, chemical, radiological, or nuclear substances. This subpart applies only to those new drug products for which: Definitive human efficacy studies cannot be conducted because it would be unethical to deliberately expose healthy human volunteers to a lethal or permanently disabling toxic biological, chemical, radiological, or nuclear substance; and field trials to study the product's effectiveness after an accidental or hostile exposure have not been feasible. This subpart does not apply to products that can be approved based on efficacy standards described elsewhere in FDA's regulations (e.g., accelerated approval based on surrogate markers or clinical endpoints other than survival or irreversible morbidity), nor does it address the safety evaluation for the products to which it does apply.

Sec. 314.610 Approval based on evidence of effectiveness from studies in animals.

(a) FDA may grant marketing approval for a new drug product for which safety has been established and for which the requirements of 314.600 are met based on adequate and well-controlled animal studies when the results of those animal studies establish that the drug product is reasonably likely to produce clinical benefit in humans. In assessing the sufficiency of animal data, the agency may take into account other data, including human data, available to the agency. FDA will rely on the evidence from studies in animals to provide substantial evidence of the effectiveness of these products only when:

(1) There is a reasonably well-understood pathophysiological mechanism of the toxicity of the substance and its prevention or substantial reduction by the product;

(2) The effect is demonstrated in more than one animal species expected to react with a response predictive for humans, unless the effect is demonstrated in a single animal species that represents a sufficiently well-characterized animal model for predicting the response in humans;

(3) The animal study endpoint is clearly related to the desired benefit in humans, generally the enhancement of survival or prevention of major morbidity; and

(4) The data or information on the kinetics and pharmacodynamics of the product or other relevant data or information, in animals and humans, allows selection of an effective dose in humans.

(b) Approval under this subpart will be subject to three requirements:

(1) Postmarketing studies. The applicant must conduct postmarketing studies, such as field studies, to verify and describe the drug's clinical benefit and to assess its safety when used as indicated when such studies are feasible and ethical. Such postmarketing studies would not be feasible until an exigency arises. When such studies are feasible, the applicant must conduct such studies with due diligence. Applicants must include as part of their application a plan or approach to postmarketing study commitments in the event such studies become ethical and feasible.

(2) Approval with restrictions to ensure safe use. If FDA concludes that a drug product shown to be effective under this subpart can be safely used only if distribution or use is restricted, FDA will require such postmarketing restrictions as are needed to ensure safe use of the drug product, commensurate with the specific safety concerns presented by the drug product, such as:

(i) Distribution restricted to certain facilities or health care practitioners with special training or experience;

(ii) Distribution conditioned on the performance of specified medical procedures, including medical followup; and

(iii) Distribution conditioned on specified recordkeeping requirements.

(3) Information to be provided to patient recipients. For drug products or specific indications approved under this subpart, applicants must prepare, as part of their proposed labeling, labeling to be provided to patient recipients. The patient labeling must explain that, for ethical or feasibility reasons, the drug's approval was based on efficacy studies conducted in animals alone and must give the drug's indication(s), directions for use (dosage and administration), contraindications, a description of any reasonably foreseeable risks, adverse reactions, anticipated benefits, drug interactions, and any other relevant information required by FDA at the time of approval. The patient labeling must be available with the product to be provided to patients prior to administration or dispensing of the drug product for the use approved under this subpart, if possible.

Sec. 314.620 Withdrawal procedures.

(a) Reasons to withdraw approval. For new drugs approved under this subpart, FDA may withdraw approval, following a hearing as provided in part 15 of this chapter, as modified by this section, if:

(1) A postmarketing clinical study fails to verify clinical benefit;

(2) The applicant fails to perform the postmarketing study with due diligence;

(3) Use after marketing demonstrates that postmarketing restrictions are inadequate to ensure safe use of the drug product;

(4) The applicant fails to adhere to the postmarketing restrictions applied at the time of approval under this subpart;

(5) The promotional materials are false or misleading; or

(6) Other evidence demonstrates that the drug product is not shown to be safe or effective under its conditions of use.

(b) Notice of opportunity for a hearing. The Director of the Center for Drug Evaluation and Research (CDER) will give the applicant notice of an opportunity for a hearing on CDER's proposal to withdraw the approval of an application approved under this subpart. The notice, which will ordinarily be a letter, will state generally the reasons for the action and the proposed grounds for the order.

(c) Submission of data and information.

(1) If the applicant fails to file a written request for a hearing within 15 days of receipt of the notice, the applicant waives the opportunity for a hearing.

(2) If the applicant files a timely request for a hearing, the agency will publish a notice of hearing in theFederal Registerin accordance with 12.32(e) and 15.20 of this chapter.

(3) An applicant who requests a hearing under this section must, within 30 days of receipt of the notice of opportunity for a hearing, submit the data and information upon which the applicant intends to rely at the hearing.

(d) Separation of functions. Separation of functions (as specified in 10.55 of this chapter) will not apply at any point in withdrawal proceedings under this section.

(e) Procedures for hearings. Hearings held under this section will be conducted in accordance with the provisions of part 15 of this chapter, with the following modifications:

(1) An advisory committee duly constituted under part 14 of this chapter will be present at the hearing. The committee will be asked to review the issues involved and to provide advice and recommendations to the Commissioner of Food and Drugs.

(2) The presiding officer, the advisory committee members, up to three representatives of the applicant, and up to three representatives of CDER may question any person during or

at the conclusion of the person's presentation. No other person attending the hearing may question a person making a presentation. The presiding officer may, as a matter of discretion, permit questions to be submitted to the presiding officer for response by a person making a presentation.

(f) Judicial review. The Commissioner of Food and Drugs' decision constitutes final agency action from which the applicant may petition for judicial review. Before requesting an order from a court for a stay of action pending review, an applicant must first submit a petition for a stay of action under 10.35 of this chapter.

Sec. 314.630 Postmarketing safety reporting.

Drug products approved under this subpart are subject to the postmarketing recordkeeping and safety reporting requirements applicable to all approved drug products, as provided in 314.80 and 314.81.

Sec. 314.640 Promotional materials.

For drug products being considered for approval under this subpart, unless otherwise informed by the agency, applicants must submit to the agency for consideration during the preapproval review period copies of all promotional materials, including promotional labeling as well as advertisements, intended for dissemination or publication within 120 days following marketing approval. After 120 days following marketing approval, unless otherwise informed by the agency, the applicant must submit promotional materials at least 30 days prior to the intended time of initial dissemination of the labeling or initial publication of the advertisement.

Sec. 314.650 Termination of requirements.

If FDA determines after approval under this subpart that the requirements established in 314.610(b)(2), 314.620, and 314.630 are no longer necessary for the safe and effective use of a drug product, FDA will so notify the applicant. Ordinarily, for drug products approved under 314.610, these requirements will no longer apply when FDA determines that the postmarketing study verifies and describes the drug product's clinical benefit. For drug products approved under 314.610, the restrictions would no longer apply when FDA determines that safe use of the drug product can be ensured through appropriate labeling. FDA also retains the discretion to remove specific postapproval requirements upon review of a petition submitted by the sponsor in accordance with 10.30 of this chapter.

Authority: 21 U.S.C. 321, 331, 351, 352, 353, 355, 356, 356a, 356b, 356c, 371, 374, 379e.

Source: 50 FR 7493, Feb. 22, 1985, unless otherwise noted.

Part 320: Bioavailability and Bioequivalence Requirements

[Code of Federal Regulations]

[Title 21, Volume 5]

[Revised as of April 1, 2009]

[CITE: 21CFR320]

Title 21--Food and Drugs

Chapter I--Food and Drug Administration

Department of Health and Human Services

Subchapter D--Drugs for Human Use

Part 320 Bioavailability and Bioequivalence Requirements[1]

Subpart A--General Provisions

Sec. 320.1 Definitions.

(a) ***Bioavailability*** means the rate and extent to which the active ingredient or active moiety is absorbed from a drug product and becomes available at the site of action. For drug products that are not intended to be absorbed into the bloodstream, bioavailability may be assessed by measurements intended to reflect the rate and extent to which the active ingredient or active moiety becomes available at the site of action.

(b) ***Drug product*** means a finished dosage form, e.g., tablet, capsule, or solution, that contains the active drug ingredient, generally, but not necessarily, in association with inactive ingredients.

---

[1] Available on the FDA website at http://www.accessdata.fda.gov/scripts/cdrh/cfdocs/cfcfr/CFRSearch.cfm?CFRPart=320&showFR=1

(c) **Pharmaceutical equivalents** means drug products in identical dosage forms that contain identical amounts of the identical active drug ingredient,i.e. , the same salt or ester of the same therapeutic moiety, or, in the case of modified release dosage forms that require a reservoir or overage or such forms as prefilled syringes where residual volume may vary, that deliver identical amounts of the active drug ingredient over the identical dosing period; do not necessarily contain the same inactive ingredients; and meet the identical compendial or other applicable standard of identity, strength, quality, and purity, including potency and, where applicable, content uniformity, disintegration times, and/or dissolution rates.

(d) **Pharmaceutical alternatives** means drug products that contain the identical therapeutic moiety, or its precursor, but not necessarily in the same amount or dosage form or as the same salt or ester. Each such drug product individually meets either the identical or its own respective compendial or other applicable standard of identity, strength, quality, and purity, including potency and, where applicable, content uniformity, disintegration times and/or dissolution rates.

(e) **Bioequivalence** means the absence of a significant difference in the rate and extent to which the active ingredient or active moiety in pharmaceutical equivalents or pharmaceutical alternatives becomes available at the site of drug action when administered at the same molar dose under similar conditions in an appropriately designed study. Where there is an intentional difference in rate (e.g., in certain extended release dosage forms), certain pharmaceutical equivalents or alternatives may be considered bioequivalent if there is no significant difference in the extent to which the active ingredient or moiety from each product becomes available at the site of drug action. This applies only if the difference in the rate at which the active ingredient or moiety becomes available at the site of drug action is intentional and is reflected in the proposed labeling, is not essential to the attainment of effective body drug concentrations on chronic use, and is considered medically insignificant for the drug.

(f) **Bioequivalence requirement** means a requirement imposed by the Food and Drug Administration for in vitro and/or in vivo testing of specified drug products which must be satisfied as a condition of marketing.

(g) **Same drug product formulation** means the formulation of the drug product submitted for approval and any formulations that have minor differences in composition or method of manufacture from the formulation submitted for approval, but are similar enough to be relevant to the agency's determination of bioequivalence.

[42 FR 1634, Jan. 7, 1977, as amended at 42 FR 1648, Jan. 7, 1977; 57 FR 17997, Apr. 28, 1992; 67 FR 77672, Dec. 19, 2002; 74 FR 2861, Jan. 16, 2009]

Subpart B--Procedures for Determining the Bioavailability or Bioequivalence of Drug Products

Sec. 320.21 Requirements for submission of bioavailability and bioequivalence data.

(a) Any person submitting a full new drug application to the Food and Drug Administration (FDA) shall include in the application either:

(1) Evidence measuring the in vivo bioavailability of the drug product that is the subject of the application; or

(2) Information to permit FDA to waive the submission of evidence measuring in vivo bioavailability.

(b) Any person submitting an abbreviated new drug application to FDA shall include in the application either:

(1) Evidence demonstrating that the drug product that is the subject of the abbreviated new drug application is bioequivalent to the reference listed drug (defined in 314.3(b) of this chapter). A complete study report must be submitted for the bioequivalence study upon which the applicant relies for approval. For all other bioequivalence studies conducted on the same drug product formulation, the applicant must submit either a complete or summary report. If a summary report of a bioequivalence study is submitted and FDA determines that there may be bioequivalence issues or concerns with the product, FDA may require that the applicant submit a complete report of the bioequivalence study to FDA; or

(2) Information to show that the drug product is bioequivalent to the reference listed drug which would permit FDA to waive

the submission of evidence demonstrating in vivo
bioequivalence as provided in paragraph (f) of this section.

(c) Any person submitting a supplemental application to FDA shall
include in the supplemental application the evidence or
information set forth in paragraphs (a) and (b) of this section if
the supplemental application proposes any of the following
changes:

(1) A change in the manufacturing site or a change in the
manufacturing process, including a change in product
formulation or dosage strength, beyond the variations
provided for in the approved application.

(2) A change in the labeling to provide for a new indication for
use of the drug product, if clinical studies are required to
support the new indication for use.

(3) A change in the labeling to provide for a new dosage regimen
or for an additional dosage regimen for a special patient
population, e.g., infants, if clinical studies are required to
support the new or additional dosage regimen.

(d) FDA may approve a full new drug application, or a supplemental
application proposing any of the changes set forth in paragraph (c)
of this section, that does not contain evidence of in vivo
bioavailability or information to permit waiver of the requirement
for in vivo bioavailability data, if all of the following conditions are
met.

(1) The application is otherwise approvable.

(2) The application agrees to submit, within the time specified by
FDA, either:

(i) Evidence measuring the in vivo bioavailability and
demonstrating the in vivo bioequivalence of the drug
product that is the subject of the application; or

(ii) Information to permit FDA to waive measurement of in
vivo bioavailability.

(e) Evidence measuring the in vivo bioavailability and demonstrating
the in vivo bioequivalence of a drug product shall be obtained
using one of the approaches for determining bioavailability set
forth in 320.24.

(f) Information to permit FDA to waive the submission of evidence measuring the in vivo bioavailability or demonstrating the in vivo bioequivalence shall meet the criteria set forth in 320.22.

(g) Any person holding an approved full or abbreviated new drug application shall submit to FDA a supplemental application containing new evidence measuring the in vivo bioavailability or demonstrating the in vivo bioequivalence of the drug product that is the subject of the application if notified by FDA that:

(1) There are data demonstrating that the dosage regimen in the labeling is based on incorrect assumptions or facts regarding the pharmacokinetics of the drug product and that following this dosage regimen could potentially result in subtherapeutic or toxic levels; or

(2) There are data measuring significant intra-batch and batch-to-batch variability, e.g., plus or minus 25 percent, in the bioavailability of the drug product.

(h) The requirements of this section regarding the submission of evidence measuring the in vivo bioavailability or demonstrating the in vivo bioequivalence apply only to a full or abbreviated new drug application or a supplemental application for a finished dosage formulation.

[57 FR 17998, Apr. 28, 1992, as amended at 67 FR 77672, Dec. 19, 2002; 74 FR 2862, Jan. 16, 2009]

Sec. 320.22 Criteria for waiver of evidence of in vivo bioavailability or bioequivalence.

(a) Any person submitting a full or abbreviated new drug application, or a supplemental application proposing any of the changes set forth in 320.21(c), may request FDA to waive the requirement for the submission of evidence measuring the in vivo bioavailability or demonstrating the in vivo bioequivalence of the drug product that is the subject of the application. An applicant shall submit a request for waiver with the application. Except as provided in paragraph (f) of this section, FDA shall waive the requirement for the submission of evidence of in vivo bioavailability or bioequivalence if the drug product meets any of the provisions of paragraphs (b), (c), (d), or (e) of this section.

Part 320

(b) For certain drug products, the in vivo bioavailability or bioequivalence of the drug product may be self-evident. FDA shall waive the requirement for the submission of evidence obtained in vivo measuring the bioavailability or demonstrating the bioequivalence of these drug products. A drug product's in vivo bioavailability or bioequivalence may be considered self-evident based on other data in the application if the product meets one of the following criteria:

(1) The drug product:

    (i) Is a parenteral solution intended solely for administration by injection, or an ophthalmic or otic solution; and

    (ii) Contains the same active and inactive ingredients in the same concentration as a drug product that is the subject of an approved full new drug application or abbreviated new drug application.

(2) The drug product:

    (i) Is administered by inhalation as a gas, e.g., a medicinal or an inhalation anesthetic; and

    (ii) Contains an active ingredient in the same dosage form as a drug product that is the subject of an approved full new drug application or abbreviated new drug application.

(3) The drug product:

    (i) Is a solution for application to the skin, an oral solution, elixir, syrup, tincture, a solution for aerosolization or nebulization, a nasal solution, or similar other solubilized form; and

    (ii) Contains an active drug ingredient in the same concentration and dosage form as a drug product that is the subject of an approved full new drug application or abbreviated new drug application; and

    (iii) Contains no inactive ingredient or other change in formulation from the drug product that is the subject of the approved full new drug application or abbreviated new drug application that may significantly affect absorption of the active drug ingredient or active moiety for products that are systemically absorbed, or that may significantly affect systemic or local availability for products intended to act locally.

(c) FDA shall waive the requirement for the submission of evidence measuring the in vivo bioavailability or demonstrating the in vivo bioequivalence of a solid oral dosage form (other than a delayed release or extended release dosage form) of a drug product determined to be effective for at least one indication in a Drug Efficacy Study Implementation notice or which is identical, related, or similar to such a drug product under 310.6 of this chapter unless FDA has evaluated the drug product under the criteria set forth in 320.33, included the drug product in the Approved Drug Products with Therapeutic Equivalence Evaluations List, and rated the drug product as having a known or potential bioequivalence problem. A drug product so rated reflects a determination by FDA that an in vivo bioequivalence study is required.

(d) For certain drug products, bioavailability may be measured or bioequivalence may be demonstrated by evidence obtained in vitro in lieu of in vivo data. FDA shall waive the requirement for the submission of evidence obtained in vivo measuring the bioavailability or demonstrating the bioequivalence of the drug product if the drug product meets one of the following criteria:

Part 320

    (1) [Reserved]

    (2) The drug product is in the same dosage form, but in a different strength, and is proportionally similar in its active and inactive ingredients to another drug product for which the same manufacturer has obtained approval and the conditions in paragraphs (d)(2)(i) through (d)(2)(iii) of this section are met:

      (i) The bioavailability of this other drug product has been measured;

      (ii) Both drug products meet an appropriate in vitro test approved by FDA; and

      (iii) The applicant submits evidence showing that both drug products are proportionally similar in their active and inactive ingredients.

      (iv) Paragraph (d) of this section does not apply to delayed release or extended release products.

    (3) The drug product is, on the basis of scientific evidence submitted in the application, shown to meet an in vitro test that has been correlated with in vivo data.

(4) The drug product is a reformulated product that is identical, except for a different color, flavor, or preservative that could not affect the bioavailability of the reformulated product, to another drug product for which the same manufacturer has obtained approval and the following conditions are met:

(i) The bioavailability of the other product has been measured; and

(ii) Both drug products meet an appropriate in vitro test approved by FDA.

(e) FDA, for good cause, may waive a requirement for the submission of evidence of in vivo bioavailability or bioequivalence if waiver is compatible with the protection of the public health. For full new drug applications, FDA may defer a requirement for the submission of evidence of in vivo bioavailability if deferral is compatible with the protection of the public health.

(f) FDA, for good cause, may require evidence of in vivo bioavailability or bioequivalence for any drug product if the agency determines that any difference between the drug product and a listed drug may affect the bioavailability or bioequivalence of the drug product.

[57 FR 17998, Apr. 28, 1992, as amended at 67 FR 77673, Dec. 19, 2002]

Sec. 320.23 Basis for measuring in vivo bioavailability or demonstrating bioequivalence.

(a)(1) The in vivo bioavailability of a drug product is measured if the product's rate and extent of absorption, as determined by comparison of measured parameters, e.g., concentration of the active drug ingredient in the blood, urinary excretion rates, or pharmacological effects, do not indicate a significant difference from the reference material's rate and extent of absorption. For drug products that are not intended to be absorbed into the bloodstream, bioavailability may be assessed by measurements intended to reflect the rate and extent to which the active ingredient or active moiety becomes available at the site of action.

(2) Statistical techniques used shall be of sufficient sensitivity to detect differences in rate and extent of absorption that are not attributable to subject variability.

(3) A drug product that differs from the reference material in its rate of absorption, but not in its extent of absorption, may be considered to be bioavailable if the difference in the rate of absorption is intentional, is appropriately reflected in the labeling, is not essential to the attainment of effective body drug concentrations on chronic use, and is considered medically insignificant for the drug product.

(b) Two drug products will be considered bioequivalent drug products if they are pharmaceutical equivalents or pharmaceutical alternatives whose rate and extent of absorption do not show a significant difference when administered at the same molar dose of the active moiety under similar experimental conditions, either single dose or multiple dose. Some pharmaceutical equivalents or pharmaceutical alternatives may be equivalent in the extent of their absorption but not in their rate of absorption and yet may be considered bioequivalent because such differences in the rate of absorption are intentional and are reflected in the labeling, are not essential to the attainment of effective body drug concentrations on chronic use, and are considered medically insignificant for the particular drug product studied.

[57 FR 17999, Apr. 28, 1992, as amended at 67 FR 77673, Dec. 19, 2002]

Sec. 320.24 Types of evidence to measure bioavailability or establish bioequivalence.

(a) Bioavailability may be measured or bioequivalence may be demonstrated by several in vivo and in vitro methods. FDA may require in vivo or in vitro testing, or both, to measure the bioavailability of a drug product or establish the bioequivalence of specific drug products. Information on bioequivalence requirements for specific products is included in the current edition of FDA's publication "Approved Drug Products with Therapeutic Equivalence Evaluations" and any current supplement to the publication. The selection of the method used to meet an in vivo or in vitro testing requirement depends upon the purpose of the study, the analytical methods available, and the nature of the drug product. Applicants shall conduct bioavailability and bioequivalence testing using the most accurate, sensitive, and reproducible approach available among those set forth in paragraph (b) of this section. The method used must be capable of measuring bioavailability or establishing bioequivalence, as appropriate, for the product being tested.

Part 320

(b) The following in vivo and in vitro approaches, in descending order of accuracy, sensitivity, and reproducibility, are acceptable for determining the bioavailability or bioequivalence of a drug product.

(1)(i) An in vivo test in humans in which the concentration of the active ingredient or active moiety, and, when appropriate, its active metabolite(s), in whole blood, plasma, serum, or other appropriate biological fluid is measured as a function of time. This approach is particularly applicable to dosage forms intended to deliver the active moiety to the bloodstream for systemic distribution within the body; or

(ii) An in vitro test that has been correlated with and is predictive of human in vivo bioavailability data; or

(2) An in vivo test in humans in which the urinary excretion of the active moiety, and, when appropriate, its active metabolite(s), are measured as a function of time. The intervals at which measurements are taken should ordinarily be as short as possible so that the measure of the rate of elimination is as accurate as possible. Depending on the nature of the drug product, this approach may be applicable to the category of dosage forms described in paragraph (b)(1)(i) of this section. This method is not appropriate where urinary excretion is not a significant mechanism of elimination.

(3) An in vivo test in humans in which an appropriate acute pharmacological effect of the active moiety, and, when appropriate, its active metabolite(s), are measured as a function of time if such effect can be measured with sufficient accuracy, sensitivity, and reproducibility. This approach is applicable to the category of dosage forms described in paragraph (b)(1)(i) of this section only when appropriate methods are not available for measurement of the concentration of the moiety, and, when appropriate, its active metabolite(s), in biological fluids or excretory products but a method is available for the measurement of an appropriate acute pharmacological effect. This approach may be particularly applicable to dosage forms that are not intended to deliver the active moiety to the bloodstream for systemic distribution.

(4) Well-controlled clinical trials that establish the safety and effectiveness of the drug product, for purposes of measuring

bioavailability, or appropriately designed comparative clinical trials, for purposes of demonstrating bioequivalence. This approach is the least accurate, sensitive, and reproducible of the general approaches for measuring bioavailability or demonstrating bioequivalence. For dosage forms intended to deliver the active moiety to the bloodstream for systemic distribution, this approach may be considered acceptable only when analytical methods cannot be developed to permit use of one of the approaches outlined in paragraphs (b)(1)(i) and (b)(2) of this section, when the approaches described in paragraphs (b)(1)(ii), (b)(1)(iii), and (b)(3) of this section are not available. This approach may also be considered sufficiently accurate for measuring bioavailability or demonstrating bioequivalence of dosage forms intended to deliver the active moiety locally, e.g., topical preparations for the skin, eye, and mucous membranes; oral dosage forms not intended to be absorbed, e.g., an antacid or radiopaque medium; and bronchodilators administered by inhalation if the onset and duration of pharmacological activity are defined.

(5) A currently available in vitro test acceptable to FDA (usually a dissolution rate test) that ensures human in vivo bioavailability.

(6) Any other approach deemed adequate by FDA to measure bioavailability or establish bioequivalence.

(c) FDA may, notwithstanding prior requirements for measuring bioavailability or establishing bioequivalence, require in vivo testing in humans of a product at any time if the agency has evidence that the product:

(1) May not produce therapeutic effects comparable to a pharmaceutical equivalent or alternative with which it is intended to be used interchangeably;

(2) May not be bioequivalent to a pharmaceutical equivalent or alternative with which it is intended to be used interchangeably; or

(3) Has greater than anticipated potential toxicity related to pharmacokinetic or other characteristics.

[57 FR 17999, Apr. 28, 1992; 57 FR 29354, July 1, 1992, as amended at 67 FR 77673, Dec. 19, 2002]

Sec. 320.25 Guidelines for the conduct of an in vivo bioavailability study.

(a) Guiding principles.

(1) The basic principle in an in vivo bioavailability study is that no unnecessary human research should be done.

(2) An in vivo bioavailability study is generally done in a normal adult population under standardized conditions. In some situations, an in vivo bioavailability study in humans may preferably and more properly be done in suitable patients. Critically ill patients shall not be included in an in vivo bioavailability study unless the attending physician determines that there is a potential benefit to the patient.

(b) Basic design. The basic design of an in vivo bioavailability study is determined by the following:

(1) The scientific questions to be answered.

(2) The nature of the reference material and the dosage form to be tested.

(3) The availability of analytical methods.

(4) Benefit-risk considerations in regard to testing in humans.

(c) Comparison to a reference material. In vivo bioavailability testing of a drug product shall be in comparison to an appropriate reference material unless some other approach is more appropriate for valid scientific reasons.

(d) Previously unmarketed active drug ingredients or therapeutic moieties.

(1) An in vivo bioavailability study involving a drug product containing an active drug ingredient or therapeutic moiety that has not been approved for marketing can be used to measure the following pharmacokinetic data:

(i) The bioavailability of the formulation proposed for marketing; and

(ii) The essential pharmacokinetic characteristics of the active drug ingredient or therapeutic moiety, such as the rate of absorption, the extent of absorption, the half-life of the therapeutic moiety in vivo, and the rate of excretion and/or metabolism. Dose proportionality of the active drug ingredient or the therapeutic moiety needs to be established after single-dose administration and in certain instances after multiple-dose administration. This characterization is a necessary part of the investigation of the drug to support drug labeling.

(2) The reference material in such a bioavailability study should be a solution or suspension containing the same quantity of the active drug ingredient or therapeutic moiety as the formulation proposed for marketing.

(3) The reference material should be administered by the same route as the formulation proposed for marketing unless an alternative or additional route is necessary to answer the scientific question under study. For example, in the case of an active drug ingredient or therapeutic moiety that is poorly absorbed after oral administration, it may be necessary to compare the oral dosage form proposed for marketing with the active drug ingredient or therapeutic moiety administered in solution both orally and intravenously.

(e) New formulations of active drug ingredients or therapeutic moieties approved for marketing.

(1) An in vivo bioavailability study involving a drug product that is a new dosage form, or a new salt or ester of an active drug ingredient or therapeutic moiety that has been approved for marketing can be used to:

(i) Measure the bioavailability of the new formulation, new dosage form, or new salt or ester relative to an appropriate reference material; and

(ii) Define the pharmacokinetic parameters of the new formulation, new dosage form, or new salt or ester to establish dosage recommendation.

(2) The selection of the reference material(s) in such a bioavailability study depends upon the scientific questions to be answered, the data needed to establish comparability to a currently marketed drug product, and the data needed to establish dosage recommendations.

(3) The reference material should be taken from a current batch of a drug product that is the subject of an approved new drug application and that contains the same active drug ingredient

Part 320

or therapeutic moiety, if the new formulation, new dosage form, or new salt or ester is intended to be comparable to or to meet any comparative labeling claims made in relation to the drug product that is the subject of an approved new drug application.

(f) Extended release formulations.

    (1) The purpose of an in vivo bioavailability study involving a drug product for which an extended release claim is made is to determine if all of the following conditions are met:

        (i) The drug product meets the extended release claims made for it.

        (ii) The bioavailability profile established for the drug product rules out the occurrence of any dose dumping.

        (iii) The drug product's steady-state performance is equivalent to a currently marketed nonextended release or extended release drug product that contains the same active drug ingredient or therapeutic moiety and that is subject to an approved full new drug application.

        (iv) The drug product's formulation provides consistent pharmacokinetic performance between individual dosage units.

    (2) The reference material(s) for such a bioavailability study shall be chosen to permit an appropriate scientific evaluation of the extended release claims made for the drug product. The reference material shall be one of the following or any combination thereof:

        (i) A solution or suspension of the active drug ingredient or therapeutic moiety.

        (ii) A currently marketed noncontrolled release drug product containing the same active drug ingredient or therapeutic moiety and administered according to the dosage recommendations in the labeling of the noncontrolled release drug product.

        (iii) A currently marketed extended release drug product subject to an approved full new drug application containing the same active drug ingredient or therapeutic moiety and administered according to the dosage recommendations in the labeling proposed for the extended release drug product.

(iv) A reference material other than one set forth in paragraph (f)(2) (i), (ii) or (iii) of this section that is appropriate for valid scientific reasons.

(g) Combination drug products.

(1) Generally, the purpose of an in vivo bioavailability study involving a combination drug product is to determine if the rate and extent of absorption of each active drug ingredient or therapeutic moiety in the combination drug product is equivalent to the rate and extent of absorption of each active drug ingredient or therapeutic moiety administered concurrently in separate single-ingredient preparations.

(2) The reference material in such a bioavailability study should be two or more currently marketed, single-ingredient drug products each of which contains one of the active drug ingredients or therapeutic moieties in the combination drug product. The Food and Drug Administration may, for valid scientific reasons, specify that the reference material shall be a combination drug product that is the subject of an approved new drug application.

(3) The Food and Drug Administration may permit a bioavailability study involving a combination drug product to determine the rate and extent of absorption of selected, but not all, active drug ingredients or therapeutic moieties in the combination drug product. The Food and Drug Administration may permit this determination if the pharmacokinetics and the interactions of the active drug ingredients or therapeutic moieties in the combination drug product are well known and the therapeutic activity of the combination drug product is generally recognized to reside in only one of the active drug ingredients or therapeutic moieties, e.g., ampicillin in an ampicillin-probenecid combination drug product.

(h) Use of a placebo as the reference material. Where appropriate or where necessary to demonstrate the sensitivity of the test, the reference material in a bioavailability study may be a placebo if:

(1) The study measures the therapeutic or acute pharmacological effect of the active drug ingredient or therapeutic moiety; or

Part 320

(2) The study is a clinical trial to establish the safety and effectiveness of the drug product.

(i) Standards for test drug product and reference material. (1) Both the drug product to be tested and the reference material, if it is another drug product, shall be shown to meet all compendial or other applicable standards of identity, strength, quality, and purity, including potency and, where applicable, content uniformity, disintegration times, and dissolution rates.

(2) Samples of the drug product to be tested shall be manufactured using the same equipment and under the same conditions as those used for full-scale production.

[42 FR 1648, Jan. 7, 1977, as amended at 67 FR 77674, Dec. 19, 2002]

Sec. 320.26 Guidelines on the design of a single-dose in vivo bioavailability or bioequivalence study.

(a) Basic principles.

(1) An in vivo bioavailability or bioequivalence study should be a single-dose comparison of the drug product to be tested and the appropriate reference material conducted in normal adults.

(2) The test product and the reference material should be administered to subjects in the fasting state, unless some other approach is more appropriate for valid scientific reasons.

(b) Study design.

(1) A single-dose study should be crossover in design, unless a parallel design or other design is more appropriate for valid scientific reasons, and should provide for a drug elimination period.

(2) Unless some other approach is appropriate for valid scientific reasons, the drug elimination period should be either:

(i) At least three times the half-life of the active drug ingredient or therapeutic moiety, or its metabolite(s), measured in the blood or urine; or

(ii) At least three times the half-life of decay of the acute pharmacological effect.

(c) Collection of blood samples.

    (1) When comparison of the test product and the reference material is to be based on blood concentration time curves, unless some other approach is more appropriate for valid scientific reasons, blood samples should be taken with sufficient frequency to permit an estimate of both:

        (i) The peak concentration in the blood of the active drug ingredient or therapeutic moiety, or its metabolite(s), measured; and

        (ii) The total area under the curve for a time period at least three times the half-life of the active drug ingredient or therapeutic moiety, or its metabolite(s), measured.

    (2) In a study comparing oral dosage forms, the sampling times should be identical.

    (3) In a study comparing an intravenous dosage form and an oral dosage form, the sampling times should be those needed to describe both:

        (i) The distribution and elimination phase of the intravenous dosage form; and

        (ii) The absorption and elimination phase of the oral dosage form.

    (4) In a study comparing drug delivery systems other than oral or intravenous dosage forms with an appropriate reference standard, the sampling times should be based on valid scientific reasons.

(d) Collection of urine samples. When comparison of the test product and the reference material is to be based on cumulative urinary excretion-time curves, unless some other approach is more appropriate for valid scientific reasons, samples of the urine should be collected with sufficient frequency to permit an estimate of the rate and extent of urinary excretion of the active drug ingredient or therapeutic moiety, or its metabolite(s), measured.

(e) Measurement of an acute pharmacological effect.

    (1) When comparison of the test product and the reference material is to be based on acute pharmacological effect-time curves, measurements of this effect should be made with sufficient frequency to permit a reasonable estimate of the

Part 320

total area under the curve for a time period at least three times the half-life of decay of the pharmacological effect, unless some other approach is more appropriate for valid scientific reasons.

(2) The use of an acute pharmacological effect to determine bioavailability may further require demonstration of dose-related response. In such a case, bioavailability may be determined by comparison of the dose-response curves as well as the total area under the acute pharmacological effect-time curves for any given dose.

[42 FR 1648, Jan. 7, 1977, as amended at 67 FR 77674, Dec. 19, 2002]

Sec. 320.27 Guidelines on the design of a multiple-dose in vivo bioavailability study.

(a) Basic principles.

(1) In selected circumstances it may be necessary for the test product and the reference material to be compared after repeated administration to determine steady-state levels of the active drug ingredient or therapeutic moiety in the body.

(2) The test product and the reference material should be administered to subjects in the fasting or nonfasting state, depending upon the conditions reflected in the proposed labeling of the test product.

(3) A multiple-dose study may be required to determine the bioavailability of a drug product in the following circumstances:

(i) There is a difference in the rate of absorption but not in the extent of absorption.

(ii) There is excessive variability in bioavailability from subject to subject.

(iii) The concentration of the active drug ingredient or therapeutic moiety, or its metabolite(s), in the blood resulting from a single dose is too low for accurate determination by the analytical method.

(iv) The drug product is an extended release dosage form.

(b) Study design.

(1) A multiple-dose study should be crossover in design, unless a parallel design or other design is more appropriate for valid scientific reasons, and should provide for a drug elimination period if steady-state conditions are not achieved.

(2) A multiple-dose study is not required to be of crossover design if the study is to establish dose proportionality under a multiple-dose regimen or to establish the pharmacokinetic profile of a new drug product, a new drug delivery system, or an extended release dosage form.

(3) If a drug elimination period is required, unless some other approach is more appropriate for valid scientific reasons, the drug elimination period should be either:

    (i) At least five times the half-life of the active drug ingredient or therapeutic moiety, or its active metabolite(s), measured in the blood or urine; or

    (ii) At least five times the half-life of decay of the acute pharmacological effect.

(c) Achievement of steady-state conditions. Whenever a multiple-dose study is conducted, unless some other approach is more appropriate for valid scientific reasons, sufficient doses of the test product and reference material should be administered in accordance with the labeling to achieve steady-state conditions.

(d) Collection of blood or urine samples.

(1) Whenever comparison of the test product and the reference material is to be based on blood concentration-time curves at steady state, appropriate dosage administration and sampling should be carried out to document attainment of steady state.

(2) Whenever comparison of the test product and the reference material is to be based on cumulative urinary excretion-time curves at steady state, appropriate dosage administration and sampling should be carried out to document attainment of steady state.

(3) A more complete characterization of the blood concentration or urinary excretion rate during the absorption and elimination phases of a single dose administered at steady-state is encouraged to permit estimation of the total area under concentration-time curves or cumulative urinary excretion-time curves and to obtain pharmacokinetic

Part 320

information, e.g., half-life or blood clearance, that is essential in preparing adequate labeling for the drug product.

(e) Steady-state parameters.

(1) In certain instances, e.g., in a study involving a new drug entity, blood clearances at steady-state obtained in a multiple-dose study should be compared to blood clearances obtained in a single-dose study to support adequate dosage recommendations.

(2) In a linear system, the area under the blood concentration-time curve during a dosing interval in a multiple-dose steady-state study is directly proportional to the fraction of the dose absorbed and is equal to the corresponding "zero to infinity" area under the curve for a single-dose study. Therefore, when steady-state conditions are achieved, a comparison of blood concentrations during a dosing interval may be used to define the fraction of the active drug ingredient or therapeutic moiety absorbed.

(3) Other methods based on valid scientific reasons should be used to determine the bioavailability of a drug product having dose-dependent kinetics (non-linear system).

(f) Measurement of an acute pharmacological effect. When comparison of the test product and the reference material is to be based on acute pharmacological effect-time curves, measurements of this effect should be made with sufficient frequency to demonstrate a maximum effect and a lack of significant difference between the test product and the reference material.

[42 FR 1648, Jan. 7, 1977, as amended at 67 FR 77674, Dec. 19, 2002]

Sec. 320.28 Correlation of bioavailability with an acute pharmacological effect or clinical evidence.

Correlation of in vivo bioavailability data with an acute pharmacological effect or clinical evidence of safety and effectiveness may be required if needed to establish the clinical significance of a special claim, e.g., in the case of an extended release preparation.

[42 FR 1648, Jan. 7, 1977, as amended at 67 FR 77674, Dec. 19, 2002]

Sec. 320.29 Analytical methods for an in vivo bioavailability or bioequivalence study.

(a) The analytical method used in an in vivo bioavailability or bioequivalence study to measure the concentration of the active drug ingredient or therapeutic moiety, or its active metabolite(s), in body fluids or excretory products, or the method used to measure an acute pharmacological effect shall be demonstrated to be accurate and of sufficient sensitivity to measure, with appropriate precision, the actual concentration of the active drug ingredient or therapeutic moiety, or its active metabolite(s), achieved in the body.

(b) When the analytical method is not sensitive enough to measure accurately the concentration of the active drug ingredient or therapeutic moiety, or its active metabolite(s), in body fluids or excretory products produced by a single dose of the test product, two or more single doses may be given together to produce higher concentration if the requirements of 320.31 are met.

[42 FR 1648, Jan. 7, 1977, as amended at 67 FR 77674, Dec. 19, 2002]

Part 320

Sec. 320.30 Inquiries regarding bioavailability and bioequivalence requirements and review of protocols by the Food and Drug Administration.

(a) The Commissioner of Food and Drugs strongly recommends that, to avoid the conduct of an improper study and unnecessary human research, any person planning to conduct a bioavailability or bioequivalence study submit the proposed protocol for the study to FDA for review prior to the initiation of the study.

(b) FDA may review a proposed protocol for a bioavailability or bioequivalence study and will offer advice with respect to whether the following conditions are met:

(1) The design of the proposed bioavailability or bioequivalence study is appropriate.

(2) The reference material to be used in the bioavailability or bioequivalence study is appropriate.

(3) The proposed chemical and statistical analytical methods are adequate.

(c)(1) General inquiries relating to in vivo bioavailability requirements and methodology shall be submitted to the Food and Drug Administration, Center for Drug Evaluation and Research, Office of Clinical Pharmacology, 10903 New Hampshire Ave., Silver Spring, MD 20993-0002.

(2) General inquiries relating to bioequivalence requirements and methodology shall be submitted to the Food and Drug Administration, Center for Drug Evaluation and Research, Division of Bioequivalence (HFD-650), 7500 Standish Pl., Rockville, MD 20855-2773.

[57 FR 18000, Apr. 28, 1992, as amended at 67 FR 77674, Dec. 19, 2002; 74 FR 13114, Mar. 26, 2009]

Sec. 320.31 Applicability of requirements regarding an "Investigational New Drug Application."

(a) Any person planning to conduct an in vivo bioavailability or bioequivalence study in humans shall submit an "Investigational New Drug Application" (IND) if:

(1) The test product contains a new chemical entity as defined in 314.108(a) of this chapter; or

(2) The study involves a radioactively labeled drug product; or

(3) The study involves a cytotoxic drug product.

(b) Any person planning to conduct a bioavailability or bioequivalence study in humans using a drug product that contains an already approved, non-new chemical entity shall submit an IND if the study is one of the following:

(1) A single-dose study in normal subjects or patients where either the maximum single or total daily dose exceeds that specified in the labeling of the drug product that is the subject of an approved new drug application or abbreviated new drug application.

(2) A multiple-dose study in normal subjects or patients where either the single or total daily dose exceeds that specified in the labeling of the drug product that is the subject of an approved new drug application or abbreviated new drug application.

(3) A multiple-dose study on an extended release product on which no single-dose study has been completed.

(c) The provisions of parts 50, 56, and 312 of this chapter are applicable to any bioavailability or bioequivalence study in humans conducted under an IND.

(d) A bioavailability or bioequivalence study in humans other than one described in paragraphs (a) through (c) of this section is exempt from the requirements of part 312 of this chapter if the following conditions are satisfied:

(1) If the study is one described under 320.38(b) or 320.63, the person conducting the study, including any contract research organization, shall retain reserve samples of any test article and reference standard used in the study and release the reserve samples to FDA upon request, in accordance with, and for the period specified in, 320.38; and

(2) An in vivo bioavailability or bioequivalence study in humans shall be conducted in compliance with the requirements for institutional review set forth in part 56 of this chapter, and informed consent set forth in part 50 of this chapter.

[57 FR 18000, Apr. 28, 1992, as amended at 58 FR 25927, Apr. 28, 1993; 67 FR 77674, Dec. 19, 2002]

Part 320

Sec. 320.32 Procedures for establishing or amending a bioequivalence requirement.

(a) The Food and Drug Administration, on its own initiative or in response to a petition by an interested person, may propose and promulgate a regulation to establish a bioequivalence requirement for a product not subject to section 505(j) of the act if it finds there is well-documented evidence that specific pharmaceutical equivalents or pharmaceutical alternatives intended to be used interchangeably for the same therapeutic effect:

(1) Are not bioequivalent drug products; or

(2) May not be bioequivalent drug products based on the criteria set forth in 320.33; or

(3) May not be bioequivalent drug products because they are members of a class of drug products that have close structural similarity and similar physicochemical or

pharmacokinetic properties to other drug products in the same class that FDA finds are not bioequivalent drug products.

(b) FDA shall include in a proposed rule to establish a bioequivalence requirement the evidence and criteria set forth in 320.33 that are to be considered in determining whether to issue the proposal. If the rulemaking is proposed in response to a petition, FDA shall include in the proposal a summary and analysis of the relevant information that was submitted in the petition as well as other available information to support the establishment of a bioequivalence requirement.

(c) FDA, on its own initiative or in response to a petition by an interested person, may propose and promulgate an amendment to a bioequivalence requirement established under this subpart.

[57 FR 18000, Apr. 28, 1992]

Sec. 320.33 Criteria and evidence to assess actual or potential bioequivalence problems.

The Commissioner of Food and Drugs shall consider the following factors, when supported by well-documented evidence, to identify specific pharmaceutical equivalents and pharmaceutical alternatives that are not or may not be bioequivalent drug products.

(a) Evidence from well-controlled clinical trials or controlled observations in patients that such drug products do not give comparable therapeutic effects.

(b) Evidence from well-controlled bioequivalence studies that such products are not bioequivalent drug products.

(c) Evidence that the drug products exhibit a narrow therapeutic ratio, e.g., there is less than a 2-fold difference in median lethal dose (LD50) and median effective dose (ED50) values, or have less than a 2-fold difference in the minimum toxic concentrations and minimum effective concentrations in the blood, and safe and effective use of the drug products requires careful dosage titration and patient monitoring.

(d) Competent medical determination that a lack of bioequivalence would have a serious adverse effect in the treatment or prevention of a serious disease or condition.

(e) Physicochemical evidence that:

   (1) The active drug ingredient has a low solubility in water, e.g., less than 5 milligrams per 1 milliliter, or, if dissolution in the stomach is critical to absorption, the volume of gastric fluids required to dissolve the recommended dose far exceeds the volume of fluids present in the stomach (taken to be 100 milliliters for adults and prorated for infants and children).

   (2) The dissolution rate of one or more such products is slow, e.g., less than 50 percent in 30 minutes when tested using either a general method specified in an official compendium or a paddle method at 50 revolutions per minute in 900 milliliters of distilled or deionized water at 37 deg. C, or differs significantly from that of an appropriate reference material such as an identical drug product that is the subject of an approved full new drug application.

   (3) The particle size and/or surface area of the active drug ingredient is critical in determining its bioavailability.

   (4) Certain physical structural characteristics of the active drug ingredient, e.g., polymorphic forms, conforms, solvates, complexes, and crystal modifications, dissolve poorly and this poor dissolution may affect absorption.

   (5) Such drug products have a high ratio of excipients to active ingredients, e.g., greater than 5 to 1.

   (6) Specific inactive ingredients, e.g., hydrophilic or hydrophobic excipients and lubricants, either may be required for absorption of the active drug ingredient or therapeutic moiety or, alternatively, if present, may interfere with such absorption.

(f) Pharmacokinetic evidence that:

   (1) The active drug ingredient, therapeutic moiety, or its precursor is absorbed in large part in a particular segment of the gastrointestinal tract or is absorbed from a localized site.

   (2) The degree of absorption of the active drug ingredient, therapeutic moiety, or its precursor is poor, e.g., less than 50 percent, ordinarily in comparison to an intravenous dose, even when it is administered in pure form, e.g., in solution.

   (3) There is rapid metabolism of the therapeutic moiety in the intestinal wall or liver during the process of absorption (first-

Part 320

class metabolism) so the therapeutic effect and/or toxicity of such drug product is determined by the rate as well as the degree of absorption.

(4) The therapeutic moiety is rapidly metabolized or excreted so that rapid dissolution and absorption are required for effectiveness.

(5) The active drug ingredient or therapeutic moiety is unstable in specific portions of the gastrointestinal tract and requires special coatings or formulations, e.g., buffers, enteric coatings, and film coatings, to assure adequate absorption.

(6) The drug product is subject to dose dependent kinetics in or near the therapeutic range, and the rate and extent of absorption are important to bioequivalence.

[42 FR 1635, Jan. 7, 1977. Redesignated and amended at 57 FR 18001, Apr. 28, 1992]

Sec. 320.34 Requirements for batch testing and certification by the Food and Drug Administration.

(a) If the Commissioner determines that individual batch testing by the Food and Drug Administration is necessary to assure that all batches of the same drug product meet an appropriate in vitro test, he shall include in the bioequivalence requirement a requirement for manufacturers to submit samples of each batch to the Food and Drug Administration and to withhold distribution of the batch until notified by the Food and Drug Administration that the batch may be introduced into interstate commerce.

(b) The Commissioner will ordinarily terminate a requirement for a manufacturer to submit samples for batch testing on a finding that the manufacturer has produced four consecutive batches that were tested by the Food and Drug Administration and found to meet the bioequivalence requirement, unless the public health requires that batch testing be extended to additional batches.

[42 FR 1635, Jan. 7, 1977. Redesignated at 57 FR 18001, Apr. 28, 1992]

Sec. 320.35 Requirements for in vitro testing of each batch.

If a bioequivalence requirement specifies a currently available in vitro test or an in vitro bioequivalence standard comparing the drug product to a reference standard, the manufacturer shall conduct the test on a sample of each batch of the drug product to assure batch-to-batch uniformity.

[42 FR 1635, Jan. 7, 1977. Redesignated at 57 FR 18001, Apr. 28, 1992]

Sec. 320.36 Requirements for maintenance of records of bioequivalence testing.

(a) All records of in vivo or in vitro tests conducted on any marketed batch of a drug product to assure that the product meets a bioequivalence requirement shall be maintained by the manufacturer for at least 2 years after the expiration date of the batch and submitted to the Food and Drug Administration on request.

(b) Any person who contracts with another party to conduct a bioequivalence study from which the data are intended to be submitted to FDA as part of an application submitted under part 314 of this chapter shall obtain from the person conducting the study sufficient accurate financial information to allow the submission of complete and accurate financial certifications or disclosure statements required under part 54 of this chapter and shall maintain that information and all records relating to the compensation given for that study and all other financial interest information required under part 54 of this chapter for 2 years after the date of approval of the application. The person maintaining these records shall, upon request for any properly authorized officer or employee of the Food and Drug Administration, at reasonable time, permit such officer or employee to have access to and copy and verify these records.

[42 FR 1635, Jan. 7, 1977. Redesignated at 57 FR 18001, Apr. 28, 1992, as amended at 63 FR 5252, Feb. 2, 1998]

Sec. 320.38 Retention of bioavailability samples.

(a) The applicant of an application or supplemental application submitted under section 505 of the Federal Food, Drug, and Cosmetic Act, or, if bioavailability testing was performed under contract, the contract research organization shall retain an appropriately identified reserve sample of the drug product for which the applicant is seeking approval (test article) and of the reference standard used to perform an in vivo bioavailability study in accordance with and for the studies described in paragraph (b) of this section that is representative of each sample of the test article and reference standard provided by the applicant for the testing.

(b) Reserve samples shall be retained for the following test articles and reference standards and for the studies described:

    (1) If the formulation of the test article is the same as the formulation(s) used in the clinical studies demonstrating substantial evidence of safety and effectiveness for the test article's claimed indications, a reserve sample of the test article used to conduct an in vivo bioavailability study comparing the test article to a reference oral solution, suspension, or injection.

    (2) If the formulation of the test article differs from the formulation(s) used in the clinical studies demonstrating substantial evidence of safety and effectiveness for the test article's claimed indications, a reserve sample of the test article and of the reference standard used to conduct an in vivo bioequivalence study comparing the test article to the formulation(s) (reference standard) used in the clinical studies.

    (3) For a new formulation, new dosage form, or a new salt or ester of an active drug ingredient or therapeutic moiety that has been approved for marketing, a reserve sample of the test article and of the reference standard used to conduct an in vivo bioequivalence study comparing the test article to a marketed product (reference standard) that contains the same active drug ingredient or therapeutic moiety.

(c) Each reserve sample shall consist of a sufficient quantity to permit FDA to perform five times all of the release tests required in the application or supplemental application.

(d) Each reserve sample shall be adequately identified so that the reserve sample can be positively identified as having come from the same sample as used in the specific bioavailability study.

(e) Each reserve sample shall be stored under conditions consistent with product labeling and in an area segregated from the area where testing is conducted and with access limited to authorized personnel. Each reserve sample shall be retained for a period of at least 5 years following the date on which the application or supplemental application is approved, or, if such application or supplemental application is not approved, at least 5 years following the date of completion of the bioavailability study in which the sample from which the reserve sample was obtained was used.

(f) Authorized FDA personnel will ordinarily collect reserve samples directly from the applicant or contract research organization at the storage site during a preapproval inspection. If authorized FDA personnel are unable to collect samples, FDA may require the applicant or contract research organization to submit the reserve samples to the place identified in the agency's request. If FDA has not collected or requested delivery of a reserve sample, or if FDA has not collected or requested delivery of any portion of a reserve sample, the applicant or contract research organization shall retain the sample or remaining sample for the 5-year period specified in paragraph (e) of this section.

(g) Upon release of the reserve samples to FDA, the applicant or contract research organization shall provide a written assurance that, to the best knowledge and belief of the individual executing the assurance, the reserve samples came from the same samples as used in the specific bioavailability or bioequivalence study identified by the agency. The assurance shall be executed by an individual authorized to act for the applicant or contract research organization in releasing the reserve samples to FDA.

(h) A contract research organization may contract with an appropriate, independent third party to provide storage of reserve samples provided that the sponsor of the study has been notified in writing of the name and address of the facility at which the reserve samples will be stored.

(i) If a contract research organization conducting a bioavailability or bioequivalence study that requires reserve sample retention under this section or 320.63 goes out of business, it shall transfer its reserve samples to an appropriate, independent third party, and shall notify in writing the sponsor of the study of the transfer and provide the study sponsor with the name and address of the facility to which the reserve samples have been transferred.

[58 FR 25927, Apr. 28, 1993, as amended at 64 FR 402, Jan. 5, 1999]

Part 320

Sec. 320.63 Retention of bioequivalence samples.

The applicant of an abbreviated application or a supplemental application submitted under section 505 of the Federal Food, Drug, and Cosmetic Act, or, if bioequivalence testing was performed under contract, the contract research organization shall retain reserve samples of any test article and reference standard used in conducting an in vivo or in vitro bioequivalence study required for approval of the abbreviated application or supplemental application. The applicant or contract research organization shall retain the reserve samples in accordance with, and for the period specified in, 320.38 and shall release the reserve samples to FDA upon request in accordance with 320.38.

[58 FR 25928, Apr. 28, 1993, as amended at 64 FR 402, Jan. 5, 1999]

Authority: 21 U.S.C. 321, 351, 352, 355, 371.

Part 511: New Animal Drugs for Investigational Use

[Code of Federal Regulations]

[Title 21, Volume 6]

[Revised as of April 1, 2009]

[CITE: 21CFR511]

Title 21--Food and Drugs

Chapter I--Food and Drug Administration

Department of Health and Human Services

Subchapter E--Animal Drugs, Feeds, and Related Products

Part 511 New Animal Drugs for Investigational Use[1]

Sec. 511.1 New animal drugs for investigational use exempt from section 512(a) of the act.

(a) New animal drugs for tests in vitro and in laboratory research animals.

    (1) A shipment or other delivery of a new animal drug or animal feed bearing or containing a new animal drug intended solely for tests in vitro or in animals used only for laboratory research purposes shall be exempt from section 512 (a) and (m) of the act if it is labeled as follows:

---

[1] Available on the FDA website at http://www.accessdata.fda.gov/scripts/cdrh/cfdocs/cfCFR/CFRSearch.cfm?CFRPart=511&showFR=1

Caution. Contains a new animal drug for investigational use only in laboratory research animals or for tests in vitro. Not for use in humans.

(2) The person distributing or causing the distribution of new animal drugs for tests in vitro or in animals used only for laboratory research purposes under this exemption shall use due diligence to assure that the consignee is regularly engaged in conducting such tests and that the shipment of the new animal drug will actually be used for tests in vitro or in animals used only for laboratory research.

(3) The person who introduced such shipment or who delivered the new animal drug for introduction into interstate commerce shall maintain adequate records showing the name and post office address of the expert or expert organization to whom the new animal drug is shipped and the date, quantity, and batch or code mark of each shipment and delivery for a period of 2 years after such shipment and delivery. Upon the request of a properly authorized employee of the Department at reasonable times, he shall make such records available for inspection and copying.

(4) The exemption allowed in this paragraph shall not apply to any new animal drug intended for in vitro use in the regular course of diagnosing or treating disease, including antibacterial sensitivity discs impregnated with any new animal drug or drugs, which discs are intended for use in determining susceptibility of microorganisms to the new animal drug or drugs.

(b) New animal drugs for clinical investigation in animals. A shipment or other delivery of a new animal drug or an animal feed containing a new animal drug intended for clinical investigational use in animals shall be exempt from section 512(a) and (m) of the act if all the following conditions are met:

(1) The label shall bear the statements:

Caution. Contains a new animal drug for use only in investigational animals in clinical trials. Not for use in humans. Edible products of investigational animals are not to be used for food unless authorization has been granted by the U.S. Food and Drug Administration or by the U.S. Department of Agriculture.

In the case of containers too small or otherwise unable to accommodate a label with sufficient space to bear the caution statements required by paragraph (a) or (b) of this section, the statements may be included on the carton label and other labeling on or within the package from which the new animal drug is to be dispensed.

(2) The person or firm distributing or causing the distribution of the new animal drug or animal feed containing a new animal drug shall use due diligence to assure that the new animal drug or animal feed containing a new animal drug will actually be used for tests in animals and is not used in humans.

(3) The person who introduced such shipment or who delivered the new animal drug or animal feed containing a new animal drug for introduction into interstate commerce shall maintain adequate records showing the name and post office address of the investigator to whom the new animal drug or animal feed containing a new animal drug is shipped and the date, quantity, and batch or code mark of each shipment and delivery for a period of 2 years after such shipment and delivery. Upon the request of a properly authorized employee of the Department at reasonable times, such records shall be made available for inspection and copying.

(4) Prior to shipment of the new animal drug for clinical tests in animals, the sponsor of the investigation shall submit in triplicate to the Food and Drug Administration a "Notice of Claimed Investigational Exemption for a New Animal Drug" including a signed statement containing the following information:

(i) The identity of the new animal drug.

(ii) All labeling and other pertinent information to be supplied to the investigators. When such pertinent information includes nonclinical laboratory studies, the information shall include, with respect to each nonclinical study, either a statement that the study was conducted in compliance with the requirements set forth in part 58 of this chapter, or, if the study was not conducted in compliance with such regulations, a brief statement of the reason for the noncompliance.

(iii) The name and address of each clinical investigator.

Part 511

(iv) The approximate number of animals to be treated (or if not available, the amount of new animal drug to be shipped).

(v) If the new animal drug is given to food-producing animals, the statement shall contain the following additional information:

(a) A commitment that the edible products from such animals shall not be used for food without prior authorization in accordance with the provisions prescribed in this section.

(b) Approximate dates of the beginning and end of the experiment or series of experiments.

(c) The maximum daily dose(s) to be administered to a given species, the size of animal, maximum duration of administration, method(s) of administration, and proposed withdrawal time, if any.

(vi) If a sponsor has transferred any obligations for the conduct of any clinical study to a contract research organization, a statement containing the name and address of the contract research organization, identification of the clinical study, and a listing of the obligations transferred. If all obligations governing the conduct of the study have been transferred, a general statement of this transfer--in lieu of a listing of the specific obligations transferred--may be submitted.

(5) Authorization for use of edible products derived from a treated food-producing animal may be granted under the provisions of this section and when the following specified conditions are met, except that in the case of an animal administered any unlicensed experimental veterinary biological product regulated under the viruses, serums, toxins statute (21 U.S.C., chapter V, sec. 151et seq.) the product shall be exempt from the requirements of this section when U.S. Department of Agriculture approval has been obtained as provided in 9 CFR 103.2. Conditional authorization may be granted in advance of identification of the name(s) and address(es) of the clinical investigator(s) as required by paragraph (b)(4)(iii) of this section. Information required for authorization shall include, in addition to all other requirements of this section, the following:

(i) Data to show that consumption of food derived from animals treated at the maximum levels with the minimum withdrawal periods, if any, specified in accordance with paragraph (b)(4)(v)(c) of this section, will not be inconsistent with the public health; or

(ii) Data to show that food derived from animals treated at the maximum levels and with the minimum withdrawal periods, if any, specified in accordance with paragraph (b)(4)(v)(c) of this section, does not contain drug residues or metabolites.

(iii) The name and location of the packing plant where the animals will be processed, except that this requirement may be waived, on request, by the terms of the authorization.

Authorizations granted under this paragraph do not exempt investigational animals and their products from compliance with other applicable inspection requirements. Any person who contests a refusal to grant such authorization shall have an opportunity for a regulatory hearing before the Food and Drug Administration pursuant to part 16 of this chapter.

(6) On written request of the Food and Drug Administration, the sponsor shall submit any additional information reported to or otherwise received by him with respect to the investigation deemed necessary to facilitate a determination whether there are grounds in the interest of public health for terminating the exemption.

(7) The sponsor shall assure himself that the new animal drug is shipped only to investigators who:

(i) Are qualified by scientific training and/experience to evaluate the safety and/or effectiveness of the new animal drug.

(ii) Shall maintain complete records of the investigations, including complete records of the receipt and disposition of each shipment or delivery of the new animal drug under investigation. Copies of all records of the investigation shall be retained by the investigator for 2 years after the termination of the investigation or approval of a new animal drug application.

Part 511

(iii) Shall furnish adequate and timely reports of the investigation to the sponsor.

(8) The sponsor:

(i) Shall retain all reports received from investigators for 2 years after the termination of the investigation or approval of a new animal drug application and make such reports available to a duly authorized employee of the Department for inspection at all reasonable times.

(ii) Shall provide for current monitoring of the investigation by a person qualified by scientific training and experience to evaluate information obtained from the investigation, and shall promptly investigate and report to the Food and Drug Administration and to all investigators any findings associated with use of the new animal drug that may suggest significant hazards pertinent to the safety of the new animal drug.

(iii) Shall not unduly prolong distribution of the new animal drug for investigational use.

(iv) Shall not, nor shall any person acting for or on behalf of the sponsor, represent that the new animal drug is safe or effective for the purposes for which it is under investigation. This requirement is not intended to restrict the full exchange of scientific information.

(v) Shall not commercially distribute nor test-market the new animal drug until a new animal drug application is approved pursuant to section 512(c) of the act.

(9) If the shipment or other delivery of the new animal drug is imported or offered for importation into the United States for clinical investigational use in animals, it shall also meet the following conditions:

(i) The importer of all such shipments or deliveries is an agent of the foreign exporter residing in the United States or the ultimate consignee, which person has, prior to such shipments and deliveries, informed the Food and Drug Administration of his intention to import the new animal drug as sponsor in compliance with the conditions prescribed in this subdivision; or

(ii) The new animal drug is shipped directly to a scientific institution with adequate facilities and qualified personnel to conduct laboratory or clinical investigations and is intended solely for use in such institutions and which institution has submitted a statement as sponsor of the investigation.

(10) The sponsor shall submit either a claim for categorical exclusion under 25.30 or 25.33 of this chapter or an environmental assessment under 25.40 of this chapter.

(c) Withdrawal of eligibility to receive investigational-use new animal drugs.

(1) Whenever the Food and Drug Administration has information indicating that an investigator has repeatedly or deliberately failed to comply with the conditions of these exempting regulations or has submitted false information either to the sponsor of the investigation or in any required report, the Center for Veterinary Medicine will furnish the investigator written notice of the matter complained of in general terms and offer him an opportunity to explain the matter in an informal conference and/or in writing. If an explanation is offered but not accepted by the Center for Veterinary Medicine, the investigator shall have an opportunity for a regulatory hearing before the Food and Drug Administration pursuant to part 16 of this chapter on the question of whether the investigator is entitled to receive investigational new animal drugs.

(2) If, after evaluating all available information, including any explanation presented by the investigator, the Commissioner determines that the investigator has repeatedly or deliberately failed to comply with the conditions of the exempting regulations in this section or has repeatedly or deliberately submitted false information to the sponsor of an investigation, the Commissioner will notify the investigator and the sponsor of any investigation in which he has been named as a participant that the investigator is not entitled to receive investigational use new animal drugs with a statement of the basis for such determination.

(3) Each "Notice of Claimed Investigational Exemption for a New Animal Drug" and each approved new animal drug application containing data reported by an investigator who has been determined to be ineligible to receive investigational-use new animal drugs will be examined to determine whether he has submitted unreliable data that are

essential to the continuation of the investigation or essential to the approval of any new animal drug application.

(4) If the Commissioner determines, after the unreliable data submitted by the investigator are eliminated from consideration, that the data remaining are inadequate to support a conclusion that it is reasonably safe to continue the investigation, he shall first notify the sponsor, who shall have an opportunity for a regulatory hearing before the Food and Drug Administration pursuant to part 16 of this chapter on whether the exemption should be terminated. If a danger to the public health exists, however, he shall terminate the exemption forthwith and notify the sponsor of the termination. In such event the sponsor shall have an opportunity for a regulatory hearing before the Food and Drug Administration pursuant to part 16 (see 42 FR 15675, March 22, 1977) of this chapter on the question of whether the exemption should be reinstated.

(5) If the Commissioner determines, after the unreliable data submitted by the investigator are eliminated from consideration, that the data remaining are such that a new animal drug application would not have been approved, he will proceed to withdraw approval of the application in accordance with section 512(e) of the act.

(6) An investigator who has been determined to be ineligible may be reinstated as eligible to receive investigational-use new animal drugs when the Commissioner determines that he has presented adequate assurance that he will employ such new animal drugs solely in compliance with the exempting regulations in this section for investigational-use new animal drugs.

(d) Termination of exemption. If the Commissioner finds that:

(1) The sponsor of the investigation has failed to comply with any of the conditions for the exemption established under this section, or

(2) The continuance of the investigation is unsafe or otherwise contrary to the public interest or the drug is being or has been used for purposes other than bona fide scientific investigation, he shall first notify the sponsor and invite his immediate correction. If the conditions of the exemption are not immediately met, the sponsor shall have an opportunity

for a regulatory hearing before the Food and Drug Administration pursuant of part 16 of this chapter on whether the exemption should be terminated. If the exemption is terminated the sponsor shall recall or have destroyed the unused supplies of the new animal drug.

(e) Statements and requests. "Notice(s) of Claimed Investigational Exemption for a New Animal Drug" and requests for authorization to use investigational animals and their products for food should be addressed to the Department of Health and Human Services, Food and Drug Administration, Center for Veterinary Medicine, 7500 Standish Pl., Rockville, MD 20855.

(f) Contract research organizations.

(1) For purposes of this part and part 514,contract research organization means a person that assumes, as an independent contractor with the sponsor, one or more of the obligations of a sponsor, e.g., design of a protocol, selection or monitoring of investigations, evaluation of reports, and preparation of materials to be submitted to the Food and Drug Administration.

(2) A sponsor may transfer responsibility for any or all of the obligations set forth in this part to a contract research organization. Any such transfer shall be in writing and, if not all obligations are transferred, shall describe each of the obligations being assumed by the contract research organization. If all obligations are transferred, a general statement that all obligations have been transferred is acceptable. Any obligation not covered by the written description shall be deemed not to have been transferred.

(3) A contract research organization that assumes any obligation of a sponsor shall comply with the specific regulations in this chapter applicable to this obligation and shall be subject to the same regulatory action as a sponsor for failure to comply with any obligation assumed under these regulations. Thus, all references tosponsor in this part apply to a contract research organization to the extent that it assumes one or more obligations of the sponsor.

(g) Index of legally marketed unapproved new animal drugs for minor species. All provisions of part 511 apply to new animal drugs for investigational use in support of indexing, as described in section 572 of the act, subject to the provisions of 516.125 of this chapter.

Part 511

[40 FR 13823, Mar. 27, 1975, as amended at 41 FR 48268, Nov. 2, 1976; 42 FR 15675, Mar. 22, 1977; 50 FR 7517, Feb. 22, 1985; 50 FR 16668, Apr. 26, 1985; 52 FR 8847, Mar. 19, 1987; 54 FR 18280, Apr. 28, 1989; 57 FR 6475, Feb. 25, 1992; 62 FR 40599, July 29, 1997; 72 FR 69121, Dec. 6, 2007]

Authority: 21 U.S.C. 321, 351, 352, 353, 360b, 371.

Part 514: New Animal Drug Applications

[Code of Federal Regulations]

[Title 21, Volume 6]

[Revised as of April 1, 2009]

[CITE: 21CFR514]

Title 21--Food and Drugs

Chapter I--Food and Drug Administration

Department of Health and Human Services

Subchapter E--Animal Drugs, Feeds, and Related Products

Part 514 New Animal Drug Applications[1]

Subpart A--General Provisions

Sec. 514.1 Applications.

(a) Applications to be filed under section 512(b) of the act shall be submitted in the form and contain the information described in paragraph (b) of this section, as appropriate to support the particular submission. If any part of the application is in a foreign language, an accurate and complete English translation shall be appended to such part. Translations of literature printed in a foreign language shall be accompanied by copies of the original publication. The application must be signed by the applicant or by an authorized attorney, agent, or official. If the applicant or such authorized representative does not reside or have a place of business within the United States, the application must also furnish the name and post office address of, and must be countersigned by, an authorized attorney, agent, or official residing

---

[1] Available on the FDA website at http://www.accessdata.fda.gov/scripts/cdrh/cfdocs/cfCFR/CFRSearch.cfm?CFRPart=514&showFR=1

or maintaining a place of business within the United States. Pertinent information may be incorporated in, and will be considered as part of, an application on the basis of specific reference to such information, including information submitted under the provisions of 511.1 of this chapter, in the files of the Food and Drug Administration; however, the reference must be specific in identifying the information. Any reference to information furnished by a person other than the applicant may not be considered unless its use is authorized in a written statement signed by the person who submitted it.

(b) Applications for new animal drugs shall be submitted in triplicate and assembled in the manner prescribed by paragraph (b)(15) of this section, and shall include the following information, as appropriate to support the particular submission:

(1) Identification. Whether the submission is an original or supplemental application; the name and the address of the applicant; the date of the application; the trade name(s) (if one has been proposed) and chemical name(s) of the new animal drug. Upon receipt, the application will be assigned a number NADA __, which shall be used for all correspondence with respect to the application.

(2) Table of contents and summary. The application shall be organized in a cohesive fashion, shall contain a table of contents which identifies the data and other material submitted, and shall contain a well-organized summary and evaluation of the data in the following form:

(i) Chemistry:

(a) Chemical structural formula or description for any new animal drug substance.

(b) Relationship to other chemically or pharmacologically related drugs.

(c) Description of dosage form and quantitative composition.

(ii) Scientific rationale and purpose the new animal drug is to serve:

(a) Clinical purpose.

(b) Highlights of laboratory studies: The reasons why certain types of studies were done or omitted as related to the proposed conditions of use and to information already known about this class of compounds. Emphasize any unusual or particularly significant pharmacological effects or toxicological findings.

(c) Highlights of clinical studies: The rationale of the clinical study plan showing why types of studies were done, amended, or omitted as related to laboratory studies and prior clinical experience.

(d) Conclusions: A short statement of conclusions combining the major points of effectiveness and safety as they relate to the use of the new animal drug.

(3) Labeling. Three copies of each piece of all labeling to be used for the article (total of 9).

(i) All labeling should be identified to show its position on, or the manner in which it is to accompany the market package.

(ii) Labeling for nonprescription new animal drugs should include adequate directions for use by the layman under all conditions of use for which the new animal drug is intended, recommended, or suggested in any of the labeling or advertising sponsored by the applicant.

(iii) Labeling for prescription veterinary drugs should bear adequate information for use under which veterinarians can use the new animal drug safely and for the purposes for which it is intended, including those purposes for which it is to be advertised or represented, in accord with 201.105 of this chapter.

(iv) All labeling for prescription or nonprescription new animal drugs shall be submitted with any necessary use restrictions prominently and conspicuously displayed.

(v) Labeling for new animal drugs intended for use in the manufacture of medicated feeds shall include:

(a) Specimens of labeling to be used for such new animal drug with adequate directions for the manufacture and use of finished feeds for all conditions for which the new animal drug is intended, recommended, or suggested in any of the

Part 514

labeling, including advertising, sponsored by the applicant. Ingredient labeling may utilize collective names as provided in 501.110 of this chapter.

(b) Representative labeling proposed to be used for Type B and Type C medicated feeds containing the new animal drug.

(vi) Draft labeling may be submitted for preliminary consideration of an application. Final printed labeling will ordinarily be required prior to approval of an application. Proposed advertising for veterinary prescription drugs may be submitted for comment or approval.

(4) Components and composition. A complete list of all articles used for production of the new animal drug including a full list of the composition of each article:

(i) A full list of the articles used as components of the new animal drug. This list should include all substances used in the synthesis, extraction, or other method of preparation of any new animal drug and in the preparation of the finished dosage form, regardless of whether they undergo chemical change or are removed in the process. Each component should be identified by its established name, if any, or complete chemical name, using structural formulas when necessary for specific identification. If any proprietary name is used, it should be followed by a complete quantitative statement of composition. Reasonable alternatives for any listed component may be specified.

(ii) A full statement of the composition of the new animal drug. The statement shall set forth the name and amount of each ingredient, whether active or not, contained in a stated quantity of the new animal drug in the form in which it is to be distributed (for example, amount per tablet or milliliter) and a batch formula representative of that to be employed for the manufacture of the finished dosage form. All components should be included in the batch formula regardless of whether they appear in the finished product. Any calculated excess of an ingredient over the label declaration should be designated as such and percent excess shown. Reasonable variation may be specified.

(iii) If it is a new animal drug produced by fermentation:

(a) Source and type of microorganism used to produce the new animal drug.

(b) Composition of media used to produce the new animal drug.

(c) Type of precursor used, if any, to guide or enhance production of the antibiotic during fermentation.

(d) Name and composition of preservative, if any, used in the broth.

(e) A complete description of the extraction and purification processes including the names and compositions of the solvents, precipitants, ion exchange resins, emulsifiers, and all other agents used.

(f) If the new animal drug is produced by a catalytic hydrogenation process (such as tetracycline from chlortetracycline), a complete description of each chemical reaction with graphic formulas used to produce the new animal drug, including the names of the catalyst used, how it is removed, and how the new animal drug is extracted and purified.

(5) Manufacturing methods, facilities, and controls. A full description of the methods used in, and the facilities and controls used for, the manufacture, processing, and packing of the new animal drug. This description should include full information with respect to any new animal drug in sufficient detail to permit evaluation of the adequacy of the described methods of manufacture, processing, and packing, and the described facilities and controls to determine and preserve the identity, strength, quality, and purity of the new animal drug, and the following:

(i) If the applicant does not himself perform all the manufacturing, processing, packaging, labeling, and control operations for any new animal drug, he shall: Identify each person who will perform any part of such operations and designate the part; and provide a signed statement from each such person fully describing, directly or by reference, the methods, facilities, and controls he will use in his part of the operation. The statement shall include a commitment that no changes will be made

without prior approval by the Food and Drug
Administration, unless permitted under 514.8.

(ii) A description of the qualifications, including educational
background and experience, of the technical and
professional personnel who are responsible for assuring
that the new animal drug has the identity, strength,
quality, and purity it purports or is represented to
possess, and a statement of their responsibilities.

(iii) A description of the physical facilities including building
and equipment used in manufacturing, processing,
packaging, labeling, storage, and control operations.

(iv) The methods used in the synthesis, extraction, isolation,
or purification of any new animal drug. When the
specifications and controls applied to such new animal
drugs are inadequate in themselves to determine its
identity, strength, quality, and purity, the methods should
be described in sufficient detail, including quantities used,
times, temperature, pH, solvents, etc., to determine these
characteristics. Alternative methods or variations in
methods within reasonable limits that do not affect such
characteristics of the new animal drug may be specified.
A flow sheet and indicated equations should be submitted
when needed to explain the process.

(v) Precautions to insure proper identity, strength, quality,
and purity of the raw materials, whether active or not,
including:

(a) The specifications for acceptance and methods of
testing for each lot of raw material.

(b) A statement as to whether or not each lot of raw
materials is given a serial number to identify it, and
the use made of such numbers in subsequent plant
operations.

(vi) The instructions used in the manufacturing, processing,
packaging, and labeling of each dosage form of the new
animal drug, including:

(a) The method of preparation of the master formula
records and individual batch records and the manner
in which these records are used.

(b) The number of individuals checking weight or volume of each individual ingredient entering into each batch of the new animal drug.

(c) A statement as to whether or not the total weight or volume of each batch is determined at any stage of the manufacturing process subsequent to making up a batch according to the formula card and, if so, at what stage and by whom it is done.

(d) The precautions used in checking the actual package yield produced from a batch of the new animal drug with the theoretical yield. This should include a description of the accounting for such items as discards, breakage, etc., and the criteria used in accepting or rejecting batches of drugs in the event of an unexplained discrepancy.

(e) The precautions used to assure that each lot of the new animal drug is packaged with the proper label and labeling, including provisions for labeling storage and inventory control.

(f) Any special precautions used in the operations.

(vii) The analytical controls used during the various stages of the manufacturing, processing, packaging, and labeling of the new animal drug, including a detailed description of the collection of samples and the analytical procedures to which they are subjected. The analytical procedures should be capable of determining the active components within a reasonable degree of accuracy and of assuring the identity of such components.

(a) A description of practicable methods of analysis of adequate sensitivity to determine the amount of the new animal drug in the final dosage form should be included. The dosage form may be a finished pharmaceutical product, a Type A medicated article, a Type B or a Type C medicated feed, or a product for use in animal drinking water. Where two or more active ingredients are included, methods should be quantitative and specific for each active ingredient.

(b) If the article is one that is represented to be sterile, the same information with regard to the manufacturing, processing, packaging, and the

Part 514

collection of samples of the drug should be given for sterility controls. Include the standards used for acceptance of each lot of the finished drug.

(viii) An explanation of the exact significance of any batch control numbers used in the manufacturing, processing, packaging, and labeling of the new animal drug, including such control numbers that may appear on the label of the finished article. State whether these numbers enable determination of the complete manufacturing history of the product. Describe any methods used to permit determination of the distribution of any batch if its recall is required.

(ix) Adequate information with respect to the characteristics of and the test methods employed for the container, closure, or other component parts of the drug package to assure their suitability for the intended use.

(x) A complete description of, and data derived from, studies of the stability of the new animal drug in the final dosage form, including information showing the suitability of the analytical methods used. A description of any additional stability studies underway or planned. Stability data for the finished dosage form of the new animal drug in the container in which it is to be marketed, including any proposed multiple dose container, and, if it is to be put into solution at the time of dispensing, for the solution prepared as directed. If the new animal drug is intended for use in the manufacture of Type C medicated feed as defined in 558.3 of this chapter, stability data derived from studies in which representative formulations of the medicated feed articles are used. Similar data may be required for Type B medicated feeds as determined by the Food and Drug Administration on a case-by-case basis. Expiration dates shall be proposed for finished pharmaceutical dosage forms and Type A medicated articles. If the data indicate that an expiration date is needed for Type B or Type C medicated feeds, the applicant shall propose such expiration date. If no expiration date is proposed for Type B or Type C medicated feeds, the applicant shall justify its absence with data.

(xi) Additional procedures employed which are designed to prevent contamination and otherwise assure proper control of the product. An application may be refused unless it includes adequate information showing that the methods used in, and the facilities and controls used for, the manufacturing, processing, and packaging of the new animal drug are adequate to preserve its identity, strength, quality, and purity in conformity with good manufacturing practice and identifies each establishment, showing the location of the plant conducting these operations.

(6) Samples. Samples of the new animal drug and articles used as components and information concerning them may be requested by the Center for Veterinary Medicine as follows:

(i) Each sample shall consist of four identical, separately packaged subdivisions, each containing at least three times the amount required to perform the laboratory test procedures described in the application to determine compliance with its control specifications for identity and assays. Each of the samples submitted shall be appropriately packaged and labeled to preserve its characteristics, to identify the material and the quantity in each subdivision of the sample, and to identify each subdivision with the name of the applicant and the new animal drug application to which it relates. Included are:

(a) A sample or samples of any reference standard and blank used in the procedures described in the application for assaying each new animal drug and other assayed components of the finished new animal drug.

(b) A representative sample or samples of each strength of the finished dosage form proposed in the application and employed in the clinical investigations and a representative sample or samples of each new animal drug from the batch(es) employed in the production of such dosage form.

(c) A representative sample or samples of finished market packages of each strength of the dosage form of the new animal drug prepared for initial marketing and, if any such sample is not from a representative commercial-scale production batch, such a sample from a representative commercial-scale production batch, and a representative sample or samples of

Part 514

each new animal drug from the batch(es) employed in the production of such dosage form, provided that in the case of new animal drugs marketed in large packages the sample should contain only three times a sufficient quantity of the new animal drug to allow for performing the control tests for drug identity and assays.

(ii) The following information shall be included for the samples when requested:

(a) For each sample submitted, full information regarding its identity and the origin of any new animal drug contained therein (including a statement whether it was produced on a laboratory, pilot-plant, or full-production scale) and detailed results of all laboratory tests made to determine the identity, strength, quality, and purity of the batch represented by the sample, including assays.

(b) For any reference standard submitted, a complete description of its preparation and the results of all laboratory tests on it. If the test methods used differed from those described in the application, full details of the methods employed in obtaining the reporting results.

(7) Analytical methods for residues. Applications shall include a description of practicable methods for determining the quantity, if any, of the new animal drug in or on food, and any substance formed in or on food because of its use, and the proposed tolerance or withdrawal period or other use restrictions to ensure that the proposed use of this drug will be safe. When data or other adequate information establish that it is not reasonable to expect the new animal drug to become a component of food at concentrations considered unsafe, a regulatory method is not required.

(i) The kind of information required by this subdivision may include: Complete experimental protocols for determining drug residue levels in the edible products, and the length of time required for residues to be eliminated from such products following the drug's use; residue studies conducted under appropriate (consistent with the proposed usage) conditions of dosage, time, and route of administration to show levels, if any, of the drug and/or its metabolites in test animals during and upon cessation of treatment and at intervals thereafter in order to establish a disappearance curve; if the drug is to be used in combination with other drugs, possible effects of interaction demonstrated by the appropriate disappearance curve or depletion patterns after drug withdrawal under appropriate (consistent with the proposed usage) conditions of dosage, time, and route of administration; if the drug is given in the feed or water, appropriate consumption records of the medicated feed or water and appropriate performance data in the treated animal; if the drug is to be used in more than one species, drug residue studies or appropriate metabolic studies conducted for each species that is food-producing. To provide these data, a sufficient number of birds or animals should be used at each sample interval. Appropriate use of labeled compounds (e.g. radioactive tracers), may be utilized to establish metabolism and depletion curves. Drug residue levels ordinarily should be determined in muscle, liver, kidney, and fat and where applicable, in skin, milk, and eggs (yolk and egg white). As a part of the metabolic studies, levels of the drug or metabolite should be determined in blood where feasible. Samples may be combined where necessary. Where residues are suspected or known to be present in litter from treated animals, it may be necessary to include data with respect to such residues becoming components of other agricultural commodities because of use of litter from treated animals.

(ii) A new animal drug that has the potential to contaminate human food with residues whose consumption could present a risk of cancer to people must satisfy the requirements of subpart E of part 500 of this chapter.

(8) Evidence to establish safety and effectiveness.

(i) An application may be refused unless it contains full reports of adequate tests by all methods reasonably applicable to show whether or not the new animal drug is safe and effective for use as suggested in the proposed labeling.

(ii) An application may be refused unless it includes substantial evidence of the effectiveness of the new animal drug as defined in 514.4.

(iii) An application may be refused unless it contains detailed reports of the investigations, including studies made on laboratory animals, in which the purpose, methods, and results obtained are clearly set forth of acute, subacute, and chronic toxicity, and unless it contains appropriate clinical laboratory results related to safety and efficacy. Such information should include identification of the person who conducted each investigation, a statement of where the investigations were conducted, and where the raw data are available in the application.

(iv) All information pertinent to an evaluation of the safety and effectiveness of the new animal drug received or otherwise obtained by the applicant from any source, including information derived from other investigations or commercial marketing (for example, outside the United States), or reports in the scientific literature, both favorable and unfavorable, involving the new animal drug that is the subject of the application and related new animal drugs shall be submitted. An adequate summary may be acceptable in lieu of a reprint of a published report that only supports other data submitted. Include any evaluation of the safety or effectiveness of the new animal drug that has been made by the applicant's veterinary or medical department, expert committee, or consultants.

(v) If the new animal drug is a combination of active ingredients or animal drugs, an application may be refused unless it includes substantial evidence of the effectiveness of the combination new animal drug as required in 514.4.

(vi) An application shall include a complete list of the names and post office addresses of all investigators who received the new animal drug. This may be incorporated in whole or in part by reference to information submitted under the provisions of 511.1 of this chapter.

(vii) Explain any omission of reports from any investigator to whom the investigational new animal drug has been made available. The unexplained omission of any reports of investigations made with the new animal drug by the applicant or submitted to him by an investigator or the unexplained omission of any pertinent reports of investigations or clinical experience received or otherwise obtained by the applicant from published literature or other sources that would bias an evaluation of the safety of the new animal drug or its effectiveness in use, constitutes grounds for the refusal or withdrawal of the approval of an application.

(viii) If a sponsor has transferred any obligations for the conduct of any clinical study to a contract research organization, the application is required to include a statement containing the name and address of the contract research organization, identifying the clinical study, and listing the obligations transferred. If all obligations governing the conduct of the study have been transferred, a general statement of this transfer--in lieu of a listing of the specific obligations transferred--may be submitted.

(ix) If original subject records were audited or reviewed by the sponsor in the course of monitoring any clinical study to verify the accuracy of the case reports submitted to the sponsor, a list identifying each clinical study so audited or reviewed.

(9) Veterinary feed directive. Three copies of a veterinary feed directive (VFD) must be submitted in the format described under 558.6(a)(4) of this chapter.

(10) Supplemental applications. If it is a supplemental application, full information shall be submitted on each proposed change concerning any statement made in the approved application.

(11) Applicant's commitment. It is understood that the labeling and advertising for the new animal drug will prescribe, recommend, or suggest its use only under the conditions stated in the labeling which is part of this application and if the article is a prescription new animal drug, it is understood that any labeling which furnishes or purports to furnish information for use or which prescribes, recommends, or suggests a dosage for use of the new animal drug will also contain, in the same language and emphasis, information for its use including indications, effects, dosages, routes, methods, and frequency and duration of administration, any relevant hazards, contraindications, side effects, and precautions contained in the labeling which is part of this application. It is understood that all representations in this

Part 514

application apply to the drug produced until changes are made in conformity with 514.8.

(12) Additional commitments.

   (i) New animal drugs as defined in 510.3 of this chapter, intended for use in the manufacture of animal feeds in any State will be shipped only to persons who may receive such drugs in accordance with 510.7 of this chapter.

   (ii) The methods, facilities, and controls described under item 5 of this application conform to the current good manufacturing practice regulations in subchapter C of this chapter.

   (iii) With respect to each nonclinical laboratory study contained in the application, either a statement that the study was conducted in compliance with the good laboratory practice regulations set forth in part 58 of this chapter, or, if the study was not conducted in compliance with such regulations, a brief statement of the reason for the noncompliance.

(13) [Reserved]

(14) Environmental assessment. The applicant is required to submit either a claim for categorical exclusion under 25.30 or 25.33 of this chapter or an environmental assessment under 25.40 of this chapter.

(15) Assembling and binding the application. Assemble and bind an original and two copies of the application as follows:

   (i) Bind the original or ribbon copy of the application as copy No. 1.

   (ii) Bind two identical copies as copy No. 2 and copy No. 3.

   (iii) Identify each front cover with the name of the applicant, new animal drug, and the copy number.

   (iv) Number each page of the application sequentially in the upper right hand corner or in another location so that the page numbers remain legible after the application has been bound, and organize the application consistent with paragraphs (b) (1) through (14) of this section. Each copy should bear the same page numbering, whether sequential in each volume or continuous and sequential throughout the application.

(v) Include complete labeling in each of the copies. It is suggested that labeling be identified by date of printing or date of preparation.

(vi) Submit separate applications for each different dosage form of the drug proposed. Repeating basic information pertinent to all dosage forms in each application is unnecessary if reference is made to the application containing such information. Include in each application information applicable to the specific dosage form, such as labeling, composition, stability data, and method of manufacture.

(vii) Submit in folders amendments, supplements, and other correspondence sent after submission of an original application. The front cover of these submissions should be identified with the name of the applicant, new animal drug, copy number, and the new animal drug application number, if known.

(c) When a new animal drug application is submitted for a new animal drug which has a stimulant, depressant, or hallucinogenic effect on the central nervous system, if it appears that the drug has a potential for abuse, the Commissioner shall forward that information to the Attorney General of the United States.

[40 FR 13825, Mar. 27, 1975]

Editorial Note: For Federal Registercitations affecting 514.1, see the List of CFR Sections Affected, which appears in the Finding Aids section of the printed volume and on GPO Access.

Sec. 514.3 Definitions.

The definition and interpretation of terms contained in this section apply to those terms as used throughout subchapter E.

Adverse drug experience is any adverse event associated with the use of a new animal drug, whether or not considered to be drug related, and whether or not the new animal drug was used in accordance with the approved labeling (i.e., used according to label directions or used in an extralabel manner, including but not limited to different route of administration, different species, different indications, or other than labeled dosage). Adverse drug experience includes, but is not limited to:

(1) An adverse event occurring in animals in the course of the use of an animal drug product by a veterinarian or by a livestock producer or other animal owner or caretaker.

(2) Failure of a new animal drug to produce its expected pharmacological or clinical effect (lack of expected effectiveness).

(3) An adverse event occurring in humans from exposure during manufacture, testing, handling, or use of a new animal drug.

ANADA is an abbreviated new animal drug application including all amendments and supplements.

Applicant is a person or entity who owns or holds on behalf of the owner the approval for an NADA or an ANADA, and is responsible for compliance with applicable provisions of the act and regulations.

Increased frequency of adverse drug experience is an increased rate of occurrence of a particular serious adverse drug event, expected or unexpected, after appropriate adjustment for drug exposure.

NADA is a new animal drug application including all amendments and supplements.

Nonapplicant is any person other than the applicant whose name appears on the label and who is engaged in manufacturing, packing, distribution, or labeling of the product.

Potential applicant means any person:

(1) Intending to investigate a new animal drug under section 512(j) of the Federal Food, Drug, and Cosmetic Act (the act),

(2) Investigating a new animal drug under section 512(j) of the act,

(3) Intending to file a new animal drug application (NADA) or supplemental NADA under section 512(b)(1) of the act, or

(4) Intending to file an abbreviated new animal drug application (ANADA) under section 512(b)(2) of the act.

Presubmission conference means one or more conferences between a potential applicant and FDA to reach a binding agreement establishing a submission or investigational requirement.

Presubmission conference agreement means that section of the memorandum of conference headed "Presubmission Conference Agreement" that records any agreement on the submission or investigational requirement reached by a potential applicant and FDA during the presubmission conference.

Product defect/manufacturing defect is the deviation of a distributed product from the standards specified in the approved application, or any significant chemical, physical, or other change, or deterioration in the distributed drug product, including any microbial or chemical contamination. A manufacturing defect is a product defect caused or aggravated by a manufacturing or related process. A manufacturing defect may occur from a single event or from deficiencies inherent to the manufacturing process. These defects are generally associated with product contamination, product deterioration, manufacturing error, defective packaging, damage from disaster, or labeling error. For example, a labeling error may include any incident that causes a distributed product to be mistaken for, or its labeling applied to, another product.

Serious adverse drug experience is an adverse event that is fatal, or life-threatening, or requires professional intervention, or causes an abortion, or stillbirth, or infertility, or congenital anomaly, or prolonged or permanent disability, or disfigurement.

Unexpected adverse drug experience is an adverse event that is not listed in the current labeling for the new animal drug and includes any event that may be symptomatically and pathophysiologically related to an event listed on the labeling, but differs from the event because of greater severity or specificity. For example, under this definition hepatic necrosis would be unexpected if the labeling referred only to elevated hepatic enzymes or hepatitis.

[68 FR 15365, Mar. 31, 2003, as amended at 69 FR 51170, Aug. 18, 2004]

Sec. 514.4 Substantial evidence.

(a) Definition of substantial evidence. Substantial evidence means evidence consisting of one or more adequate and well-controlled studies, such as a study in a target species, study in laboratory

Part 514

animals, field study, bioequivalence study, or an in vitro study, on the basis of which it could fairly and reasonably be concluded by experts qualified by scientific training and experience to evaluate the effectiveness of the new animal drug involved that the new animal drug will have the effect it purports or is represented to have under the conditions of use prescribed, recommended, or suggested in the labeling or proposed labeling thereof. Substantial evidence shall include such adequate and well-controlled studies that are, as a matter of sound scientific judgment, necessary to establish that a new animal drug will have its intended effect.

(b) Characteristics of substantial evidence –

(1) Qualifications of experts. Any study that is intended to be part of substantial evidence of the effectiveness of a new animal drug shall be conducted by experts qualified by scientific training and experience.

(2) Intended uses and conditions of use. Substantial evidence of effectiveness of a new animal drug shall demonstrate that the new animal drug is effective for each intended use and associated conditions of use for and under which approval is sought.

(i) Dose range labeling. Sponsors should, to the extent possible, provide for a dose range because it increases the utility of the new animal drug by providing the user flexibility in the selection of a safe and effective dose. In general, substantial evidence to support dose range labeling for a new animal drug intended for use in the diagnosis, cure, mitigation, treatment, or prevention of disease must consist of at least one adequate and well-controlled study on the basis of which qualified experts could fairly and reasonably conclude that the new animal drug will be effective for the intended use at the lowest dose of the dose range suggested in the proposed labeling for that intended use. Substantial evidence to support dose range labeling for a new animal drug intended to affect the structure or function of the body of an animal generally must consist of at least one adequate and well-controlled study on the basis of which qualified experts could fairly and reasonably conclude that the new animal drug will be effective for the intended use at all doses within the range suggested in the proposed labeling for the intended use.

(ii) [Reserved]

(3) Studies –

  (i) Number. Substantial evidence of the effectiveness of a new animal drug for each intended use and associated conditions of use shall consist of a sufficient number of current adequate and well-controlled studies of sufficient quality and persuasiveness to permit qualified experts:

    (A) To determine that the parameters selected for measurement and the measured responses reliably reflect the effectiveness of the new animal drug;

    (B) To determine that the results obtained are likely to be repeatable, and that valid inferences can be drawn to the target animal population; and

    (C) To conclude that the new animal drug is effective for the intended use at the dose or dose range and associated conditions of use prescribed, recommended, or suggested in the proposed labeling.

  (ii) Types. Adequate and well-controlled studies that are intended to provide substantial evidence of the effectiveness of a new animal drug may include, but are not limited to, published studies, foreign studies, studies using models, and studies conducted by or on behalf of the sponsor. Studies using models shall be validated to establish an adequate relationship of parameters measured and effects observed in the model with one or more significant effects of treatment.

(c) Substantial evidence for combination new animal drugs –

  (1) Definitions. The following definitions of terms apply to this section:

    (i) Combination new animal drug means a new animal drug that contains more than one active ingredient or animal drug that is applied or administered simultaneously in a single dosage form or simultaneously in or on animal feed or drinking water.

    (ii) Dosage form combination new animal drug means a combination new animal drug intended for use other than in animal feed or drinking water.

Part 514

(iii) Antibacterial with respect to a particular target animal species means an active ingredient or animal drug: That is approved in that species for the diagnosis, cure, mitigation, treatment, or prevention of bacterial disease; or that is approved for use in that species for any other use that is attributable to its antibacterial properties. But, antibacterial does not include ionophores or arsenicals intended for use in combination in animal feed or drinking water.

(iv) Appropriate concurrent use exists when there is credible evidence that the conditions for which the combination new animal drug is intended can occur simultaneously.

(2) Combination new animal drugs that contain only active ingredients or animal drugs that have previously been separately approved.

(i) For dosage form combination new animal drugs, except for those that contain a nontopical antibacterial, that contain only active ingredients or animal drugs that have previously been separately approved for the particular uses and conditions of use for which they are intended in combination, a sponsor shall demonstrate:

(A) By substantial evidence, as defined in this section, that any active ingredient or animal drug intended only for the same use as another active ingredient or animal drug in the combination makes a contribution to the effectiveness of the combination new animal drug;

(B) That each active ingredient or animal drug intended for at least one use that is different from all the other active ingredients or animal drugs used in the combination provides appropriate concurrent use for the intended target animal population; and

(C) That the active ingredients or animal drugs are physically compatible and do not have disparate dosing regimens if FDA, based on scientific information, has reason to believe the active ingredients or animal drugs are physically incompatible or have disparate dosing regimens.

(ii) For combination new animal drugs intended for use in animal feed or drinking water that contain only active ingredients or animal drugs that have previously been separately approved for the particular uses and conditions of use for which they are intended in combination, the sponsor shall demonstrate:

(A) By substantial evidence, as defined in this section, that any active ingredient or animal drug intended only for the same use as another active ingredient or animal drug in the combination makes a contribution to the effectiveness of the combination new animal drug;

(B) For such combination new animal drugs that contain more than one antibacterial ingredient or animal drug, by substantial evidence, as defined in this section, that each antibacterial makes a contribution to labeled effectiveness;

(C) That each active ingredient or animal drug intended for at least one use that is different from all other active ingredients or animal drugs used in the combination provides appropriate concurrent use for the intended target animal population; and

(D) That the active ingredients or animal drugs intended for use in drinking water are physically compatible if FDA, based on scientific information, has reason to believe the active ingredients or animal drugs are physically incompatible.

(3) Other combination new animal drugs. For all other combination new animal drugs, the sponsor shall demonstrate by substantial evidence, as defined in this section, that the combination new animal drug will have the effect it purports or is represented to have under the conditions of use prescribed, recommended, or suggested in the proposed labeling and that each active ingredient or animal drug contributes to the effectiveness of the combination new animal drug.

[64 FR 40756, July 28, 1999]

Sec. 514.5 Presubmission conferences.

(a) General principle underlying the conduct of a presubmission conference. The general principle underlying the conduct of any

Part 514

presubmission conference is that there should be candid, full, and open communication.

(b) Requesting a presubmission conference. A potential applicant is entitled to one or more conferences prior to the submission of an NADA, supplemental NADA, or an ANADA to reach an agreement establishing part or all of a submission or investigational requirement. A potential applicant's request for a presubmission conference must be submitted to FDA in a signed letter. The letter must include a proposed agenda that clearly outlines the scope, purpose, and objectives of the presubmission conference and must list the names and positions of the representatives who are expected to attend the presubmission conference on behalf of the applicant.

(c) Timing. A potential applicant may request one or more presubmission conferences at any time prior to the filing of a NADA, supplemental NADA, or an ANADA. A request for a presubmission conference must be received by FDA at least 30 calendar days in advance of the requested conference date. FDA will schedule the presubmission conference at a time agreeable to both FDA and the potential applicant.

(d) Advance information. The potential applicant must provide to FDA, at least 30 calendar days before a scheduled presubmission conference, a detailed agenda, a copy of any materials to be presented at the conference, a list of proposed indications and, if available, a copy of the proposed labeling for the product under consideration, and copies of materials evaluated or referenced relative to issues listed in the agenda for the conference. If the materials are not provided or are not sufficient to provide the basis for meaningful discussion, FDA may elect to postpone part or all of the meeting until sufficient materials are provided to FDA.

(e) Conduct of a presubmission conference. The potential applicant and FDA may each bring consultants to the presubmission conference. The presubmission conference(s) will be directed primarily at establishing agreement between FDA and the potential applicant regarding a submission or investigational requirement. The submission or investigational requirement may include, among other things, the number, types, and general design of studies that are necessary to demonstrate the safety and effectiveness of a new animal drug for the intended uses and conditions of use prescribed, recommended, or suggested in the proposed labeling for the new animal drug.

(f) Documentation of a presubmission conference –

(1) Memorandum of conference –

(i) Preparation. FDA will prepare a memorandum for each presubmission conference that will include, among other things, any background pertinent to the request for meeting; a summary of the key points of discussion; agreements; and action items and assignments of responsibility. That portion of the memorandum of conference that documents any agreements reached regarding all or part of a submission or investigational requirement will be included under the heading "Presubmission Conference Agreement." If the presubmission conference agreement section of the memorandum is silent on an issue, including one that was discussed in the conference or addressed by materials provided for the conference, such silence does not constitute agreement between FDA and the potential applicant on the issue.

(ii) Sending a copy to the potential applicant. FDA will send a copy of the memorandum to the potential applicant for review no later than 45 calendar days after the date of the conference

(iii) Requests for changes or clarification. If a potential applicant requests changes to, or clarification of, the substance of the memorandum, the request must be sent to FDA within 30 calendar days from the date a copy of the memorandum is sent to the applicant. If the potential applicant requests changes or clarification, FDA will send the potential applicant a response to their request no later than 45 calendar days after the date of receipt of the request.

(iv) Administrative record. A copy of FDA's original memorandum of conference and, as appropriate, a copy of an amended memorandum to correct or clarify the content of the original memorandum will be made part of the administrative file.

Part 514

(2) Field studies. If FDA requires more than one field study to establish by substantial evidence that the new animal drug is effective for its intended uses under the conditions of use prescribed, recommended, or suggested in the proposed labeling, FDA will provide written scientific justification for requiring more than one field study. Such justification must be provided no later than 25 calendar days after the date of the conference at which the requirement for more than one field study is established. If FDA does not believe more than one field study is required but the potential applicant voluntarily proposes to conduct more than one field study, FDA will not provide such written justification. If FDA requires one field study to be conducted at multiple locations, FDA will provide justification for requiring multiple locations verbally during the presubmission conference and in writing as part of the memorandum of conference.

(g) Modification of presubmission conference agreements. An agreement made under a presubmission conference requested under section 512(b)(3) of the act and documented in a memorandum of conference is binding on the potential applicant and FDA and may only be modified if:

(1) FDA and the potential applicant mutually agree to modify, in part or in whole, the agreement and such modification is documented and provided to the potential applicant as described in paragraph (f)(1) of this section; or

(2) FDA by written order determines that a substantiated scientific requirement essential to the determination of safety or effectiveness of the new animal drug appeared after the conference.

(h) When the terms of a presubmission conference agreement are not valid –

(1) A presubmission conference agreement will no longer be valid if:

(i) The potential applicant makes to FDA, before, during, or after the presubmission conference, any untrue statement of material fact; or

(ii) The potential applicant fails to follow any material term of the agreement; and

(2) A presubmission conference may no longer be valid if the potential applicant submits false or misleading data relating to a new animal drug to FDA.

(i) Dispute resolution. FDA is committed to resolving differences between a potential applicant and FDA reviewing divisions with respect to requirements for the investigation of new animal drugs and for NADAs, supplemental NADAs, and ANADAs as quickly and amicably as possible through a cooperative exchange of information and views. When administrative or procedural disputes arise, a potential applicant should first attempt to resolve the matter within the appropriate review division beginning with the individual(s) most directly assigned to the review of the application or investigational exemption. If the dispute cannot be resolved after such attempts, the dispute shall be evaluated and administered in accordance with applicable regulations (21 CFR 10.75). Dispute resolution procedures may be further explained by guidance available from the Center for Veterinary Medicine.

[69 FR 51170, Aug. 18, 2004]

Sec. 514.6 Amended applications.

The applicant may submit an amendment to an application that is pending, including changes that may alter the conditions of use, the labeling, safety, effectiveness, identity, strength, quality, or purity of the drug or the adequacy of the manufacturing methods, facilities, and controls to preserve them, in which case the unamended application may be considered as withdrawn and the amended application may be considered resubmitted on the date on which the amendment is received by the Food and Drug Administration. The applicant will be notified of such date.

Sec. 514.7 Withdrawal of applications without prejudice.

The sponsor may withdraw his pending application from consideration as a new animal drug application upon written notification to the Food and Drug Administration. Such withdrawal may be made without prejudice to a future filing. Upon resubmission, the time limitation will begin to run from the date the resubmission is received by the Food and Drug Administration. The original application will be retained by the Food and Drug Administration

Part 514

although it is considered withdrawn. The applicant shall be furnished a copy at cost on request.

Sec. 514.8 Supplements and other changes to an approved application.

(a) Definitions.

(1) The definitions and interpretations contained in section 201 of the Federal Food, Drug, and Cosmetic Act (the act) apply to those terms when used in this part.

(2) The following definitions of terms apply to this part:

(i) Assess the effects of the change means to evaluate the effects of a manufacturing change on the identity, strength, quality, purity, and potency of a drug as these factors may relate to the safety or effectiveness of the drug.

(ii) Drug substance means an active ingredient as defined under 210.3(b)(7) of this chapter.

(iii) Minor changes and stability report (MCSR) means an annual report that is submitted to the application once each year within 60 days before or after the anniversary date of the application's original approval or on a mutually agreed upon date. The report must include minor manufacturing and control changes made according to 514.8(b)(4) or state that no changes were made; and stability data generated on commercial or production batches according to an approved stability protocol or commitment.

(iv) Specification means the quality standard (i.e., tests, analytical procedures, and acceptance criteria) provided in an approved application to confirm the quality of drugs including, for example, drug substances, Type A medicated articles, drug products, intermediates, raw materials, reagents, components, in-process materials, container closure systems, and other materials used in the production of a drug. For the purpose of this definition, the term "acceptance criteria" means numerical limits, ranges, or other criteria for the tests described.

(b) Manufacturing changes to an approved application —

(1) General provisions.

  (i) The applicant must notify FDA about each change in each condition established in an approved application beyond the variations already provided for in the application. The notice is required to describe the change fully. Depending on the type of change, the applicant must notify FDA about it in a supplement under paragraph (b)(2) or (b)(3) of this section or by inclusion of the information in the annual report to the application under paragraph (b)(4) of this section.

  (ii) The holder of an approved application under section 512 of the act must assess the effects of the change before distributing a drug made with a manufacturing change.

  (iii) Notwithstanding the requirements of paragraphs (b)(2) and (b)(3) of this section, an applicant must make a change provided for in those paragraphs in accordance with a regulation or guidance that provides for a less burdensome notification of the change (for example, by submission of a supplement that does not require approval prior to distribution of the drug, or by notification in the next annual report described in paragraph (b)(4) of this section).

  (iv) In each supplement and amendment to a supplement providing for a change under paragraph (b)(2) or (b)(3) of this section, the applicant must include a statement certifying that a field copy has been provided to the appropriate FDA district office. No field copy is required for a supplement providing for a change made to a drug manufactured outside of the United States.

  (v) A supplement or annual report described in paragraph (b)(4) of this section must include a list of all changes contained in the supplement or annual report. For supplements, this list must be provided in the cover letter.

(2) Changes requiring submission and approval of a supplement prior to distribution of the drug made using the change (major changes).

  (i) A supplement must be submitted for any change in the drug, production process, quality controls, equipment, or facilities that has a substantial potential to have an

Part 514

adverse effect on the identity, strength, quality, purity, or potency of the drug as these factors may relate to the safety or effectiveness of the drug.

(ii) These changes include, but are not limited to:

(A) Except those described in paragraphs (b)(3) and (b)(4) of this section, changes in the qualitative or quantitative formulation of the drug, including inactive ingredients, or in the specifications provided in the approved application;

(B) Changes requiring completion of appropriate clinical studies to demonstrate the equivalence of the drug to the drug as manufactured without the change;

(C) Changes that may affect drug substance or drug product sterility assurance, such as changes in drug substance, drug product or component sterilization method(s) or an addition, deletion, or substitution of steps in an aseptic processing operation;

(D) Changes in the synthesis or manufacture of the drug substance that may affect the impurity profile and/or the physical, chemical, or biological properties of the drug substance;

(E) Changes in a drug product container closure system that controls the drug delivered to the animal or changes in the type or composition of a packaging component that may affect the impurity profile of the drug product;

(F) Changes solely affecting a natural product, a recombinant DNA-derived protein/polypeptide, or a complex or conjugate of a drug substance with a monoclonal antibody for the following:

(1) Changes in the virus or adventitious agent removal or inactivation method(s),

(2) Changes in the source material or cell line, and

(3) Establishment of a new master cell bank or seed;

(G) Changes to a drug under an application that is subject to a validity assessment because of significant questions regarding the integrity of the data supporting that application.

(iii) The applicant must obtain approval of a supplement from FDA prior to distribution of a drug made using a change under paragraph (b)(2) of this section. The supplement must be labeled "Prior Approval Supplement." Except for submissions under paragraph (b)(2)(v) of this section, the following information must be contained in the supplement:

(A) A completed Form FDA 356V;

(B) A detailed description of the proposed change;

(C) The drug(s) involved;

(D) The manufacturing site(s) or area(s) affected;

(E) A description of the methods used and studies performed to assess the effects of the change;

(F) The data derived from such studies;

(G) Appropriate documentation (for example, updated master batch records, specification sheets) including previously approved documentation (with the changes highlighted) or references to previously approved documentation;

(H) For a natural product, a recombinant DNA-derived protein/polypeptide, or a complex or conjugate of a drug substance with a monoclonal antibody, relevant validation protocols and standard operating procedures must be provided in addition to the requirements in paragraphs (b)(2)(iii)(E) and (b)(2)(iii)(F) of this section;

(I) For sterilization process and test methodologies related to sterilization process validation, relevant validation protocols and a list of relevant standard operating procedures must be provided in addition to the requirements in paragraphs (b)(2)(iii)(E) and (b)(2)(iii)(F) of this section; and

(J) Any other information as directed by FDA.

(iv) An applicant may ask FDA to expedite its review of a supplement for public health reasons or if a delay in making the change described in it would impose an

Part 514

extraordinary hardship on the applicant. Such a supplement and its mailing cover must be plainly marked: "Prior Approval Supplement-Expedited Review Requested."

(v) Comparability Protocols. An applicant may submit one or more protocols describing the specific tests and studies and acceptance criteria to be achieved to demonstrate the lack of adverse effect for specified types of manufacturing changes on the identity, strength, quality, purity, and potency of the drug as these factors may relate to the safety or effectiveness of the drug. Any such protocols, if not included in the approved application, or changes to an approved protocol, must be submitted as a supplement requiring approval from FDA prior to distribution of the drug produced with the manufacturing change. The supplement, if approved, may subsequently justify a reduced reporting category for the particular change because the use of the protocol for that type of change reduces the potential risk of an adverse effect. A comparability protocol supplement must be labeled "Prior Approval Supplement--Comparability Protocol."

(3) Changes requiring submission of a supplement at least 30 days prior to distribution of the drug made using the change (moderate changes).

(i) A supplement must be submitted for any change in the drug, production process, quality controls, equipment, or facilities that has a moderate potential to have an adverse effect on the identity, strength, quality, purity, or potency of the drug as these factors may relate to the safety or effectiveness of the drug.

(ii) These changes include, but are not limited to:

(A) A change in the container closure system that does not affect the quality of the drug except as otherwise described in paragraphs (b)(2) and (b)(4) of this section;

(B) Changes solely affecting a natural protein, a recombinant DNA-derived protein/polypeptide or a complex or conjugate of a drug substance with a monoclonal antibody, including:

(1) An increase or decrease in production scale during finishing steps that involves different equipment, and

(2) Replacement of equipment with that of a different design that does not affect the process methodology or process operating parameters.

(C) Relaxation of an acceptance criterion or deletion of a test to comply with an official compendium that is consistent with FDA statutory and regulatory requirements.

(iii) A supplement submitted under paragraph (b)(3)(i) or (b)(3)(vi) of this section is required to give a full explanation of the basis for the change and identify the date on which the change is made. The supplement submitted under paragraph (b)(3)(i) must be labeled "Supplement-Changes Being Effected in 30 Days."

(iv) Pending approval of the supplement by FDA and except as provided in paragraph (b)(3)(vi) of this section, distribution of the drug made using the change may begin not less than 30 days after receipt of the supplement by FDA. The information listed in paragraphs (b)(2)(iii)(A) through (b)(2)(iii)(J) of this section must be contained in the supplement.

(v) The applicant must not distribute the drug made using the change if within 30 days following FDA's receipt of the supplement, FDA informs the applicant that either:

(A) The change requires approval prior to distribution of the drug in accordance with paragraph (b)(2) of this section; or

(B) Any of the information required under paragraph (b)(3)(iv) of this section is missing. In this case, the applicant must not distribute the drug made using the change until the supplement has been amended to provide the missing information.

(vi) The agency may designate a category of changes for the purpose of providing that, in the case of a change in such category, the holder of an approved application may commence distribution of the drug involved upon receipt by the agency of a supplement for the change. The information listed in paragraphs (b)(2)(iii)(A) through

Part 514

(b)(2)(iii)(J) of this section must be contained in the supplement. The supplement must be labeled "Supplement-Changes Being Effected." These changes include, but are not limited to:

(A) Addition to a specification or changes in the methods or controls to provide increased assurance that the drug will have the characteristics of identity, strength, quality, purity, or potency that it purports or is represented to possess; and

(B) A change in the size and/or shape of a container for a nonsterile drug product, except for solid dosage forms, without a change in the labeled amount of drug product or from one container closure system to another.

(vii)   If the agency disapproves the supplemental application, it may order the manufacturer to cease distribution of the drug(s) made with the manufacturing change.

(4) Changes and updated stability data to be described and submitted in an annual report (minor changes).

(i) Changes in the drug, production process, quality controls, equipment, or facilities that have a minimal potential to have an adverse effect on the identity, strength, quality, purity, or potency of the drug as these factors may relate to the safety or effectiveness of the drug must be documented by the applicant in an annual report to the application as described under paragraph (a)(2)(iii) of this section. The report must be labeled "Minor Changes and Stability Report."

(ii) These changes include but are not limited to:

(A) Any change made to comply with a change to an official compendium, except a change in paragraph (b)(3)(ii)(C) of this section, that is consistent with FDA statutory and regulatory requirements;

(B) The deletion or reduction of an ingredient intended to affect only the color of the drug product;

(C) Replacement of equipment with that of the same design and operating principles except for those equipment changes described in paragraph (b)(3)(ii)(B)(2) of this section;

(D) A change in the size and/or shape of a container containing the same number of dosage units for a nonsterile solid dosage form drug product, without a change from one container closure system to another;

(E) A change within the container closure system for a nonsterile drug product, based upon a showing of equivalency to the approved system under a protocol approved in the application or published in an official compendium;

(F) An extension of an expiration dating period based upon full shelf-life data on production batches obtained from a protocol approved in the application;

(G) The addition or revision of an alternative analytical procedure that provides the same or increased assurance of the identity, strength, quality, purity, or potency of the drug being tested as the analytical procedure described in the approved application, or deletion of an alternative analytical procedure; and

(H) The addition by embossing, debossing, or engraving of a code imprint to a solid oral dosage form drug product other than a modified release dosage form, or a minor change in an existing code imprint.

(iii) For changes under this category, the applicant is required to submit in the annual report:

(A) A completed Form FDA 356V;

(B) A statement by the holder of the approved application that the effects of the change have been assessed;

(C) A detailed description of the change(s);

(D) The manufacturing site(s) or area(s) involved;

(E) The date each change was implemented;

(F) Data from studies and tests performed to assess the effects of the change;

Part 514

(G) For a natural product, recombinant DNA-derived protein/polypeptide, complex or conjugate of a drug substance with a monoclonal antibody, sterilization process or test methodology related to sterilization process validation, relevant validation protocols and/or standard operating procedures;

(H) Appropriate documentation (for example, updated master batch records, specification sheets, etc.) including previously approved documentation (with the changes highlighted) or references to previously approved documentation;

(I) Updated stability data generated on commercial or production batches according to an approved stability protocol or commitment; and

(J) Any other information as directed by FDA.

(c) Labeling and other changes to an approved application –

(1) General provisions. The applicant must notify FDA about each change in each condition established in an approved application beyond the variations already provided for in the application. The notice is required to describe the change fully.

(2) Labeling changes requiring the submission and approval of a supplement prior to distribution of the drug made using the change (major changes).

(i) Addition of intended uses and changes to package labeling require a supplement. These changes include, but are not limited to:

(A) Revision in labeling, such as updating information pertaining to effects, dosages, adverse reactions, contraindications, which includes information headed "adverse reactions," "warnings," "precautions," and "contraindications," except ones described in (c)(3) of this section;

(B) Addition of an intended use;

(C) If it is a prescription drug, any mailing or promotional piece used after the drug is placed on the market is labeling requiring a supplemental application, unless:

(1) The parts of the labeling furnishing directions, warnings, and information for use of the drug are the same in language and emphasis as labeling approved or permitted; and

(2) Any other parts of the labeling are consistent with and not contrary to such approved or permitted labeling.

(3) Prescription drug labeling not requiring an approved supplemental application is submitted in accordance with 514.80(b)(5)(ii).

(D) Any other changes in labeling, except ones described in paragraph (c)(3) of this section.

(ii) The applicant must obtain approval of the supplement from FDA prior to distribution of the drug. The supplement must contain the following:

(A) A completed Form FDA 356V;

(B) A detailed description of the proposed change;

(C) The drug(s) involved;

(D) The data derived from studies in support of the change; and

(E) Any other information as directed by FDA.

(3) Labeling changes to be placed into effect prior to receipt of a written notice of approval of a supplemental application.

(i) Labeling changes of the following kinds that increase the assurance of drug safety proposed in supplemental applications must be placed into effect immediately:

(A) The addition to package labeling, promotional labeling, or prescription drug advertising of additional warning, contraindication, adverse reaction, and precaution information;

(B) The deletion from package labeling, promotional labeling, or drug advertising of false, misleading, or unsupported intended uses or claims for effectiveness; and

(C) Any other changes as directed by FDA.

Part 514

(ii) Labeling changes (for example, design and style) that do not decrease safety of drug use proposed in supplemental applications may be placed into effect prior to written notice of approval from FDA of a supplemental application.

(iii) A supplement submitted under paragraph (c)(3) of this section must include the following information:

(A) A full explanation of the basis for the changes, the date on which such changes are being effected, and plainly marked on the mailing cover and on the supplement, "Supplement--Labeling Changes Being Effected";

(B) Two sets of printed copies of any revised labeling to be placed in use, identified with the new animal drug application number; and

(C) A statement by the applicant that all promotional labeling and all drug advertising will promptly be revised consistent with the changes made in the labeling on or within the new animal drug package no later than upon approval of the supplemental application.

(iv) If the supplemental application is not approved and the drug is being distributed with the proposed labeling, FDA may initiate an enforcement action because the drug is misbranded under section 502 of the act and/or adulterated under section 501 of the act. In addition, under section 512(e) of the act, FDA may, after due notice and opportunity for a hearing, issue an order withdrawing approval of the application.

(4) Changes providing for additional distributors to be reported under Records and reports concerning experience with approved new animal drugs (514.80). Supplemental applications as described under paragraph (c)(2) of this section will not be required for an additional distributor to distribute a drug that is the subject of an approved new animal drug application or abbreviated new animal drug application if the conditions described under 514.80(b)(5)(iii) are met.

(d) Patent information. The applicant must comply with the patent information requirements under section 512(c)(3) of the act.

(e) Claimed exclusivity. If an applicant claims exclusivity under section 512(c)(2)(F) of the act upon approval of a supplemental application for a change in its previously approved drug, the applicant must include such a statement.

(f) Good laboratory practice for nonclinical laboratory studies. A supplemental application that contains nonclinical laboratory studies must include, with respect to each nonclinical study, either a statement that the study was conducted in compliance with the requirements set forth in part 58 of this chapter, or, if the study was not conducted in compliance with such regulations, a brief statement of the reason for the noncompliance.

[71 FR 74782, Dec. 13, 2006]

Sec. 514.11 Confidentiality of data and information in a new animal drug application file.

(a) For purposes of this section theNADA file includes all data and information submitted with or incorporated by reference in the NADA, INAD's incorporated into the NADA, supplemental NADA's, reports under 514.80 and 510.301 of this chapter, master files, and other related submissions. The availability for public disclosure of any record in the NADA file shall be handled in accordance with the provisions of this section.

(b) The existence of an NADA file will not be disclosed by the Food and Drug Administration before an approval has been published in theFederal Register,unless it has previously been publicly disclosed or acknowledged.

(c) If the existence of an NADA file has not been publicly disclosed or acknowledged, no data or information in the NADA file is available for public disclosure.

(d) If the existence of an NADA file has been publicly disclosed or acknowledged before an approval has been published in theFederal Register,no data or information contained in the file is available for public disclosure before such approval is published, but the Commissioner may, in his discretion, disclose a summary of such selected portions of the safety and effectiveness data as are appropriate for public consideration of a specific pending issue, e.g., at an open session of a Food and Drug Administration

Part 514

advisory committee or pursuant to an exchange of important regulatory information with a foreign government.

(e) After an approval has been published in the Federal Register, the following data and information in the NADA file are immediately available for public disclosure unless extraordinary circumstances are shown:

(1) All safety and effectiveness data and information previously disclosed to the public, as defined in 20.81 of this chapter.

(2) A summary or summaries of the safety and effectiveness data and information submitted with or incorporated by reference in the NADA file. Such summaries do not constitute the full reports of investigations under section 512(b)(1) of the act (21 U.S.C. 360b(b)(1)) on which the safety or effectiveness of the drug may be approved. Such summaries shall consist of the following:

(i) For an NADA approved prior to July 1, 1975, internal agency records that describe such data and information, e.g., a summary of basis for approval or internal reviews of the data and information, after deletion of:

(a) Names and any information that would identify the investigators.

(b) Any inappropriate gratuitous comments unnecessary to an objective analysis of the data and information.

(ii) For an NADA approved on or after July 1, 1975, a summary of such data and information prepared in one of the following two alternative ways shall be publicly released when the approval is published in the Federal Register.

(a) The Center for Veterinary Medicine may at an appropriate time prior to approval of the NADA require the applicant to prepare a summary of such data and information, which will be reviewed and, where appropriate, revised by the Center.

(b) The Center for Veterinary Medicine may prepare its own summary of such data and information.

(3) A protocol for a test or study, unless it is shown to fall within the exemption established for trade secrets and confidential commercial information in 20.61 of this chapter.

(4) Adverse reaction reports, product experience reports, consumer complaints, and other similar data and information, after deletion of:

    (i) Names and any information that would identify the person using the product.

    (ii) Names and any information that would identify any third party involved with the report, such as a physician, hospital, or other institution.

(5) A list of all active ingredients and any inactive ingredients previously disclosed to the public as defined in 20.81 of this chapter.

(6) An assay method or other analytical method, unless it serves no regulatory or compliance purpose and is shown to fall within the exemption established in 20.61 of this chapter.

(7) All correspondence and written summaries of oral discussions relating to the NADA, in accordance with the provisions of part 20 of this chapter.

(f) All safety and effectiveness data and information not previously disclosed to the public are available for public disclosure at the time any one of the following events occurs unless extraordinary circumstances are known:

(1) The NADA has been abandoned and no further work is being undertaken with respect to it.

(2) A final determination is made that the NADA is not approvable, and all legal appeals have been exhausted.

(3) Approval of the NADA is withdrawn, and all legal appeals have been exhausted.

(4) A final determination has been made that the animal drug is not a new animal drug.

(5) A final determination has been made that the animal drug may be marketed without submission of such safety and/or effectiveness data and information.

(g) The following data and information in an NADA file are not available for public disclosure unless they have been previously disclosed to the public as defined in 20.81 of this chapter or they relate to a product or ingredient that has been abandoned and they

Part 514

---

no longer represent a trade secret or confidential commercial or financial information as defined in 20.61 of this chapter:

(1) Manufacturing methods or processes, including quality control procedures.

(2) Production, sales, distribution, and similar data and information, except that any compilation of such data and information aggregated and prepared in a way that does not reveal data or information which is not available for public disclosure under this provision is available for public disclosure.

(3) Quantitative or semiquantitative formulas.

(h) For purposes of this regulation, safety and effectiveness data include all studies and tests of an animal drug on animals and all studies and tests on the animal drug for identity, stability, purity, potency, and bioavailability.

[40 FR 13825, Mar. 27, 1975, as amended at 42 FR 3109, Jan. 14, 1977; 42 FR 15675, Mar. 22, 1977; 54 FR 18280, Apr. 28, 1989; 68 FR 15365, Mar. 31, 2003]

Sec. 514.12 Confidentiality of data and information in an investigational new animal drug notice.

(a) The existence of an INAD notice will not be disclosed by the Food and Drug Administration unless it has previously been publicly disclosed or acknowledged.

(b) The availability for public disclosure of all data and information in an INAD file shall be handled in accordance with provisions established in 514.11.

Sec. 514.15 Untrue statements in applications.

Among the reasons why an application for a new animal drug or animal feed bearing or containing a new animal drug may contain an untrue statement of a material fact are:

(a) Differences in:

(1) Conditions of use prescribed, recommended, or suggested by the applicant for the product from the conditions of such use stated in the application;

(2) Articles used as components of the product from those listed in the application;

(3) Composition of the product from that stated in the application;

(4) Methods used in or the facilities and controls used for the manufacture, processing, or packing of the product from such methods, facilities, and controls described in the application;

(5) Labeling from the specimens contained in the application; or

(b) The unexplained omission in whole or in part from an application or from an amendment or supplement to an application or from any record or report required under the provisions of section 512 of the act and 514.80 or 510.301 of this chapter of any information obtained from:

(1) Investigations as to the safety, effectiveness, identity, strength, quality, or purity of the drug, made by the applicant on the drug, or

(2) Investigations or experience with the product that is the subject of the application, or any related product, available to the applicant from any source if such information is pertinent to an evaluation of the safety, effectiveness, identity, strength, quality, or purity of the drug, when such omission would bias an evaluation of the safety or effectiveness of the product.

(c) Any nonclinical laboratory study contained in the application was not conducted in compliance with the good laboratory practice regulations as set forth in part 58 of this chapter, and the application fails to include a brief statement of the reason for the noncompliance.

[40 FR 13825, Mar. 27, 1975, as amended at 49 FR 7226, Feb. 28, 1984; 50 FR 7517, Feb. 22, 1985; 68 FR 15365, Mar. 31, 2003]

Part 514

Subpart B--Administrative Actions on Applications

Sec. 514.80 Records and reports concerning experience with approved new animal drugs.

The following table outlines the purpose for each paragraph of this section:

Purpose	21 CFR Paragraph and Title
What information must be reported concerning approved NADAs or ANADAs?	514.80(a) Applicability.
What authority does FDA have for requesting records and reports?Who is required to establish, maintain, and report required information relating to experiences with a new animal drug?Is information from foreign sources required?	514.80(a)(1).
What records must be established and maintained and what reports filed with FDA?	514.80(a)(2).
What is FDA's purpose for requiring reports?	514.80(a)(3).
Do applicants of Type A medicated articles have to establish, maintain, and report information required under 514.80?	514.80(a)(4).
How do the requirements under 514.80 relate to current good manufacturing practices?	514.80(a)(5).
	514.80(b) Reporting requirements.
What are the requirements for reporting product/manufacturing defects?	514.80(b)(1) Three-day NADA/ANADA field alert report.
	514.80(b)(2) Fifteen-day NADA/ANADA alert report.
What are the requirements for reporting serious and unexpected adverse drug experiences?	514.80(b)(2)(i) Initial report.
What are the requirements for followup reporting of serious and unexpected adverse drug experiences?	514.80(b)(2)(ii) Followup report.
What are the requirements for nonapplicants for reporting adverse drug experiences?	514.80(b)(3) Nonapplicant report.
What are the general requirements for submission of periodic drug experience reports, e.g., forms to be submitted, submission date and frequency, when is it to be submitted, how many copies?How do I petition to change	514.80(b)(4) Periodic drug experience report.

Purpose	21 CFR Paragraph and Title
the date of submission or frequency of submissions?	
What must be submitted in the periodic drug experience reports?	514.80(b)(4)(i) through (b)(4)(iv).
What distribution data must be submitted?How should the distribution data be submitted?	514.80(b)(4)(i) Distribution data.
What labeling materials should be submitted?How do I report changes to the labeling materials since the last report?	514.80(b)(4)(ii) Labeling.
	514.80(b)(4)(iii) Nonclinical laboratory studies and clinical data not previously reported.
What are the requirements for submission of nonclinical laboratory studies?	514.80(b)(4)(iii)(A).
What are the requirements for submission of clinical laboratory data?	514.80(b)(4)(iii)(B).
When must results of clinical trials conducted by or for the applicant be reported?	514.80(b)(4)(iii)(C).
	514.80(b)(4)(iv) Adverse drug experiences.
How do I report product/manufacturing defects and adverse drug experiences not previously reported to FDA?	514.80(b)(4)(iv)(A).
What are the requirements for submitting adverse drug experiences cited in literature?	514.80(b)(4)(iv)(B).
What are the requirements for submitting adverse drug experiences in postapproval studies and clinical trials?	514.80(b)(4)(iv)(C).
What are the requirements for reporting increases in the frequency of serious, expected, and unexpected adverse drug experiences?	514.80(b)(4)(v) Summary report of increased frequency of adverse drug experience.
	514.80(b)(5) Other reporting.
Can FDA request that an applicant submit information at different times than stated specifically in this regulation?	514.80(b)(5)(i) Special drug experience report.
What are the requirements for submission of advertisement and promotional labeling to FDA?	514.80(b)(5)(ii) Advertisements and promotional labeling.
What are the requirements for adding a new distributor to the approved application?	514.80(b)(5)(iii) Distributor's statement.
What labels and how many labels need to be submitted for review?	514.80(b)(5)(iii)(A).

Part 514

Purpose	21 CFR Paragraph and Title
What changes are required and allowed to distributor labeling?	514.80(b)(5)(iii)(A)(1).
What are the requirements for making other changes to the distributor labeling?	514.80(b)(5)(iii)(A)(2).
What information should be included in each new distributor's signed statement?	514.80(b)(5)(iii)(B)(1) through (b)(5)(iii)(B)(5).
What are the conditions for submitting information that is common to more than one application? (i.e., can I submit common information to one application?)	514.80(c) Multiple applications.
What information has to be submitted to the common application and related application?	514.80(c)(1) through (c)(4).
What forms do I need?What are Forms FDA 1932 and 2301?How can I get them?Can I use computer-generated equivalents?	514.80(d) Reporting forms.
How long must I maintain Form FDA 1932 and records and reports of other required information, i.e., how long do I need to maintain this information?	514.80(e) Records to be maintained.
What are the requirements for allowing access to these records and reports, and copying by authorized FDA officer or employee?	514.80(f) Access to records and reports.
How do I obtain Forms FDA 1932 and 2301?Where do I mail FDA's required forms, records, and reports?	514.80(g) Mailing addresses.
What happens if the applicant fails to establish, maintain, or make the required reports?What happens if the applicant refuses to allow FDA access to, and/or copying and/or verify records and reports?	514.80(h) Withdrawal of approval.
Does an adverse drug experience reflect a conclusion that the report or information constitutes an admission that the drug caused an adverse effect?	514.80(i) Disclaimer.

(a) Applicability.

(1) Each applicant must establish and maintain indexed and complete files containing full records of all information pertinent to safety or effectiveness of a new animal drug that has not been previously submitted as part of the NADA or ANADA. Such records must include information from domestic as well as foreign sources. Each nonapplicant must establish and maintain indexed and complete files containing

full records of all information pertinent to safety or effectiveness of a new animal drug that is received or otherwise obtained by the nonapplicant. Such records must include information from domestic as well as foreign sources.

(2) Each applicant must submit reports of data, studies, and other information concerning experience with new animal drugs to the Food and Drug Administration (FDA) for each approved NADA and ANADA, as required in this section. A nonapplicant must submit data, studies, and other information concerning experience with new animal drugs to the appropriate applicant, as required in this section. The applicant, in turn, must report the nonapplicant's data, studies, and other information to FDA. Applicants and nonapplicants must submit data, studies, and other information described in this section from domestic, as well as foreign sources.

(3) FDA reviews the records and reports required in this section to facilitate a determination under section 512(e) of the Federal Food, Drug, and Cosmetic Act (21 U.S.C. 360b(e)) as to whether there may be grounds for suspending or withdrawing approval of the NADA or ANADA.

(4) The requirements of this section also apply to any approved Type A medicated article. In addition, the requirements contained in 514.80(b)(1), (b)(2), (b)(4)(iv), and (b)(4)(v) apply to any approved Type A medicated article incorporated in animal feeds.

(5) The records and reports referred to in this section are in addition to those required by the current good manufacturing practice regulations in parts 211, 225, and 226 of this chapter.

(b) Reporting requirements –

(1) Three-day NADA/ANADA field alert report. This report provides information pertaining to product and manufacturing defects that may result in serious adverse drug events. The applicant (or nonapplicant through the applicant) must submit the report to the appropriate FDA District Office or local FDA resident post within 3 working days of first becoming aware that a defect may exist. The information initially may be provided by telephone or other telecommunication means, with prompt written followup using Form FDA 1932 "Veterinary Adverse Drug Reaction,

Part 514

Lack of Effectiveness, Product Defect Report." The mailing cover for these reports must be plainly marked "3-Day NADA/ANADA Field Alert Report."

(2) Fifteen-day NADA/ANADA alert report –

(i) Initial report. This report provides information on each serious, unexpected adverse drug event, regardless of the source of the information. The applicant (or nonapplicant through the applicant) must submit the report to FDA within 15 working days of first receiving the information. The report must be submitted on Form FDA 1932, and its mailing cover must be plainly marked "15-Day NADA/ANADA Alert Report."

(ii) Followup report. The applicant must promptly investigate all adverse drug events that are the subject of 15-day NADA/ANADA alert reports. If this investigation reveals significant new information, a followup report must be submitted within 15 working days of receiving such information. A followup report must be submitted on Form FDA 1932, and its mailing cover must be plainly marked "15-Day NADA/ANADA Alert Report Followup." The followup report must state the date of the initial report and provide the additional information. If additional information is sought but not obtained within 3 months of the initial report, a followup report is required describing the steps taken and why additional information was not obtained.

(3) Nonapplicant report. Nonapplicants must forward reports of adverse drug experiences to the applicant within 3 working days of first receiving the information. The applicant must then submit the report(s) to FDA as required in this section. The nonapplicant must maintain records of all nonapplicant reports, including the date the nonapplicant received the information concerning adverse drug experiences, the name and address of the applicant, and a copy of the adverse drug experience report including the date such report was submitted to the applicant. If the nonapplicant elects to also report directly to FDA, the nonapplicant should submit the report on Form FDA 1932 within 15 working days of first receiving the information.

(4) Periodic drug experience report. This report must be accompanied by a completed Form FDA 2301 "Transmittal

of Periodic Reports and Promotional Materials for New Animal Drugs." It must be submitted every 6 months for the first 2 years following approval of an NADA or ANADA and yearly thereafter. Reports required by this section must contain data and information for the full reporting period. The 6-month periodic drug experience reports must be submitted within 30 days following the end of the 6-month reporting period. The yearly periodic drug experience reports must be submitted within 60 days of the anniversary date of the approval of the NADA or ANADA. Any previously submitted information contained in the report must be identified as such. For yearly (annual) periodic drug experience reports, the applicant may petition FDA to change the date of submission or frequency of reporting, and after approval of such petition, file such reports on the new filing date or at the new reporting frequency. Also, FDA may require a report at different times or more frequently. The periodic drug experience report must contain the following:

(i) Distribution data. Information about the distribution of each new animal drug product, including information on any distributor-labeled product. This information must include the total number of distributed units of each size, strength, or potency (e.g., 100,000 bottles of 100 5-milligram tablets; 50,000 10-milliliter vials of 5-percent solution). This information must be presented in two categories: Quantities distributed domestically and quantities exported.

(ii) Labeling. Applicant and distributor current package labeling, including package inserts (if any). For large-size package labeling or large shipping cartons, a representative copy must be submitted (e.g., a photocopy of pertinent areas of large feed bags). A summary of any changes in labeling made since the last report (listed by date of implementation) must be included with the labeling or if there have been no changes, a statement of such fact must be included with the labeling.

(iii) Nonclinical laboratory studies and clinical data not previously reported.

(A) Copies of in vitro studies (e.g., mutagenicity) and other nonclinical laboratory studies conducted by or otherwise obtained by the applicant.

Part 514

(B) Copies of published clinical trials of the new animal drug (or abstracts of them) including clinical trials on safety and effectiveness, clinical trials on new uses, and reports of clinical experience pertinent to safety conducted by or otherwise obtained by the applicant. Review articles, papers, and abstracts in which the drug is used as a research tool, promotional articles, press clippings, and papers that do not contain tabulations or summaries of original data are not required to be reported.

(C) Descriptions of completed clinical trials conducted by or for the applicant must be submitted no later than 1 year after completion of research. Supporting information is not to be reported.

(iv) Adverse drug experiences.

(A) Product/manufacturing defects and adverse drug experiences not previously reported under 514.80(b)(1) and (b)(2) must be reported individually on Form FDA 1932.

(B) Reports of adverse drug experiences in the literature must be noted in the periodic drug experience report. A bibliography of pertinent references must be included with the report. Upon FDA's request, the applicant must provide a full text copy of these publications.

(C) Reports of previously not reported adverse drug experiences that occur in postapproval studies must be reported separately from other experiences in the periodic drug experience report and clearly marked or highlighted.

(v) Summary report of increased frequency of adverse drug experience. The applicant must periodically review the incidence of reports of adverse drug experiences to determine if there has been an increased frequency of serious (expected and unexpected) adverse drug events. The applicant must evaluate the increased frequency of serious (expected or unexpected) adverse drug events at least as often as reporting of periodic drug experience reports. The applicant must report the increased frequency of serious (expected and unexpected) adverse drug events in the periodic drug experience report.

Summaries of reports of increased frequency of adverse drug events must be submitted in narrative form. The summaries must state the time period on which the increased frequency is based, time period comparisons in determining increased frequency, references to any previously submitted Form FDA 1932, the method of analysis, and the interpretation of the results. The summaries must be submitted in a separate section within the periodic drug experience report.

(5) Other reporting –

(i) Special drug experience report. Upon written request, FDA may require that the applicant submit a report required under 514.80 at different times or more frequently than the timeframes stated in 514.80.

(ii) Advertisements and promotional labeling. The applicant must submit at the time of initial dissemination one set of specimens of mailing pieces and other labeling for prescription and over-the-counter new animal drugs. For prescription new animal drugs, the applicant must also submit one set of specimens of any advertisement at the time of initial publication or broadcast. Mailing pieces and labeling designed to contain product samples must be complete except that product samples may be omitted. Each submission of promotional labeling or advertisements must be accompanied by a completed Form FDA 2301.

(iii) Distributor's statement. At the time of initial distribution of a new animal drug product by a distributor, the applicant must submit a special drug experience report accompanied by a completed Form FDA 2301 containing the following:

(A) The distributor's current product labeling.

(1) The distributor's labeling must be identical to that in the approved NADA/ANADA except for a different and suitable proprietary name (if used) and the name and address of the distributor. The name and address of the distributor must be preceded by an appropriate qualifying phrase as permitted by the regulations such as "manufactured for" or "distributed by."

    (2) Other labeling changes must be the subject of a supplemental NADA or ANADA as described under 514.8.

  (B) A signed statement by the distributor stating:

    (1) The category of the distributor's operations (e.g., wholesale or retail),

    (2) That the distributor will distribute the new animal drug only under the approved labeling,

    (3) That the distributor will promote the product only for use under the conditions stated in the approved labeling,

    (4) That the distributor will adhere to the records and reports requirements of this section, and

    (5) That the distributor is regularly and lawfully engaged in the distribution or dispensing of prescription products if the product is a prescription new animal drug.

(c) Multiple applications. Whenever an applicant is required to submit a periodic drug experience report under the provisions of 514.80(b)(4) with respect to more than one approved NADA or ANADA for preparations containing the same new animal drug so that the same information is required to be reported for more than one application, the applicant may elect to submit as a part of the report for one such application (the primary application) all the information common to such applications in lieu of reporting separately and repetitively on each. If the applicant elects to do this, the applicant must do the following:

  (1) State when a report applies to multiple applications and identify all related applications for which the report is submitted by NADA or ANADA number.

  (2) Ensure that the primary application contains a list of the NADA or ANADA numbers of all related applications.

  (3) Submit a completed Form FDA 2301 to the primary application and each related application with reference to the primary application by NADA/ANADA number and submission date for the complete report of the common information.

(4) All other information specific to a particular NADA/ANADA must be included in the report for that particular NADA/ANADA.

(d) *Reporting forms.* Applicant must report adverse drug experiences and product/manufacturing defects on Form FDA 1932, "Veterinary Adverse Drug Reaction, Lack of Effectiveness, Product Defect Report." Periodic drug experience reports and special drug experience reports must be accompanied by a completed Form FDA 2301 "Transmittal of Periodic Reports and Promotional Material for New Animal Drugs," in accordance with directions provided on the forms. Computer-generated equivalents of Form FDA 1932 or Form FDA 2301, approved by FDA before use, may be used. Form FDA 1932 and Form FDA 2301 may be obtained on the Internet athttp://www.fda.gov/cvm/forms/forms.html, by telephoning the Division of Surveillance (HFV-210), or by submitting a written request to the following address: Food and Drug Administration, Center for Veterinary Medicine, Division of Surveillance (HFV-210), 7500 Standish Pl., Rockville, MD 20855-2764.

(e) *Records to be maintained.* The applicants and nonapplicants must maintain records and reports of all information required by this section for a period of 5 years after the date of submission.

(f) *Access to records and reports.* The applicant and nonapplicant must, upon request from any authorized FDA officer or employee, at all reasonable times, permit such officer or employee to have access to copy and to verify all such required records and reports.

(g) *Mailing addresses.* Completed 15-day alert reports, periodic drug experience reports, and special drug experience reports must be submitted to the following address: Food and Drug Administration, Center for Veterinary Medicine, Document Control Unit (HFV-199), 7500 Standish Pl., Rockville, MD 20855-2764. Three-day alert reports must be submitted to the appropriate FDA district office or local FDA resident post. Addresses for district offices and resident posts may be obtained from the Internet athttp://www.fda.gov (click on "Contact FDA," then "FDA Field Offices").

(h) *Withdrawal of approval.* If FDA finds that the applicant has failed to establish the required records, or has failed to maintain those

Part 514

records, or failed to make the required reports, or has refused access to an authorized FDA officer or employee to copy or to verify such records or reports, FDA may withdraw approval of the application to which such records or reports relate. If FDA determines that withdrawal of the approval is necessary, the agency shall give the applicant notice and opportunity for hearing, as provided in 514.200, on the question of whether to withdraw approval of the application.

(i) Disclaimer. Any report or information submitted under this section and any release of that report or information by FDA will be without prejudice and does not necessarily reflect a conclusion that the report or information constitutes an admission that the drug caused or contributed to an adverse event. A person need not admit, and may deny, that the report or information constitutes an admission that a drug caused or contributed to an adverse event.

[68 FR 15365, Mar. 31, 2003]

Sec. 514.100 Evaluation and comment on applications.

(a) After the filed application has been evaluated, the applicant will be furnished written comment on any apparent deficiencies in the application.

(b) When the description of the methods used in, and the facilities and controls used for, the manufacture, processing, and packing of such new animal drug appears adequate on its face, but it is not feasible to reach a conclusion as to the safety and effectiveness of the new animal drug solely from consideration of this description, the applicant may be notified that an establishment inspection is required to verify their adequacy.

(c) A request for samples of a new animal drug or any edible tissues and byproducts of animals treated with such a drug, shall specify the quantity deemed adequate to permit tests of analytical methods to determine their adequacy for regulatory purposes. The request should be made as early in the 180-day period as possible to assure timely completion. The date used for computing the 180-day limit for the purposes of section 512(c) of the act shall be moved forward 1 day for each day after the mailing date of the request until all of the requested samples are received. If the samples are not received within 90 days after the request, the application will be considered withdrawn without prejudice.

(d) The information contained in an application may be insufficient to determine whether a new animal drug is safe or effective in use if it fails to include (among other things) a statement showing whether such drug is to be limited to prescription sale and exempt under section 502(f) of the act from the requirement that its labeling bear adequate directions for lay use. If such drug is to be exempt, the information may also be insufficient if:

(1) The specimen labeling proposed fails to bear adequate information for professional use including indications, effects, dosages, routes, methods, and frequency and duration of administration and any relevant hazards, contraindications, side effects, and precautions under which practitioners licensed by law to administer such drug can use the drug for the purposes for which it is intended, including all purposes for which it is to be advertised, or represented, in accordance with 201.105 of this chapter, and information concerning hazards, contraindications, side effects, and precautions relevant with respect to any uses for which such drug is to be prescribed.

(2) The application fails to show that the labeling and advertising of such drug will offer the drug for use only under those conditions for which it is offered in the labeling that is part of the application.

(3) The application fails to show that all labeling that furnishes or purports to furnish information for professional use of such drug will contain, in the same language and emphasis, the information for use including indications, effects, dosages, routes, methods, and frequency and duration of administration and any relevant warnings, hazards, contraindications, side effects, and precautions, which is contained in the labeling that is part of the application in accordance with 201.105 of this chapter.

(e) The information contained in an application will be considered insufficient to determine whether a new animal drug is safe and effective for use when there is a refusal or failure upon written notice to furnish inspectors authorized by the Food and Drug Administration an adequate opportunity to inspect the facilities, controls, and records pertinent to the application.

Part 514

(f) On the basis of preliminary consideration of an application or supplemental application containing typewritten or other draft labeling in lieu of final printed labeling, an applicant may be informed that such application is approvable when satisfactory final printed labeling identical in content to such draft copy is submitted.

(g) When an application has been found incomplete on the basis of a need for the kind of information described in 514.6, such application shall be considered withdrawn without prejudice to future filing on the date of issuance of the letter citing the inadequacies contained in the application, unless within 30 days the sponsor chooses to avail himself of the opportunity for hearing as prescribed by 514.111.

Sec. 514.105 Approval of applications.

(a) The Commissioner shall forward for publication in theFederal Registera regulation prescribing the conditions under which the new animal drug may be used, including the name and address of the applicant; the conditions and indications for use covered by the application; any tolerance, withdrawal period, or other use restrictions; any tolerance required for the new animal drug substance or its metabolites in edible products of food-producing animals; and, if such new animal drug is intended for use in animal feed, appropriate purposes and conditions of use (including special labeling requirements) applicable to any animal feed; and such other information the Commissioner deems necessary to assure safe and effective use.

(b) He shall notify the applicant by sending him a copy of the proposed publication as described in paragraph (a)(1) of this section.

[40 FR 13825, Mar. 27, 1975, as amended at 51 FR 7392, Mar. 3, 1986; 64 FR 63203, Nov. 19, 1999]

Sec. 514.106 Approval of supplemental applications.

(a) Within 180 days after a supplement to an approved application is filed pursuant to 514.8, the Commissioner shall approve the supplemental application in accordance with procedures set forth in 514.105(a)(1) and (2) if he/she determines that the application satisfies the requirements of applicable statutory provisions and regulations.

(b) The Commissioner will assign a supplemental application to its proper category to ensure processing of the application.

  (1) Category I. Supplements that ordinarily do not require a reevaluation of any of the safety or effectiveness data in the parent application. Category I supplements include the following:

  (i) A corporate change that alters the identity or address of the sponsor of the new animal drug application (NADA).

  (ii) The sale, purchase, or construction of manufacturing facilities.

  (iii) The sale or purchase of an NADA.

  (iv) A change in container, container style, shape, size, or components.

  (v) A change in approved labeling (color, style, format, addition, deletion, or revision of certain statements, e.g., trade name, storage, expiration dates, etc).

  (vi) A change in promotional material for a prescription new animal drug not exempted by 514.8(c)(2)(i)(C)(1) through (c)(2)(i)(C)(3).

  (vii) Changes in manufacturing processes that do not alter the method of manufacture or change the final dosage form.

  (viii) A change in bulk drug shipments.

  (ix) A change in an analytical method or control procedures that do not alter the approved standards.

  (x) A change in an expiration date.

  (xi) Addition of an alternate manufacturer, repackager, or relabeler of the drug product.

  (xii) Addition of an alternate supplier of the new drug substance.

  (xiii) A change permitted in advance of approval as described under 514.8(b)(3).

Part 514

(2) Category II. Supplements that may require a reevaluation of certain safety or effectiveness data in the parent application. Category II supplements include the following:

(i) A change in the active ingredient concentration or composition of the final product.

(ii) A change in quality, purity, strength, and identity specifications of the active or inactive ingredients.

(iii) A change in dose (amount of drug administered per dose).

(iv) A change in the treatment regimen (schedule of dosing).

(v) Addition of a new therapeutic claim to the approved uses of the product.

(vi) Addition of a new or revised animal production claim.

(vii) Addition of a new species.

(viii) A change in the prescription or over-the-counter status of a drug product.

(ix) A change in statements regarding side effects, warnings, precautions, and contraindications, except the addition of approved statements to container, package, and promotional labeling, and prescription drug advertising.

(x) A change in the drug withdrawal period prior to slaughter or in the milk discard time.

(xi) A change in the tolerance for drug residues.

(xii) A change in analytical methods for drug residues.

(xiii) A revised method of synthesis or fermentation of the new drug substance.

(xiv) Updating or changes in the manufacturing process of the new drug substance and/or final dosage form (other than a change in equipment that does not alter the method of manufacture of a new animal drug, or a change from one commercial batch size to another without any change in manufacturing procedure), or changes in the methods, facilities, or controls used for the manufacture, processing, packaging, or holding of the new animal drug (other than use of an establishment not covered by the approval that is in effect) that give increased assurance that the drug will have the characteristics of identity, strength, quality, and purity which it purports or is represented to possess.

[55 FR 46052, Nov. 1, 1990; 55 FR 49973, Dec. 3, 1990; 56 FR 12422, Mar. 25, 1991; 71 FR 74785, Dec. 13, 2006]

Sec. 514.110 Reasons for refusing to file applications.

(a) The date of receipt of an application for a new animal drug shall be the date on which the application shall be deemed to be filed.

(b) An application for a new animal drug shall not be considered acceptable for filing for any of the following reasons:

 (1) It does not contain complete and accurate English translations of any pertinent part in a foreign language.

 (2) Fewer than three copies are submitted.

 (3) It is incomplete on its face in that it is not properly organized and indexed.

 (4) On its face the information concerning required matter is so inadequate that the application is clearly not approvable.

 (5) The new animal drug is to be manufactured, prepared, propagated, compounded, or processed in whole or in part in any State in an establishment that has not been registered or exempted from registration under the provisions of section 510 of the act.

 (6) The sponsor does not reside or maintain a place of business within the United States and the application has not been countersigned by an attorney, agent, or other representative of the applicant, which representative resides in the United States and has been duly authorized to act on behalf of the applicant and to receive communications on all matters pertaining to the application.

 (7) The new animal drug is a drug subject to licensing under the animal virus, serum, and toxin law of March 4, 1913 (37 Stat. 832; 21 U.S.C. 151et seq.). Such applications will be referred to the U.S. Department of Agriculture for action.

 (8) It fails to include, with respect to each nonclinical laboratory study contained in the application, either a statement that the study was conducted in compliance with the good laboratory practice regulations set forth in part 58 of this chapter, or, if

Part 514

the study was not conducted in compliance with such regulations, a brief statement of the reasons for the noncompliance.

(9) [Reserved]

(10) The applicant fails to submit a complete environmental assessment under 25.40 of this chapter or fails to provide sufficient information to establish that the requested action is subject to categorical exclusion under 25.30 or 25.33 of this chapter.

(c) If an application is determined not to be acceptable for filing, the applicant shall be notified within 30 days of receipt of the application and shall be given the reasons therefore.

(d) If the applicant disputes the findings that his application is not acceptable for filing, he may make written request that the application be filed over protest, in which case it will be filed as of the day originally received.

[40 FR 13825, Mar. 27, 1975, as amended at 50 FR 7517, Feb. 22, 1985; 50 FR 16668, Apr. 26, 1985; 62 FR 40600, July 29, 1997]

Sec. 514.111 Refusal to approve an application.

(a) The Commissioner shall, within 180 days after the filing of the application, inform the applicant in writing of his intention to issue a notice of opportunity for a hearing on a proposal to refuse to approve the application, if the Commissioner determines upon the basis of the application, or upon the basis of other information before him with respect to a new animal drug, that:

(1) The reports of investigations required to be submitted pursuant to section 512(b) of the act do not include adequate tests by all methods reasonably applicable to show whether or not such drug is safe for use under the conditions prescribed, recommended, or suggested in the proposed labeling thereof; or

(2) The results of such tests show that such drug is unsafe for use under such conditions or do not show that such drug is safe for use under such conditions; or

(3) The methods used in and the facilities and controls used for the manufacture, processing, and packing of such drug are

inadequate to preserve its identity, strength, quality, and purity; or

(4) Upon the basis of the information submitted to the Food and Drug Administration as part of the application, or upon the basis of any other information before it with respect to such drug, it has insufficient information to determine whether such drug is safe for use under such conditions. In making this determination the Commissioner shall consider, among other relevant factors:

(i) The probable consumption of such drug and of any substance formed in or on food because of the use of such drug;

(ii) The cumulative effect on man or animal of such drug, taking into account any chemically or pharmacologically related substances;

(iii) Safety factors which, in the opinion of experts qualified by scientific training and experience to evaluate the safety of such drugs, are appropriate for the use of animal experimentation data; and

(iv) Whether the conditions of use prescribed, recommended, or suggested in the proposed labeling are reasonably certain to be followed in practice; or

(5) Evaluated on the basis of information submitted as part of the application and any other information before the Food and Drug Administration with respect to such drug, there is lack of substantial evidence as defined in 514.4.

(6) Failure to include an appropriate proposed tolerance for residues in edible products derived from animals or a withdrawal period or other restrictions for use of such drug if any tolerance or withdrawal period or other restrictions for use are required in order to assure that the edible products derived from animals treated with such drug will be safe.

(7) Based on a fair evaluation of all material facts, the labeling is false or misleading in any particular; or

(8) Such drug induces cancer when ingested by man or animal or, after appropriate tests for evaluation of the safety of such drug, induces cancer in man or animal, except that this subparagraph shall not apply with respect to such drug if the Commissioner finds that, under the conditions of use

Part 514

specified in proposed labeling and reasonably certain to be followed in practice:

(i) Such drug will not adversely affect the animal for which it is intended; and

(ii) No residue of such drug will be found (by methods of examination prescribed or approved by the Commissioner by regulations) in any edible portion of such animal after slaughter or in any food yielded by, or derived from the living animals.

(9) The applicant fails to submit an adequate environmental assessment under 25.40 of this chapter or fails to provide sufficient information to establish that the requested action is subject to categorical exclusion under 25.30 or 25.33 of this chapter.

(10) The drug fails to satisfy the requirements of subpart E of part 500 of this chapter.

(11) Any nonclinical laboratory study that is described in the application and that is essential to show that the drug is safe for use under the conditions prescribed, recommended, or suggested in its proposed labeling, was not conducted in compliance with the good laboratory practice regulations as set forth in part 58 of this chapter and no reason for the noncompliance is provided or, if it is, the differences between the practices used in conducting the study and the good laboratory practice regulations do not support the validity of the study.

(b) The Commissioner, as provided in 514.200 of this chapter, shall expeditiously notify the applicant of an opportunity for a hearing on the question of whether such application is approvable, unless by the 30th day following the date of issuance of the letter informing the applicant of the intention to issue a notice of opportunity for a hearing the applicant:

(1) Withdraws the application; or

(2) Waives the opportunity for a hearing; or

(3) Agrees with the Commissioner on an additional period to precede issuance of such notice of hearing.

[40 FR 13825, Mar. 27, 1975, as amended at 43 FR 22675, May 26, 1978; 44 FR 16007, Mar. 16, 1979; 50 FR 7517, Feb. 22, 1985; 50 FR 16668, Apr. 26, 1985; 52 FR 49588, Dec. 31, 1987; 54 FR 18280, Apr. 28, 1989; 62 FR 40600, July 29,

1997; 63 FR 10770, Mar. 5, 1998; 64 FR 40757, July 28, 1999; 64 FR 63204, Nov. 19, 1999]

Sec. 514.115 Withdrawal of approval of applications.

(a) The Secretary may suspend approval of an application approved pursuant to section 512(c) of the act and give the applicant prompt notice of his action and afford the applicant the opportunity for an expedited hearing on a finding that there is an imminent hazard to the health of man or of the animals for which such new animal drug or animal feed is intended.

(b) The Commissioner shall notify in writing the person holding an application approved pursuant to section 512(c) of the act and afford an opportunity for a hearing on a proposal to withdraw approval of such application if he finds:

(1) That the application contains any untrue statement of a material fact; or

(2) That the applicant has made any changes from the standpoint of safety or effectiveness beyond the variations provided for in the application unless he has supplemented the application by filing with the Secretary adequate information respecting all such changes and unless there is in effect an approval of the supplemental application, or such changes are those for which written authorization or approval is not required as provided for in 514.8. The supplemental application shall be treated in the same manner as the original application.

(3) That in the case of an application for use of a new animal drug approved or deemed approved pursuant to section 512(c) of the act:

   (i) Experience or scientific data show that such drug is unsafe for use under the conditions of use upon the basis of which the application was approved; or

   (ii) New evidence not contained in such application or not available to the Secretary until after such application was approved, or tests by new methods, or tests by methods not deemed reasonably applicable when such application was approved, evaluated together with the evidence available to the Secretary when the application was approved, shows that such drug is not shown to be safe for use under the conditions of use upon the basis of

Part 514

which the application was approved or that section 512
(d)(1)(H) of the act applies to such drug; or

(iii) On the basis of new information before him with respect
to such drug, evaluated together with the evidence
available to him when the application was approved,
there is a lack of substantial evidence that such drug will
have the effect it purports or is represented to have under
the conditions of use prescribed, recommended, or
suggested in the labeling thereof.

(4) That any nonclinical laboratory study that is described in the
application and that is essential to show that the drug is safe
for use under the conditions prescribed, recommended, or
suggested in its proposed labeling, was not conducted in
compliance with the good laboratory practice regulations as
set forth in part 58 of this chapter and no reason for the
noncompliance is provided or, if it is, the differences between
the practices used in conducting the study and the good
laboratory practice regulations do not support the validity of
the study.

(c) The Commissioner may notify in writing the person holding an
application approved pursuant to section 512(c) of the act and
afford an opportunity for a hearing on a proposal to withdraw
approval of such application if he finds:

(1) That the applicant has failed to establish a system for
maintaining required records, or has repeatedly or deliberately
failed to maintain such records or to make required reports in
accordance with a regulation or order under section 512(l)(1)
of the act, or the applicant has refused to permit access to, or
copying, or verification of, such records as required by
section 512(l)(2) of the act; or

(2) That on the basis of new information before him evaluated
together with the evidence before him when the application
was approved, the methods used in, or the facilities and
controls used for, the manufacture, processing, and packing
of such drug or animal feed are inadequate to assure and
preserve its identity, strength, quality, and purity and were not
made adequate within a reasonable time after receipt of
written notice from the Secretary specifying the matter
complained of; or

(3) That on the basis of new information before him, evaluated together with the evidence before him when the application was approved, the labeling of such drug, based on a fair evaluation of all material facts, is false or misleading in any particular and was not corrected within a reasonable time after receipt of written notice from the Secretary specifying the matter complained of.

(d) Approval of an application pursuant to section 512(c) of the act will be withdrawn on the basis of a request for its withdrawal submitted in writing by a person holding an approved new animal drug application on the grounds that the drug subject to such application is no longer being marketed and information is included in support of this finding, provided none of the conditions cited in paragraphs (a), (b), and (c) of this section pertain to the subject drug. A written request for such withdrawal shall be construed as a waiver of the opportunity for a hearing as otherwise provided for in this section. Withdrawal of approval of an application under the provisions of this paragraph shall be without prejudice.

(e) On the basis of the withdrawal of approval of an application for a new animal drug approved pursuant to section 512(c) of the act, the regulation published pursuant to section 512(i) of the act covering the conditions of use of such drug as provided for in the application shall be revoked.

[40 FR 13825, Mar. 27, 1975, as amended at 50 FR 7517, Feb. 22, 1985; 64 FR 63204, Nov. 19, 1999]

Sec. 514.116 Notice of withdrawal of approval of application.

When an approval of an application submitted pursuant to section 512 of the act is withdrawn by the Commissioner, he will give appropriate public notice of such action by publication in theFederal Register.

Sec. 514.117 Adequate and well-controlled studies.

(a) Purpose. The primary purpose of conducting adequate and well-controlled studies of a new animal drug is to distinguish the effect of the new animal drug from other influences, such as spontaneous change in the course of the disease, normal animal production performance, or biased observation. One or more adequate and well-controlled studies are required to establish, by substantial evidence, that a new animal drug is effective. The

Part 514

characteristics described in paragraph (b) of this section have been developed over a period of years and are generally recognized as the essentials of an adequate and well-controlled study. Well controlled, as used in the phrase adequate and well controlled, emphasizes an important aspect of adequacy. The Food and Drug Administration (FDA) considers these characteristics in determining whether a study is adequate and well controlled for purposes of section 512 of the Federal Food, Drug, and Cosmetic Act (the act) (21 U.S.C. 360b). Adequate and well-controlled studies, in addition to providing a basis for determining whether a new animal drug is effective, may also be relied upon to support target animal safety. The report of an adequate and well-controlled study should provide sufficient details of study design, conduct, and analysis to allow critical evaluation and a determination of whether the characteristics of an adequate and well-controlled study are present.

(b) Characteristics. An adequate and well-controlled study has the following characteristics:

(1) The protocol for the study (protocol) and the report of the study results (study report) must include a clear statement of the study objective(s).

(2) The study is conducted in accordance with an appropriate standard of conduct that addresses, among other issues, study conduct, study personnel, study facilities, and study documentation. The protocol contains a statement acknowledging the applicability of, and intention to follow, a standard of conduct acceptable to FDA. The study report contains a statement describing adherence to the standard.

(3) The study is conducted with a new animal drug that is produced in accordance with appropriate manufacturing practices, which include, but are not necessarily limited to, the manufacture, processing, packaging, holding, and labeling of the new animal drug such that the critical characteristics of identity, strength, quality, purity, and physical form of the new animal drug are known, recorded, and reproducible, to permit meaningful evaluations of and comparisons with other studies conducted with the new animal drug. The physical form of a new animal drug includes the formulation and physical characterization (including delivery systems thereof, if any) of the new animal drug as presented to the animal. The protocol and study report must include an identification

number which can be correlated with the specific formulation and production process used to manufacture the new animal drug used in the study.

(4) The study uses a design that permits a valid comparison with one or more controls to provide a quantitative evaluation of drug effects. The protocol and the study report must describe the precise nature of the study design, e.g., duration of treatment periods, whether treatments are parallel, sequential, or crossover, and the determination of sample size. Within the broad range of studies conducted to support a determination of the effectiveness of a new animal drug, certain of the controls listed below would be appropriate and preferred depending on the study conducted:

(i) Placebo concurrent control. The new animal drug is compared with an inactive preparation designed to resemble the new animal drug as far as possible.

(ii) Untreated concurrent control. The new animal drug is compared with the absence of any treatment. The use of this control may be appropriate when objective measurements of effectiveness, not subject to observer bias, are available.

(iii) Active treatment concurrent control. The new animal drug is compared with known effective therapy. The use of this control is appropriate when the use of a placebo control or of an untreated concurrent control would unreasonably compromise the welfare of the animals. Similarity of the new animal drug and the active control drug can mean either that both drugs were effective or that neither was effective. The study report should assess the ability of the study to have detected a difference between treatments. The evaluation of the study should explain why the new animal drugs should be considered effective in the study, for example, by reference to results in previous placebo-controlled studies of the active control.

(iv) Historical control. The results of treatment with the new animal drug are quantitatively compared with experience historically derived from the adequately documented natural history of the disease or condition, or with a regimen (therapeutic, diagnostic, prophylactic) whose effectiveness is established, in comparable animals.

Part 514

Because historical control populations usually cannot be as well assessed with respect to pertinent variables as can concurrent control populations, historical control designs are usually reserved for special circumstances. Examples include studies in which the effect of the new animal drug is self-evident or studies of diseases with high and predictable mortality, or signs and symptoms of predictable duration or severity, or, in the case of prophylaxis, predictable morbidity.

(5) The study uses a method of selecting animals that provides adequate assurances that the animals are suitable for the purposes of the study. For example, the animals can reasonably be expected to have animal production characteristics typical of the class(es) of animals for which the new animal drug is intended, there is adequate assurance that the animals have the disease or condition being studied, or, in the case of prophylactic agents, evidence of susceptibility and exposure to the condition against which prophylaxis is desired has been provided. The protocol and the study report describe the method of selecting animals for the study.

(6) The study uses a method to assign a treatment or a control to each experimental unit of animals that is random and minimizes bias. Experimental units of animals are groups of animals that are comparable with respect to pertinent variables such as age, sex, class of animal, severity of disease, duration of disease, dietary regimen, level of animal production, and use of drugs or therapy other than the new animal drug. The protocol and the study report describe the method of assignment of animals to an experimental unit to account for pertinent variables and method of assignment of a treatment or a control to the experimental units. When the effect of such variables is accounted for by an appropriate design, and when, within the same animal, effects due to the test drug can be obtained free of the effects of such variables, the same animal may be used for both the test drug and the control using the controls set forth in paragraph (b)(4) of this section.

(7) The study uses methods to minimize bias on the part of observers and analysts of the data that are adequate to prevent undue influences on the results and interpretation of the study data. The protocol and study report explain the methods of observation and recording of the animal response

variables and document the methods, such as "blinding" or "masking," used in the study for excluding or minimizing bias in the observations.

(8) The study uses methods to assess animal response that are well defined and reliable. The protocol and study report describe the methods for conducting the study, including any appropriate analytical and statistical methods, used to collect and analyze the data resulting from the conduct of the study, describe the criteria used to assess response, and, when appropriate, justify the selection of the methods to assess animal response.

(9) There is an analysis and evaluation of the results of the study in accord with the protocol adequate to assess the effects of the new animal drug. The study report evaluates the methods used to conduct, and presents and evaluates the results of, the study as to their adequacy to assess the effects of the new animal drug. This evaluation of the results of the study assesses, among other items, the comparability of treatment and control groups with respect to pertinent variables and the effects of any interim analyses performed.

(c) Field studies.

(1) Field conditions as used in this section refers to conditions which closely approximate the conditions under which the new animal drug, if approved, is intended to be applied or administered.

(2) Studies of a new animal drug conducted under field conditions shall, consistent with generally recognized scientific principles and procedures, use an appropriate control that permits comparison, employ procedures to minimize bias, and have the characteristics generally described in paragraph (b) of this section. However, because field studies are conducted under field conditions, it is recognized that the level of control over some study conditions need not or should not be the same as the level of control in laboratory studies. While not all conditions relating to a field study need to be or should be controlled, observations of the conditions under which the new animal drug is tested shall be recorded in sufficient detail to permit evaluation of the study. Adequate and well-controlled field studies shall balance the need to control study conditions

Part 514

with the need to observe the true effect of the new animal drug under closely approximated actual use conditions.

(d) Waiver. The Director of the Center for Veterinary Medicine (the Director) may, on the Director's own initiative or on the petition of an interested person, waive in whole or in part any of the criteria in paragraph (b) of this section with respect to a specific study. A petition for a waiver is required to set forth clearly and concisely the specific criteria from which waiver is sought, why the criteria are not reasonably applicable to the particular study, what alternative procedures, if any, are to be, or have been employed, and what results have been obtained. The petition is also required to state why the studies so conducted will yield, or have yielded, substantial evidence of effectiveness, notwithstanding nonconformance with the criteria for which waiver is requested.

(e) Uncontrolled studies. Uncontrolled studies or partially controlled studies are not acceptable as the sole basis for the approval of claims of effectiveness or target animal safety. Such studies, carefully conducted and documented, may provide corroborative support of adequate and well-controlled studies regarding effectiveness and may yield valuable data regarding safety of the new animal drug. Such studies will be considered on their merits in light of the characteristics listed here. Isolated case reports, random experience, and reports lacking the details which permit scientific evaluation will not be considered.

[63 FR 10770, Mar. 5, 1998]

Sec. 514.120 Revocation of order refusing to approve an application or suspending or withdrawing approval of an application.

The Commissioner, upon his own initiative or upon request of an applicant stating reasonable grounds therefor and if he finds that the facts so require, may issue an order approving an application that previously has had its approval refused, suspended, or withdrawn.

Sec. 514.121 Service of notices and orders.

All notices and orders under this subchapter E and section 512 of the act pertaining to new animal drug applications shall be served:

(a) In person by any officer or employee of the Department designated by the Commissioner; or

(b) By mailing the order by certified mail addressed to the applicant or respondent at his last known address in the records of the Food and Drug Administration.

Subpart C--Hearing Procedures

Sec. 514.200 Contents of notice of opportunity for a hearing.

(a) The notice to the applicant of opportunity for a hearing on a proposal by the Commissioner to refuse to approve an application or to withdraw the approval of an application will specify the grounds upon which he proposes to issue his order. On request of the applicant, the Commissioner will explain the reasons for his action. The notice of opportunity for a hearing will be published in theFederal Registerand will specify that the applicant has 30 days after issuance of the notice within which he is required to file a written appearance electing whether:

   (1) To avail himself of the opportunity for a hearing; or

   (2) Not to avail himself of the opportunity for a hearing.

(b) If the applicant fails to file a written appearance in answer to the notice of opportunity for hearing, his failure will be construed as an election not to avail himself of the opportunity for the hearing, and the Commissioner without further notice may enter a final order.

(c) If the applicant elects to avail himself of the opportunity for a hearing, he is required to file a written appearance requesting the hearing within 30 days after the publication of the notice, giving the reason why the application should not be refused or should not be withdrawn, together with a well-organized and full-factual analysis of the clinical and other investigational data he is prepared to prove in support of his opposition to the Commissioner's proposal. A request for a hearing may not rest upon mere allegations or denials, but must set forth specific facts showing there is a genuine and substantial issue of fact that requires a hearing. When it clearly appears from the data in the application and from the reasons and a factual analysis in the request for the hearing that no genuine and substantial issue of fact precludes the refusal to approve the application or the withdrawal of approval of the application (for example, no adequate and well-controlled clinical investigations to support the claims of effectiveness have been identified), the Commissioner will enter an order on this

Part 514

data, stating his findings and conclusions. If a hearing is requested and is justified by the applicant's response to the notice of opportunity for a hearing, the issues will be defined, an Administrative Law Judge will be named, and he shall issue a written notice of the time and place at which the hearing will commence. In the case of denial of approval, such time shall be not more than 90 days after the expiration of such 30 days unless the Administrative Law Judge and the applicant otherwise agree; and, in the case of withdrawal of approval, such time shall be as soon as practicable.

(d) The hearing will be open to the public; however, if the Commissioner finds that portions of the application which serve as a basis for the hearing contain information concerning a method or process entitled to protection as a trade secret, the part of the hearing involving such portions will not be public, unless the respondent so specifies in his appearance.

[40 FR 13825, Mar. 27, 1975, as amended at 43 FR 1941, Jan. 13, 1978]

Sec. 514.201 Procedures for hearings.

Hearings relating to new animal drugs under section 512(d) and (e) of the act shall be governed by part 12 of this chapter.

[64 FR 63204, Nov. 19, 1999]

Subparts D-E [Reserved]

Subpart F--Judicial Review

Sec. 514.235 Judicial review.

(a) The transcript and record shall be certified by the Commissioner. In any case in which the Commissioner enters an order without a hearing pursuant to 314.200(g) of this chapter, the request(s) for hearing together with the data and information submitted and the Commissioner's findings and conclusions shall be included in the record certified by the Commissioner.

(b) Judicial review of an order withdrawing approval of a new drug application, whether or not a hearing has been held, may be sought by a manufacturer or distributor of an identical, related, or similar drug product, as defined in 310.6 of this chapter, in a

United States court of appeals pursuant to section 505(h) of the act.

[42 FR 4717, Jan. 25, 1977]

Authority: 21 U.S.C. 321, 331, 351, 352, 356a, 360b, 371, 379e, 381.

Source: 40 FR 13825, Mar. 27, 1975, unless otherwise noted.

Part 514

Part 601: Licensing

[Code of Federal Regulations]

[Title 21, Volume 7]

[Revised as of April 1, 2009]

[CITE: 21CFR601]

Title 21--Food and Drugs

Chapter I--Food and Drug Administration

Department of Health and Human Services

Subchapter F--Biologics

Part 601 Licensing[1]

Subpart A--General Provisions

Sec. 601.2 Applications for biologics licenses; procedures for filing.

(a) General. To obtain a biologics license under section 351 of the Public Health Service Act for any biological product, the manufacturer shall submit an application to the Director, Center for Biologics Evaluation and Research or the Director, Center for Drug Evaluation and Research (see mailing addresses in 600.2 of this chapter), on forms prescribed for such purposes, and shall submit data derived from nonclinical laboratory and clinical studies which demonstrate that the manufactured product meets prescribed requirements of safety, purity, and potency; with respect to each nonclinical laboratory study, either a statement that the study was conducted in compliance with the requirements set forth in part 58 of this chapter, or, if the study was not conducted

---

[1] Available on the FDA website at http://www.accessdata.fda.gov/scripts/cdrh/cfdocs/cfCFR/CFRSearch.cfm?CFRPart=601&showFR=1

in compliance with such regulations, a brief statement of the reason for the noncompliance; statements regarding each clinical investigation involving human subjects contained in the application, that it either was conducted in compliance with the requirements for institutional review set forth in part 56 of this chapter; or was not subject to such requirements in accordance with 56.104 or 56.105, and was conducted in compliance with requirements for informed consent set forth in part 50 of this chapter. A full description of manufacturing methods; data establishing stability of the product through the dating period; sample(s) representative of the product for introduction or delivery for introduction into interstate commerce; summaries of results of tests performed on the lot(s) represented by the submitted sample(s); specimens of the labels, enclosures, and containers, and if applicable, any Medication Guide required under part 208 of this chapter proposed to be used for the product; and the address of each location involved in the manufacture of the biological product shall be listed in the biologics license application. The applicant shall also include a financial certification or disclosure statement(s) or both for clinical investigators as required by part 54 of this chapter. An application for a biologics license shall not be considered as filed until all pertinent information and data have been received by the Food and Drug Administration. The applicant shall also include either a claim for categorical exclusion under 25.30 or 25.31 of this chapter or an environmental assessment under 25.40 of this chapter. The applicant, or the applicant's attorney, agent, or other authorized official shall sign the application. An application for any of the following specified categories of biological products subject to licensure shall be handled as set forth in paragraph (c) of this section:

(1) Therapeutic DNA plasmid products;

(2) Therapeutic synthetic peptide products of 40 or fewer amino acids;

(3) Monoclonal antibody products for in vivo use; and

(4) Therapeutic recombinant DNA-derived products.

(b) [Reserved]

(c)(1) To obtain marketing approval for a biological product subject to licensure which is a therapeutic DNA plasmid product, therapeutic synthetic peptide product of 40 or fewer amino acids, monoclonal antibody product for in vivo use, or therapeutic recombinant DNA-derived product, an applicant shall submit a biologics license application in accordance with paragraph (a) of this section except that the following sections in parts 600 through 680 of this chapter shall not be applicable to such products: 600.10(b) and (c), 600.11, 600.12, 600.13, 610.11, 610.53, and 610.62 of this chapter.

(2) To the extent that the requirements in this paragraph (c) conflict with other requirements in this subchapter, this paragraph (c) shall supersede other requirements.

(d) Approval of a biologics license application or issuance of a biologics license shall constitute a determination that the establishment(s) and the product meet applicable requirements to ensure the continued safety, purity, and potency of such products. Applicable requirements for the maintenance of establishments for the manufacture of a product subject to this section shall include but not be limited to the good manufacturing practice requirements set forth in parts 210, 211, 600, 606, and 820 of this chapter.

(e) Any establishment and product license for a biological product issued under section 351 of the Public Health Service Act (42 U.S.C. 201et seq.) that has not been revoked or suspended as of December 20, 1999, shall constitute an approved biologics license application in effect under the same terms and conditions set forth in such product license and such portions of the establishment license relating to such product.

[64 FR 56450, Oct. 20, 1999, as amended at 70 FR 14983, Mar. 24, 2005]

Sec. 601.3 Complete response letter to the applicant.

(a) Complete response letter. The Food and Drug Administration will send the biologics license applicant or supplement applicant a complete response letter if the agency determines that it will not approve the biologics license application or supplement in its present form.

(1) Description of specific deficiencies. A complete response letter will describe all of the deficiencies that the agency has identified in a biologics license application or supplement, except as stated in paragraph (a)(2) of this section.

Part 601

(2) Inadequate data. If FDA determines, after a biologics license application or supplement is filed, that the data submitted are inadequate to support approval, the agency might issue a complete response letter without first conducting required inspections, testing submitted product lots, and/or reviewing proposed product labeling.

(3) Recommendation of actions for approval. When possible, a complete response letter will recommend actions that the applicant might take to place its biologics license application or supplement in condition for approval.

(b) Applicant actions. After receiving a complete response letter, the biologics license applicant or supplement applicant must take either of the following actions:

(1) Resubmission. Resubmit the application or supplement, addressing all deficiencies identified in the complete response letter.

(2) Withdrawal. Withdraw the application or supplement. A decision to withdraw the application or supplement is without prejudice to a subsequent submission.

(c) Failure to take action.

(1) FDA may consider a biologics license applicant or supplement applicant's failure to either resubmit or withdraw the application or supplement within 1 year after issuance of a complete response letter to be a request by the applicant to withdraw the application or supplement, unless the applicant has requested an extension of time in which to resubmit the application or supplement. FDA will grant any reasonable request for such an extension. FDA may consider an applicant's failure to resubmit the application or supplement within the extended time period or request an additional extension to be a request by the applicant to withdraw the application.

(2) If FDA considers an applicant's failure to take action in accordance with paragraph (c)(1) of this section to be a request to withdraw the application, the agency will notify the applicant in writing. The applicant will have 30 days from the date of the notification to explain why the application or supplement should not be withdrawn and to request an extension of time in which to resubmit the application or

supplement. FDA will grant any reasonable request for an extension. If the applicant does not respond to the notification within 30 days, the application or supplement will be deemed to be withdrawn.

[73 FR 39611, July 10, 2008]

Sec. 601.4 Issuance and denial of license.

(a) A biologics license shall be issued upon a determination by the Director, Center for Biologics Evaluation and Research or the Director, Center for Drug Evaluation and Research that the establishment(s) and the product meet the applicable requirements established in this chapter. A biologics license shall be valid until suspended or revoked.

(b) If the Commissioner determines that the establishment or product does not meet the requirements established in this chapter, the biologics license application shall be denied and the applicant shall be informed of the grounds for, and of an opportunity for a hearing on, the decision. If the applicant so requests, the Commissioner shall issue a notice of opportunity for hearing on the matter pursuant to 12.21(b) of this chapter.

[42 FR 4718, Jan. 25, 1977, as amended at 42 FR 15676, Mar. 22, 1977; 42 FR 19142, Apr. 12, 1977; 64 FR 56450, Oct. 20, 1999; 70 FR 14983, Mar. 24, 2005]

Sec. 601.5 Revocation of license.

(a) A biologics license shall be revoked upon application of the manufacturer giving notice of intention to discontinue the manufacture of all products manufactured under such license or to discontinue the manufacture of a particular product for which a license is held and waiving an opportunity for a hearing on the matter.

(b)(1) The Commissioner shall notify the licensed manufacturer of the intention to revoke the biologics license, setting forth the grounds for, and offering an opportunity for a hearing on the proposed revocation if the Commissioner finds any of the following:

(i) Authorized Food and Drug Administration employees after reasonable efforts have been unable to gain access to an establishment or a location for the purpose of

Part 601

carrying out the inspection required under 600.21 of this chapter,

(ii) Manufacturing of products or of a product has been discontinued to an extent that a meaningful inspection or evaluation cannot be made,

(iii) The manufacturer has failed to report a change as required by 601.12 of this chapter,

(iv) The establishment or any location thereof, or the product for which the license has been issued, fails to conform to the applicable standards established in the license and in this chapter designed to ensure the continued safety, purity, and potency of the manufactured product,

(v) The establishment or the manufacturing methods have been so changed as to require a new showing that the establishment or product meets the requirements established in this chapter in order to protect the public health, or

(vi) The licensed product is not safe and effective for all of its intended uses or is misbranded with respect to any such use.

(2) Except as provided in 601.6 of this chapter, or in cases involving willfulness, the notification required in this paragraph shall provide a reasonable period for the licensed manufacturer to demonstrate or achieve compliance with the requirements of this chapter, before proceedings will be instituted for the revocation of the license. If compliance is not demonstrated or achieved and the licensed manufacturer does not waive the opportunity for a hearing, the Commissioner shall issue a notice of opportunity for hearing on the matter under 12.21(b) of this chapter.

[64 FR 56451, Oct. 20, 1999]

Sec. 601.6 Suspension of license.

(a) Whenever the Commissioner has reasonable grounds to believe that any of the grounds for revocation of a license exist and that by reason thereof there is a danger to health, the Commissioner may notify the licensed manufacturer that the biologics license is suspended and require that the licensed manufacturer do the following:

(1) Notify the selling agents and distributors to whom such product or products have been delivered of such suspension, and

(2) Furnish to the Center for Biologics Evaluation and Research or the Center for Drug Evaluation and Research, complete records of such deliveries and notice of suspension.

(b) Upon suspension of a license, the Commissioner shall either:

(1) Proceed under the provisions of 601.5(b) of this chapter to revoke the license, or

(2) If the licensed manufacturer agrees, hold revocation in abeyance pending resolution of the matters involved.

[64 FR 56451, Oct. 20, 1999, as amended at 70 FR 14983, Mar. 24, 2005]

Sec. 601.7 Procedure for hearings.

(a) A notice of opportunity for hearing, notice of appearance and request for hearing, and grant or denial of hearing for a biological drug pursuant to this part, for which the exemption from the Federal Food, Drug, and Cosmetic Act in 310.4 of this chapter has been revoked, shall be subject to the provisions of 314.200 of this chapter except to the extent that the notice of opportunity for hearing on the matter issued pursuant to 12.21(b) of this chapter specifically provides otherwise.

(b) Hearings pursuant to 601.4 through 601.6 shall be governed by part 12 of this chapter.

(c) When a license has been suspended pursuant to 601.6 and a hearing request has been granted, the hearing shall proceed on an expedited basis.

[42 FR 4718, Jan. 25, 1977, as amended at 42 FR 15676, Mar. 22, 1977; 42 FR 19143, Apr. 12, 1977]

Sec. 601.8 Publication of revocation.

The Commissioner, following revocation of a biologics license under 21 CFR 601.5(b), will publish a notice in theFederal Registerwith a statement of the specific grounds for the revocation.

[74 FR 20585, May 5, 2009]

Part 601

Sec. 601.9 Licenses; reissuance.

(a) Compliance with requirements. A biologics license, previously suspended or revoked, may be reissued or reinstated upon a showing of compliance with requirements and upon such inspection and examination as may be considered necessary by the Director, Center for Biologics Evaluation and Research or the Director, Center for Drug Evaluation and Research.

(b) Exclusion of noncomplying location. A biologics license, excluding a location or locations that fail to comply with the requirements in this chapter, may be issued without further application and concurrently with the suspension or revocation of the license for noncompliance at the excluded location or locations.

(c) Exclusion of noncomplying product(s). In the case of multiple products included under a single biologics license application, a biologics license may be issued, excluding the noncompliant product(s), without further application and concurrently with the suspension or revocation of the biologics license for a noncompliant product(s).

[64 FR 56451, Oct. 20, 1999, as amended at 70 FR 14983, Mar. 24, 2005]

Subpart B [Reserved]

Subpart C--Biologics Licensing

Sec. 601.12 Changes to an approved application.

(a) General.

(1) As provided by this section, an applicant must inform the Food and Drug Administration (FDA) (see mailing addresses in 600.2 of this chapter) about each change in the product, production process, quality controls, equipment, facilities, responsible personnel, or labeling established in the approved license application(s).

(2) Before distributing a product made using a change, an applicant must assess the effects of the change and demonstrate through appropriate validation and/or other clinical and/or nonclinical laboratory studies the lack of

adverse effect of the change on the identity, strength, quality, purity, or potency of the product as they may relate to the safety or effectiveness of the product.

(3) Notwithstanding the requirements of paragraphs (b), (c), and (f) of this section, an applicant must make a change provided for in those paragraphs in accordance with a regulation or guidance that provides for a less burdensome notification of the change (for example, by submission of a supplement that does not require approval prior to distribution of the product or in an annual report).

(4) The applicant must promptly revise all promotional labeling and advertising to make it consistent with any labeling change implemented in accordance with paragraphs (f)(1) and (f)(2) of this section.

(5) A supplement or annual report must include a list of all changes contained in the supplement or annual report. For supplements, this list must be provided in the cover letter.

(b) Changes requiring supplement submission and approval prior to distribution of the product made using the change (major changes).

(1) A supplement shall be submitted for any change in the product, production process, quality controls, equipment, facilities, or responsible personnel that has a substantial potential to have an adverse effect on the identity, strength, quality, purity, or potency of the product as they may relate to the safety or effectiveness of the product.

(2) These changes include, but are not limited to:

(i) Except as provided in paragraphs (c) and (d) of this section, changes in the qualitative or quantitative formulation, including inactive ingredients, or in the specifications provided in the approved application;

(ii) Changes requiring completion of an appropriate human study to demonstrate the equivalence of the identity, strength, quality, purity, or potency of the product as they may relate to the safety or effectiveness of the product;

(iii) Changes in the virus or adventitious agent removal or inactivation method(s);

(iv) Changes in the source material or cell line;

Part 601

    (v) Establishment of a new master cell bank or seed; and

    (vi) Changes which may affect product sterility assurance, such as changes in product or component sterilization method(s), or an addition, deletion, or substitution of steps in an aseptic processing operation.

(3) The applicant must obtain approval of the supplement from FDA prior to distribution of the product made using the change. Except for submissions under paragraph (e) of this section, the following shall be contained in the supplement:

    (i) A detailed description of the proposed change;

    (ii) The product(s) involved;

    (iii) The manufacturing site(s) or area(s) affected;

    (iv) A description of the methods used and studies performed to evaluate the effect of the change on the identity, strength, quality, purity, or potency of the product as they may relate to the safety or effectiveness of the product;

    (v) The data derived from such studies;

    (vi) Relevant validation protocols and data; and

    (vii) A reference list of relevant standard operating procedures (SOP's).

(4) An applicant may ask FDA to expedite its review of a supplement for public health reasons or if a delay in making the change described in it would impose an extraordinary hardship on the applicant. Such a supplement and its mailing cover should be plainly marked: "Prior Approval Supplement-Expedited Review Requested.

(c) Changes requiring supplement submission at least 30 days prior to distribution of the product made using the change.

(1) A supplement shall be submitted for any change in the product, production process, quality controls, equipment, facilities, or responsible personnel that has a moderate potential to have an adverse effect on the identity, strength, quality, purity, or potency of the product as they may relate to the safety or effectiveness of the product. The supplement shall be labeled "Supplement--Changes Being Effected in 30 Days" or, if applicable under paragraph (c)(5) of this section, "Supplement--Changes Being Effected."

(2) These changes include, but are not limited to:

    (i) [Reserved]

    (ii) An increase or decrease in production scale during finishing steps that involves different equipment; and

    (iii) Replacement of equipment with that of similar, but not identical, design and operating principle that does not affect the process methodology or process operating parameters.

    (iv) Relaxation of an acceptance criterion or deletion of a test to comply with an official compendium that is consistent with FDA statutory and regulatory requirements.

(3) Pending approval of the supplement by FDA, and except as provided in paragraph (c)(5) of this section, distribution of the product made using the change may begin not less than 30 days after receipt of the supplement by FDA. The information listed in paragraph (b)(3)(i) through (b)(3)(vii) of this section shall be contained in the supplement.

(4) If within 30 days following FDA's receipt of the supplement, FDA informs the applicant that either:

    (i) The change requires approval prior to distribution of the product in accordance with paragraph (b) of this section; or

    (ii) Any of the information required under paragraph (c)(3) of this section is missing; the applicant shall not distribute the product made using the change until FDA determines that compliance with this section is achieved.

(5) In certain circumstances, FDA may determine that, based on experience with a particular type of change, the supplement for such change is usually complete and provides the proper information, and on particular assurances that the proposed change has been appropriately submitted, the product made using the change may be distributed immediately upon receipt of the supplement by FDA. These circumstances may include substantial similarity with a type of change regularly involving a "Supplement--Changes Being Effected" supplement or a situation in which the applicant presents evidence that the proposed change has been validated in accordance with an approved protocol for such change under paragraph (e) of this section.

Part 601

(6) If the agency disapproves the supplemental application, it may order the manufacturer to cease distribution of the products made with the manufacturing change.

(d) Changes to be described in an annual report (minor changes).

(1) Changes in the product, production process, quality controls, equipment, facilities, or responsible personnel that have a minimal potential to have an adverse effect on the identity, strength, quality, purity, or potency of the product as they may relate to the safety or effectiveness of the product shall be documented by the applicant in an annual report submitted each year within 60 days of the anniversary date of approval of the application. The Director, Center for Biologics Evaluation and Research or the Director, Center for Drug Evaluation and Research, may approve a written request for an alternative date to combine annual reports for multiple approved applications into a single annual report submission.

(2) These changes include, but are not limited to:

(i) Any change made to comply with a change to an official compendium, except a change described in paragraph (c)(2)(iv) of this section, that is consistent with FDA statutory and regulatory requirements.

(ii) The deletion or reduction of an ingredient intended only to affect the color of the product, except that a change intended only to affect Blood Grouping Reagents requires supplement submission and approval prior to distribution of the product made using the change in accordance with the requirements set forth in paragraph (b) of this section;

(iii) An extension of an expiration dating period based upon full shelf life data on production batches obtained from a protocol approved in the application;

(iv) A change within the container closure system for a nonsterile product, based upon a showing of equivalency to the approved system under a protocol approved in the application or published in an official compendium;

(v) A change in the size and/or shape of a container containing the same number of dosage units for a nonsterile solid dosage form product, without a change from one container closure system to another;

(vi) The addition by embossing, debossing, or engraving of a code imprint to a solid dosage form biological product other than a modified release dosage form, or a minor change in an existing code imprint; and

(vii) The addition or revision of an alternative analytical procedure that provides the same or increased assurance of the identity, strength, quality, purity, or potency of the material being tested as the analytical procedure described in the approved application, or deletion of an alternative analytical procedure.

(3) The following information for each change shall be contained in the annual report:

(i) A list of all products involved; and

(ii) A full description of the manufacturing and controls changes including: the manufacturing site(s) or area(s) involved; the date the change was made; a cross-reference to relevant validation protocols and/or SOP's; and relevant data from studies and tests performed to evaluate the effect of the change on the identity, strength, quality, purity, or potency of the product as they may relate to the safety or effectiveness of the product.

(iii) A statement by the holder of the approved application or license that the effects of the change have been assessed.

(4) The applicant shall submit the report to the FDA office responsible for reviewing the application. The report shall include all the information required under this paragraph for each change made during the annual reporting interval which ends on the anniversary date in the order in which they were implemented.

(e) An applicant may submit one or more protocols describing the specific tests and validation studies and acceptable limits to be achieved to demonstrate the lack of adverse effect for specified types of manufacturing changes on the identity, strength, quality, purity, or potency of the product as they may relate to the safety or effectiveness of the product. Any such protocols, or change to a protocol, shall be submitted as a supplement requiring approval from FDA prior to distribution of the product which, if approved, may justify a reduced reporting category for the particular change

Part 601

because the use of the protocol for that type of change reduces the potential risk of an adverse effect.

(f) Labeling changes.

    (1) Labeling changes requiring supplement submission--FDA approval must be obtained before distribution of the product with the labeling change. Except as described in paragraphs (f)(2) and (f)(3) of this section, an applicant shall submit a supplement describing a proposed change in the package insert, package label, container label, or, if applicable, a Medication Guide required under part 208 of this chapter, and include the information necessary to support the proposed change. An applicant cannot use paragraph (f)(2) of this section to make any change to the information required in 201.57(a) of this chapter. An applicant may report the minor changes to the information specified in paragraph (f)(3)(i)(D) of this section in an annual report. The supplement shall clearly highlight the proposed change in the labeling. The applicant shall obtain approval from FDA prior to distribution of the product with the labeling change.

    (2) Labeling changes requiring supplement submission--product with a labeling change that may be distributed before FDA approval.

        (i) An applicant shall submit, at the time such change is made, a supplement for any change in the package insert, package label, or container label to reflect newly acquired information, except for changes to the package insert required in 201.57(a) of this chapter (which must be made under paragraph (f)(1) of this section), to accomplish any of the following:

            (A) To add or strengthen a contraindication, warning, precaution, or adverse reaction for which the evidence of a causal association satisfies the standard for inclusion in the labeling under 201.57(c) of this chapter;

            (B) To add or strengthen a statement about abuse, dependence, psychological effect, or overdosage;

            (C) To add or strengthen an instruction about dosage and administration that is intended to increase the safety of the use of the product; and

(D) To delete false, misleading, or unsupported indications for use or claims for effectiveness.

(E) Any labeling change normally requiring a supplement submission and approval prior to distribution of the product that FDA specifically requests be submitted under this provision.

(ii) Pending approval of the supplement by FDA, the applicant may distribute a product with a package insert, package label, or container label bearing such change at the time the supplement is submitted. The supplement shall clearly identify the change being made and include necessary supporting data. The supplement and its mailing cover shall be plainly marked: "Special Labeling Supplement--Changes Being Effected."

(3) Labeling changes requiring submission in an annual report.

(i) An applicant shall submit any final printed package insert, package label, container label, or Medication Guide required under part 208 of this chapter incorporating the following changes in an annual report submitted to FDA each year as provided in paragraph (d)(1) of this section:

(A) Editorial or similar minor changes;

(B) A change in the information on how the product is supplied that does not involve a change in the dosage strength or dosage form;

(C) A change in the information specified in 208.20(b)(8)(iii) and (b)(8)(iv) of this chapter for a Medication Guide; and

(D) A change to the information required in 201.57(a) of this chapter as follows:

(1) Removal of a listed section(s) specified in 201.57(a)(5) of this chapter; and

(2) Changes to the most recent revision date of the labeling as specified in 201.57(a)(15) of this chapter.

(E) A change made pursuant to an exception or alternative granted under 201.26 or 610.68 of this chapter.

Part 601

(ii) The applicant may distribute a product with a package insert, package label, or container label bearing such change at the time the change is made.

(4) Advertisements and promotional labeling. Advertisements and promotional labeling shall be submitted to the Center for Biologics Evaluation and Research or Center for Drug Evaluation and Research in accordance with the requirements set forth in 314.81(b)(3)(i) of this chapter, except that Form FDA-2567 (Transmittal of Labels and Circulars) or an equivalent form shall be used.

(5) The submission and grant of a written request for an exception or alternative under 201.26 or 610.68 of this chapter satisfies the requirements in paragraphs (f)(1) through (f)(2) of this section.

(6) For purposes of paragraph (f)(2) of this section, information will be considered newly acquired if it consists of data, analyses, or other information not previously submitted to the agency, which may include (but are not limited to) data derived from new clinical studies, reports of adverse events, or new analyses of previously submitted data (e.g., meta-analyses) if the studies, events or analyses reveal risks of a different type or greater severity or frequency than previously included in submissions to FDA.

(g) Failure to comply. In addition to other remedies available in law and regulations, in the event of repeated failure of the applicant to comply with this section, FDA may require that the applicant submit a supplement for any proposed change and obtain approval of the supplement by FDA prior to distribution of the product made using the change.

(h) Administrative review. Under 10.75 of this chapter, an applicant may request internal FDA review of FDA employee decisions under this section.

[62 FR 39901, July 24, 1997, as amended at 63 FR 66399, Dec. 1, 1998. Redesignated at 65 FR 59718, Oct. 6, 2000, and amended at 69 FR 18766, Apr. 8, 2004; 70 FR 14983, Mar. 24, 2005; 71 FR 3997, Jan. 24, 2006; 72 FR 73600, Dec. 28, 2007; 73 FR 49609, Aug. 22, 2008; 73 FR 68333, Nov. 18, 2008]

Sec. 601.14 Regulatory submissions in electronic format.

(a) General. Electronic format submissions must be in a form that FDA can process, review, and archive. FDA will periodically issue guidance on how to provide the electronic submission (e.g., method of transmission, media, file formats, preparation and organization of files.)

(b) Labeling. The content of labeling required under 201.100(d)(3) of this chapter (commonly referred to as the package insert or professional labeling), including all text, tables, and figures, must be submitted to the agency in electronic format as described in paragraph (a) of this section. This requirement is in addition to the provisions of 601.2(a) and 601.12(f) that require applicants to submit specimens of the labels, enclosures, and containers, or to submit other final printed labeling. Submissions under this paragraph must be made in accordance with part 11 of this chapter except for the requirements of 11.10(a), (c) through (h), and (k), and the corresponding requirements of 11.30.

[68 FR 69020, Dec. 11, 2003]

Sec. 601.15 Foreign establishments and products: samples for each importation.

Random samples of each importation, obtained by the District Director of Customs and forwarded to the Director, Center for Biologics Evaluation and Research or the Director, Center for Drug Evaluation and Research (see mailing addresses in 600.2 of this chapter) must be at least two final containers of each lot of product. A copy of the associated documents which describe and identify the shipment must accompany the shipment for forwarding with the samples to the Director, Center for Biologics Evaluation and Research or the Director, Center for Drug Evaluation and Research (see mailing addresses in 600.2). For shipments of 20 or less final containers, samples need not be forwarded, provided a copy of an official release from the Center for Biologics Evaluation and Research or Center for Drug Evaluation and Research accompanies each shipment.

[70 FR 14983, Mar. 24, 2005]

Sec. 601.20 Biologics licenses; issuance and conditions.

(a) Examination--compliance with requirements. A biologics license application shall be approved only upon examination of the product and upon a determination that the product complies with the standards established in the biologics license application and the requirements prescribed in the regulations in this chapter including but not limited to the good manufacturing practice requirements set forth in parts 210, 211, 600, 606, and 820 of this chapter.

(b) Availability of product. No biologics license shall be issued unless:

(1) The product intended for introduction into interstate commerce is available for examination, and

(2) Such product is available for inspection during all phases of manufacture.

(c) Manufacturing process--impairment of assurances. No product shall be licensed if any part of the process of or relating to the manufacture of such product, in the judgment of the Director, Center for Biologics Evaluation and Research or the Director, Center for Drug Evaluation and Research, would impair the assurances of continued safety, purity, and potency as provided by the regulations contained in this chapter.

(d) Inspection--compliance with requirements. A biologics license shall be issued or a biologics license application approved only after inspection of the establishment(s) listed in the biologics license application and upon a determination that the establishment(s) complies with the standards established in the biologics license application and the requirements prescribed in applicable regulations.

(e) One biologics license to cover all locations. One biologics license shall be issued to cover all locations meeting the establishment standards identified in the approved biologics license application and each location shall be subject to inspection by FDA officials.

[64 FR 56451, Oct. 20, 1999, as amended at 70 FR 14983, Mar. 24, 2005]

Sec. 601.21 Products under development.

A biological product undergoing development, but not yet ready for a biologics license, may be shipped or otherwise delivered from one State or possession into another State or possession provided such shipment or delivery is not for introduction or delivery for introduction into interstate commerce, except as provided in sections

505(i) and 520(g) of the Federal Food, Drug, and Cosmetic Act, as amended, and the regulations thereunder (21 CFR parts 312 and 812).

[64 FR 56451, Oct. 20, 1999]

Sec. 601.22 Products in short supply; initial manufacturing at other than licensed location.

A biologics license issued to a manufacturer and covering all locations of manufacture shall authorize persons other than such manufacturer to conduct at places other than such locations the initial, and partial manufacturing of a product for shipment solely to such manufacturer only to the extent that the names of such persons and places are registered with the Commissioner of Food and Drugs and it is found upon application of such manufacturer, that the product is in short supply due either to the peculiar growth requirements of the organism involved or to the scarcity of the animal required for manufacturing purposes, and such manufacturer has established with respect to such persons and places such procedures, inspections, tests or other arrangements as will ensure full compliance with the applicable regulations of this subchapter related to continued safety, purity, and potency. Such persons and places shall be subject to all regulations of this subchapter except 601.2 to 601.6, 601.9, 601.10, 601.20, 601.21 to 601.33, and 610.60 to 610.65 of this chapter. For persons and places authorized under this section to conduct the initial and partial manufacturing of a product for shipment solely to a manufacturer of a product subject to licensure under 601.2(c), the following additional regulations shall not be applicable: 600.10(b) and (c), 600.11, 600.12, 600.13, 610.11, and 610.53 of this chapter. Failure of such manufacturer to maintain such procedures, inspections, tests, or other arrangements, or failure of any person conducting such partial manufacturing to comply with applicable regulations shall constitute a ground for suspension or revocation of the authority conferred pursuant to this section on the same basis as provided in 601.6 to 601.8 with respect to the suspension and the revocation of licenses.

[42 FR 4718, Jan. 25, 1977, as amended at 61 FR 24233, May 14, 1996; 64 FR 56452, Oct. 20, 1999]

Part 601

Part 601:
Licensing

Sec. 601.25 Review procedures to determine that licensed biological products are safe, effective, and not misbranded under prescribed, recommended, or suggested conditions of use.

For purposes of reviewing biological products that have been licensed prior to July 1, 1972, to determine that they are safe and effective and not misbranded, the following regulations shall apply. Prior administrative action exempting biological products from the provisions of the Federal Food, Drug, and Cosmetic Act is superseded to the extent that these regulations result in imposing requirements pursuant to provisions therein for a designated biological product or category of products.

(a) Advisory review panels. The Commissioner of Food and Drugs shall appoint advisory review panels

(1) to evaluate the safety and effectiveness of biological products for which a license has been issued pursuant to section 351 of the Public Health Service Act,

(2) to review the labeling of such biological products, and

(3) to advise him on which of the biological products under review are safe, effective, and not misbranded. An advisory review panel shall be established for each designated category of biological product. The members of a panel shall be qualified experts, appointed by the Commissioner, and shall include persons from lists submitted by organizations representing professional, consumer, and industry interests. Such persons shall represent a wide divergence of responsible medical and scientific opinion. The Commissioner shall designate the chairman of each panel, and summary minutes of all meetings shall be made.

(b) Request for data and views.

(1) The Commissioner of Food and Drugs will publish a notice in theFederal Registerrequesting interested persons to submit, for review and evaluation by an advisory review panel, published and unpublished data and information pertinent to a designated category of biological products.

(2) Data and information submitted pursuant to a published notice, and falling within the confidentiality provisions of 18 U.S.C. 1905, 5 U.S.C. 552(b), or 21 U.S.C. 331(j), shall be

handled by the advisory review panel and the Food and Drug Administration as confidential until publication of a proposed evaluation of the biologics under review and the full report or reports of the panel. Thirty days thereafter such data and information shall be made publicly available and may be viewed at the Division of Dockets Management of the Food and Drug Administration, except to the extent that the person submitting it demonstrates that it still falls within the confidentiality provisions of one or more of those statutes.

(3) To be considered, 12 copies of the submission on any marketed biological product within the class shall be submitted, preferably bound, indexed, and on standard sized paper, approximately 81/2* 11 inches. The time allotted for submissions will be 60 days, unless otherwise indicated in the specific notice requesting data and views for a particular category of biological products. When requested, abbreviated submissions should be sent. All submissions shall be in the following format, indicating "none" or "not applicable" where appropriate, unless changed in theFederal Register notice:

Biological Products Review Information

I. Label or labels and all other labeling (preferably mounted. Facsimile labeling is acceptable in lieu of actual container labeling), including labeling for export.

II. Representative advertising used during the past 5 years.

III. The complete quantitative composition of the biological product.

IV. Animal safety data.

    A. Individual active components.

        1. Controlled studies.

        2. Partially controlled or uncontrolled studies.

    B. Combinations of the individual active components.

        1. Controlled studies.

        2. Partially controlled or uncontrolled studies.

    C. Finished biological product.

        1. Controlled studies.

Part 601

    2.   Partially controlled or uncontrolled studies.

V. Human safety data.

   A. Individual active components.

     1.   Controlled studies.

     2.   Partially controlled or uncontrolled studies.

     3.   Documented case reports.

     4.   Pertinent marketing experiences that may influence a determination as to the safety of each individual active component.

     5.   Pertinent medical and scientific literature.

   B. Combinations of the individual active components.

     1.   Controlled studies.

     2.   Partially controlled or uncontrolled studies.

     3.   Documented case reports.

     4.   Pertinent marketing experiences that may influence a determination as to the safety of combinations of the individual active components.

     5.   Pertinent medical and scientific literature.

   C. Finished biological product.

     1.   Controlled studies.

     2.   Partially controlled or uncontrolled studies.

     3.   Documented case reports.

     4.   Pertinent marketing experiences that may influence a determination as to the safety of the finished biological product.

     5.   Pertinent medical and scientific literature.

VI. Efficacy data.

   A. Individual active components.

     1.   Controlled studies.

     2.   Partially controlled or uncontrolled studies.

     3.   Documented case reports.

4. Pertinent marketing experiences that may influence a determination on the efficacy of each individual active component.

5. Pertinent medical and scientific literature.

B. Combinations of the individual active components.

1. Controlled studies.

2. Partially controlled or uncontrolled studies.

3. Documented case reports.

4. Pertinent marketing experiences that may influence a determination as to the effectiveness of combinations of the individual active components.

5. Pertinent medical and scientific literature.

C. Finished biological product.

1. Controlled studies.

2. Partially controlled or uncontrolled studies.

3. Documented case reports.

4. Pertinent marketing experiences that may influence a determination as to the effectiveness of the finished biological product.

5. Pertinent medical and scientific literature.

VII. A summary of the data and views setting forth the medical rational and purpose (or lack thereof) for the biological product and its components and the scientific basis (or lack thereof) for the conclusion that the biological product, including its components, has been proven safe and effective and is properly labeled for the intended use or uses. If there is an absence of controlled studies in the materials submitted, an explanation as to why such studies are not considered necessary or feasible shall be included.

VIII. If the submission is by a licensed manufacturer, a statement signed by the authorized official of the licensed manufacturer shall be included, stating that to the best of his or her knowledge and belief, it includes all information, favorable and unfavorable, pertinent to an

Part 601

evaluation of the safety, effectiveness, and labeling of the
product, including information derived from
investigation, commercial marketing, or published
literature. If the submission is by an interested person
other than a licensed manufacturer, a statement signed by
the person responsible for such submission shall be
included, stating that to the best of his knowledge and
belief, it fairly reflects a balance of all the available
information, favorable and unfavorable available to him,
pertinent to an evaluation of the safety, effectiveness, and
labeling of the product.

(c) Deliberations of an advisory review panel. An advisory review
panel will meet as often and for as long as is appropriate to review
the data submitted to it and to prepare a report containing its
conclusions and recommendations to the Commissioner of Food
and Drugs with respect to the safety, effectiveness, and labeling of
the biological products in the designated category under review.

(1) A panel may also consult any individual or group.

(2) Any interested person may request in writing an opportunity
to present oral views to the panel. Such written requests for
oral presentations should include a summarization of the data
to be presented to the panel. Such request may be granted or
denied by the panel.

(3) Any interested person may present written data and views
which shall be considered by the panel. This information shall
be presented to the panel in the format set forth in paragraph
(b)(3) of this section and within the time period established
for the biological product category in the notice for review by
a panel.

(d) Standards for safety, effectiveness, and labeling. The advisory
review panel, in reviewing the submitted data and preparing the
panel's conclusions and recommendations, and the Commissioner
of Food and Drugs, in reviewing and implementing the
conclusions and recommendations of the panel, shall apply the
following standards to determine that a biological product is safe
and effective and not misbranded.

(1) Safety means the relative freedom from harmful effect to
persons affected, directly or indirectly, by a product when
prudently administered, taking into consideration the
character of the product in relation to the condition of the

recipient at the time. Proof of safety shall consist of adequate tests by methods reasonably applicable to show the biological product is safe under the prescribed conditions of use, including results of significant human experience during use.

(2) Effectiveness means a reasonable expectation that, in a significant proportion of the target population, the pharmacological or other effect of the biological product, when used under adequate directions, for use and warnings against unsafe use, will serve a clinically significant function in the diagnosis, cure, mitigation, treatment, or prevention of disease in man. Proof of effectiveness shall consist of controlled clinical investigations as defined in 314.126 of this chapter, unless this requirement is waived on the basis of a showing that it is not reasonably applicable to the biological product or essential to the validity of the investigation, and that an alternative method of investigation is adequate to substantiate effectiveness. Alternate methods, such as serological response evaluation in clinical studies and appropriate animal and other laboratory assay evaluations may be adequate to substantiate effectiveness where a previously accepted correlation between data generated in this way and clinical effectiveness already exists. Investigations may be corroborated by partially controlled or uncontrolled studies, documented clinical studies by qualified experts, and reports of significant human experience during marketing. Isolated case reports, random experience, and reports lacking the details which permit scientific evaluation will not be considered.

(3) The benefit-to-risk ratio of a biological product shall be considered in determining safety and effectiveness.

(4) A biological product may combine two or more safe and effective active components: (i) When each active component makes a contribution to the claimed effect or effects; (ii) when combining of the active ingredients does not decrease the purity, potency, safety, or effectiveness of any of the individual active components; and (iii) if the combination, when used under adequate directions for use and warnings against unsafe use, provides rational concurrent preventive therapy or treatment for a significant proportion of the target population.

(5) Labeling shall be clear and truthful in all respects and may not be false or misleading in any particular. It shall comply with

Part 601

section 351 of the Public Health Service Act and sections 502 and 503 of the Federal Food, Drug, and Cosmetic Act, and in particular with the applicable requirements of 610.60 through 610.65 and subpart D of part 201 of this chapter.

(e) Advisory review panel report to the Commissioner. An advisory review panel shall submit to the Commissioner of Food and Drugs a report containing the panel's conclusions and recommendations with respect to the biological products falling within the category covered by the panel. Included within this report shall be:

(1) A statement which designates those biological products determined by the panel to be safe and effective and not misbranded. This statement may include any condition relating to active components, labeling, tests required prior to release of lots, product standards, or other conditions necessary or appropriate for their safety and effectiveness.

(2) A statement which designates those biological products determined by the panel to be unsafe or ineffective, or to be misbranded. The statement shall include the panel's reasons for each such determination.

(3) A statement which designates those biological products determined by the panel not to fall within either paragraph (e) (1) or (2) of this section on the basis of the panel's conclusion that the available data are insufficient to classify such biological products, and for which further testing is therefore required. The report shall recommend with as must specificity as possible the type of further testing required and the time period within which it might reasonably be concluded. The report shall also recommend whether the product license should or should not be revoked, thus permitting or denying continued manufacturing and marketing of the biological product pending completion of the testing. This recommendation will be based on an assessment of the present evidence of the safety and effectiveness of the product and the potential benefits and risks likely to result from the continued use of the product for a limited period of time while the questions raised concerning the product are being resolved by further study.2

(f) Proposed order. After reviewing the conclusions and recommendations of the advisory review panel, the Commissioner of Food and Drugs shall publish in theFederal Registera proposed order containing:

(1) A statement designating the biological products in the category under review that are determined by the Commissioner of Food and Drugs to be safe and effective and not misbranded. This statement may include any condition relating to active components, labeling, tests required prior to release of lots, product standards, or other conditions necessary or appropriate for their safety and effectiveness, and may propose corresponding amendments in other regulations under this subchapter F.

(2) A statement designating the biological products in the category under review that are determined by the Commissioner of Food and Drugs to be unsafe or ineffective, or to be misbranded, together with the reasons therefor. All licenses for such products shall be proposed to be revoked.

(3) A statement designating the biological products not included in either of the above two statements on the basis of the Commissioner of Food and Drugs determination that the available data are insufficient to classify such biological products under either paragraph (f) (1) or (2) of this section. Licenses for such products may be proposed to be revoked or to remain in effect on an interim basis. Where the Commissioner determines that the potential benefits outweigh the potential risks, the proposed order shall provide that the biologics license for any biological product, falling within this paragraph, will not be revoked but will remain in effect on an interim basis while the data necessary to support its continued marketing are being obtained for evaluation by the Food and Drug Administration. The tests necessary to resolve whatever safety or effectiveness questions exist shall be described.2

(4) The full report or reports of the panel to the Commissioner of Food and Drugs.

The summary minutes of the panel meeting or meetings shall be made available to interested persons upon request. Any interested person may within 90 days after publication of the proposed order in theFederal Register,file with the Hearing Clerk of the Food and Drug Administration written comments in quintuplicate. Comments may be accompanied by a memorandum or brief in support thereof. All comments

may be reviewed at the office of the Division of Dockets
Management during regular working hours, Monday through
Friday.

(g) Final order. After reviewing the comments, the Commissioner of
Food and Drugs shall publish in theFederal Registera final order
on the matters covered in the proposed order. The final order
shall become effective as specified in the order.

(h) [Reserved]

(i) Court Appeal. The final order(s) published pursuant to paragraph
(g) of this section, and any notice published pursuant to paragraph
(h) of this section, constitute final agency action from which
appeal lies to the courts. The Food and Drug Administration will
request consolidation of all appeals in a single court. Upon court
appeal, the Commissioner of Food and Drugs may, at his
discretion, stay the effective date for part or all of the final order
or notice, pending appeal and final court adjudication.

2As of November 4, 1982, the provisions under paragraphs (e)(3) and
(f)(3) of this section for the interim marketing of certain biological
products pending completion of additional studies have been
superseded by the review and reclassification procedures under 601.26
of this chapter. The superseded text is included for the convenience of
the user only.

[38 FR 32052, Nov. 20, 1973, as amended at 39 FR 11535, Mar. 29, 1974; 40
FR 13498, Mar. 27, 1975; 43 FR 44838, Sept. 29, 1978; 47 FR 44071, Oct. 5,
1982; 47 FR 50211, Nov. 5, 1982; 51 FR 15607, Apr. 25, 1986; 55 FR 11014,
Mar. 26, 1990; 62 FR 53538, Oct. 15, 1997; 64 FR 56452, Oct. 20, 1999]

Sec. 601.26 Reclassification procedures to determine that licensed biological products are safe, effective, and not misbranded under prescribed, recommended, or suggested conditions of use.

This regulation establishes procedures for the reclassification of all
biological products that have been classified into Category IIIA. A
Category IIIA biological product is one for which an advisory review
panel has recommended under 601.25(e)(3), the Commissioner of
Food and Drugs (Commissioner) has proposed under 601.25(f)(3), or
the Commissioner has finally decided under 601.25(g) that available
data are insufficient to determine whether the product license should
be revoked or affirmed and which may be marketed pending the

completion of further testing. All of these Category IIIA products will either be reclassified into Category I (safe, effective, and not misbranded) or Category II (unsafe, ineffective, or misbranded) in accordance with the procedures set forth below.

(a) Advisory review panels. The Commissioner will appoint advisory review panels and use existing advisory review panels to (1) evaluate the safety and effectiveness of all Category IIIA biological products; (2) review the labeling of such products; and (3) advise the Commissioner on which Category IIIA biological products are safe, effective, and not misbranded. These advisory review panels will be established in accordance with procedures set forth in 601.25(a).

(b) Deliberations of advisory review panels. The deliberations of advisory review panels will be conducted in accordance with 601.25(d).

(c) Advisory review panel report to the Commissioner. An advisory review panel shall submit to the Commissioner a report containing the panel's conclusions and recommendations with respect to the biological products falling within the category of products reviewed by the panel. The panel report shall include:

(1) A statement designating the biological products in the category under review in accordance with either 601.25(e)(1) or 601.25(e)(2).

(2) A statement identifying those biological products designated under 601.25(e)(2) that the panel recommends should be designated as safe and presumptively effective and should remain on the market pending completion of further testing because there is a compelling medical need and no suitable alternative therapeutic, prophylactic, or diagnostic agent that is available in sufficient quantities to meet current medical needs. For the products or categories of products so recommended, the report shall include:

(i) A description and evaluation of the available evidence concerning effectiveness and an explanation why the evidence shows that the product has any benefit; and

(ii) A description of the alternative therapeutic, prophylactic, or diagnostic agents considered and a statement of why such alternatives are not suitable. In making this recommendation the panel shall also take into account the seriousness of the condition intended to be treated, prevented, or diagnosed by the product, the risks involved in the continued use of the product, and the likelihood that, based upon existing data, the effectiveness of the product can eventually be established by further testing and new test development. The report shall also recommend with as much specificity as possible the type of further testing required and the time period within which it might reasonably be concluded.

(d) Proposed order. After reviewing the conclusions and recommendations of the advisory review panels, the Commissioner shall publish in theFederal Registera proposed order containing:

(1) A statement designating the biological products in the category under review in accordance with either 601.25(e)(1) or 601.25(e)(2);

(2) A notice of availability of the full panel report or reports. The full panel report or reports shall be made publicly available at the time of publication of the proposed order.

(3) A proposal to accept or reject the findings of the advisory review panel required by 601.26(c)(2)(i) and (ii).

(4) A statement identifying those biological products that the Commissioner proposes should be designated as safe and presumptively effective under 601.26(c)(2) and should be permitted to remain on the market pending completion of further testing because there is a compelling medical need and no suitable alternative therapeutic, prophylactic, or diagnostic agent for the product that is available in sufficient quantities to meet current medical needs. In making this proposal, the Commissioner shall take into account the seriousness of the condition to be treated, prevented, or diagnosed by the product, the risks involved in the continued use of the product, and the likelihood that, based upon existing data, the effectiveness of the product can eventually be established by further testing.

(e) Final order. After reviewing the comments on the proposed order, the Commissioner shall publish in theFederal Registera final order on the matters covered in the proposed order. Where the Commissioner determines that there is a compelling medical need and no suitable alternative therapeutic, prophylactic, or diagnostic agent for any biological product that is available in sufficient quantities to meet current medical needs, the final order shall provide that the biologics license application for that biological product will not be revoked, but will remain in effect on an interim basis while the data necessary to support its continued marketing are being obtained for evaluation by the Food and Drug Administration. The final order shall describe the tests necessary to resolve whatever effectiveness questions exist.

(f) Additional studies and labeling.

(1) Within 60 days following publication of the final order, each licensed manufacturer for a biological product designated as requiring further study to justify continued marketing on an interim basis, under paragraph (e) of this section, shall submit to the Commissioner a written statement intended to show that studies adequate and appropriate to resolve the questions raised about the product have been undertaken. The Federal Government may undertake the studies. Any study involving a clinical investigation that involves human subjects shall be conducted in compliance with the requirements for informed consent under part 50 of this chapter. Such a study is also subject to the requirements for institutional review under part 56 of this chapter unless exempt under 56.104 or 56.105. The Commissioner may extend this 60-day period if necessary, either to review and act on proposed protocols or upon indication from the licensed manufacturer that the studies will commence at a specified reasonable time. If no such commitment is made, or adequate and appropriate studies are not undertaken, the biologics license or licenses shall be revoked.

(2) A progress report shall be filed on the studies by January 1 and July 1 until completion. If the progress report is inadequate or if the Commissioner concludes that the studies are not being pursued promptly and diligently, or if interim results indicate the product is not a medical necessity, the biologics license or licenses shall be revoked.

(3) Promptly upon completion of the studies undertaken on the product, the Commissioner will review all available data and will either retain or revoke the biologics license or licenses involved. In making this review the Commissioner may again consult the advisory review panel which prepared the report on the product, or other advisory committees, professional

organizations, or experts. The Commissioner shall take such action by notice published in theFederal Register.

(4) Labeling and promotional material for those biological products requiring additional studies shall bear a box statement in the following format:

> Based on a review by the (insert name of appropriate advisory review panel) and other information, the Food and Drug Administration has directed that further investigation be conducted before this product is conclusively determined to be effective for labeled indication(s).

(5) A written informed consent shall be obtained from participants in any additional studies required under paragraph (f)(1) of this section, explaining the nature of the product and the investigation. The explanation shall consist of such disclosure and be made so that intelligent and informed consent be given and that a clear opportunity to refuse is presented.

(g) Court appeal. The final order(s) published pursuant to paragraph (e) of this section constitute final agency action from which appeal lies to the courts. The Food and Drug Administration will request consolidation of all appeals in a single court. Upon court appeal, the Commissioner of Food and Drugs may, at the Commissioner's discretion, stay the effective date for part or all of the final order or notice, pending appeal and final court adjudication.

(h) [Reserved]

(i) Institutional review and informed consent. Information and data submitted under this section after July 27, 1981, shall include statements regarding each clinical investigation involving human subjects, that it was conducted in compliance with the requirements for informed consent under part 50 of this chapter. Such a study is also subject to the requirements for institutional review under part 56 of this chapter, unless exempt under 56.104 or 56.105.

[47 FR 44071, Oct. 5, 1982, as amended at 64 FR 56452, Oct. 20, 1999]

Sec. 601.27 Pediatric studies.

(a) Required assessment. Except as provided in paragraphs (b), (c), and (d) of this section, each application for a new active ingredient, new indication, new dosage form, new dosing regimen, or new route of administration shall contain data that are adequate to assess the safety and effectiveness of the product for the claimed indications in all relevant pediatric subpopulations, and to support dosing and administration for each pediatric subpopulation for which the product is safe and effective. Where the course of the disease and the effects of the product are similar in adults and pediatric patients, FDA may conclude that pediatric effectiveness can be extrapolated from adequate and well-controlled effectiveness studies in adults, usually supplemented with other information in pediatric patients, such as pharmacokinetic studies. In addition, studies may not be needed in each pediatric age group, if data from one age group can be extrapolated to another. Assessments required under this section for a product that represents a meaningful therapeutic benefit over existing treatments must be carried out using appropriate formulations for the age group(s) for which the assessment is required.

(b) Deferred submission.

(1) FDA may, on its own initiative or at the request of an applicant, defer submission of some or all assessments of safety and effectiveness described in paragraph (a) of this section until after licensing of the product for use in adults. Deferral may be granted if, among other reasons, the product is ready for approval in adults before studies in pediatric patients are complete, pediatric studies should be delayed until additional safety or effectiveness data have been collected. If an applicant requests deferred submission, the request must provide an adequate justification for delaying pediatric studies, a description of the planned or ongoing studies, and evidence that the studies are being or will be conducted with due diligence and at the earliest possible time.

(2) If FDA determines that there is an adequate justification for temporarily delaying the submission of assessments of pediatric safety and effectiveness, the product may be licensed for use in adults subject to the requirement that the applicant submit the required assessments within a specified time.

(c) Waivers –

(1) General. FDA may grant a full or partial waiver of the requirements of paragraph (a) of this section on its own initiative or at the request of an applicant. A request for a waiver must provide an adequate justification.

(2) Full waiver. An applicant may request a waiver of the requirements of paragraph (a) of this section if the applicant certifies that:

(i) The product does not represent a meaningful therapeutic benefit over existing therapies for pediatric patients and is not likely to be used in a substantial number of pediatric patients;

(ii) Necessary studies are impossible or highly impractical because, e.g., the number of such patients is so small or geographically dispersed; or

(iii) There is evidence strongly suggesting that the product would be ineffective or unsafe in all pediatric age groups.

(3) Partial waiver. An applicant may request a waiver of the requirements of paragraph (a) of this section with respect to a specified pediatric age group, if the applicant certifies that:

(i) The product does not represent a meaningful therapeutic benefit over existing therapies for pediatric patients in that age group, and is not likely to be used in a substantial number of patients in that age group;

(ii) Necessary studies are impossible or highly impractical because, e.g., the number of patients in that age group is so small or geographically dispersed;

(iii) There is evidence strongly suggesting that the product would be ineffective or unsafe in that age group; or

(iv) The applicant can demonstrate that reasonable attempts to produce a pediatric formulation necessary for that age group have failed.

(4) FDA action on waiver. FDA shall grant a full or partial waiver, as appropriate, if the agency finds that there is a reasonable basis on which to conclude that one or more of the grounds for waiver specified in paragraphs (c)(2) or (c)(3) of this section have been met. If a waiver is granted on the ground that it is not possible to develop a pediatric

formulation, the waiver will cover only those pediatric age groups requiring that formulation. If a waiver is granted because there is evidence that the product would be ineffective or unsafe in pediatric populations, this information will be included in the product's labeling.

(5) Definition of "meaningful therapeutic benefit". For purposes of this section, a product will be considered to offer a meaningful therapeutic benefit over existing therapies if FDA estimates that:

(i) If approved, the product would represent a significant improvement in the treatment, diagnosis, or prevention of a disease, compared to marketed products adequately labeled for that use in the relevant pediatric population. Examples of how improvement might be demonstrated include, e.g., evidence of increased effectiveness in treatment, prevention, or diagnosis of disease; elimination or substantial reduction of a treatment-limiting drug reaction; documented enhancement of compliance; or evidence of safety and effectiveness in a new subpopulation; or

(ii) The product is in a class of products or for an indication for which there is a need for additional therapeutic options.

(d) Exemption for orphan drugs. This section does not apply to any product for an indication or indications for which orphan designation has been granted under part 316, subpart C, of this chapter.

[63 FR 66671, Dec. 2, 1998]

Sec. 601.28 Annual reports of postmarketing pediatric studies.

Sponsors of licensed biological products shall submit the following information each year within 60 days of the anniversary date of approval of each product under the license to the Director, Center for Biologics Evaluation and Research or the Director, Center for Drug Evaluation and Research (see mailing addresses in 600.2 of this chapter):

(a) Summary. A brief summary stating whether labeling supplements for pediatric use have been submitted and whether new studies in

Part 601

the pediatric population to support appropriate labeling for the pediatric population have been initiated. Where possible, an estimate of patient exposure to the drug product, with special reference to the pediatric population (neonates, infants, children, and adolescents) shall be provided, including dosage form.

(b) Clinical data. Analysis of available safety and efficacy data in the pediatric population and changes proposed in the labeling based on this information. An assessment of data needed to ensure appropriate labeling for the pediatric population shall be included.

(c) Status reports. A statement on the current status of any postmarketing studies in the pediatric population performed by, or on behalf of, the applicant. The statement shall include whether postmarketing clinical studies in pediatric populations were required or agreed to, and, if so, the status of these studies shall be reported to FDA in annual progress reports of postmarketing studies under 601.70 rather than under this section.

[65 FR 59718, Oct. 6, 2000, as amended at 65 FR 64618, Oct. 30, 2000; 70 FR 14984, Mar. 24, 2005]

Sec. 601.29 Guidance documents.

(a) FDA has made available guidance documents under 10.115 of this chapter to help you comply with certain requirements of this part.

(b) The Center for Biologics Evaluation and Research (CBER) maintains a list of guidance documents that apply to the center's regulations. The lists are maintained on the Internet and are published annually in theFederal Register.You may request a copy of the CBER list from the Office of Communication, Training, and Manufacturers Assistance (HFM-40), Center for Biologics Evaluation and Research, Food and Drug Administration (see mailing addresses in 600.2 of this chapter).

[65 FR 56480, Sept. 19, 2000, as amended at 70 FR 14984, Mar. 24, 2005]

Subpart D--Diagnostic Radiopharmaceuticals

Sec. 601.30 Scope.

This subpart applies to radiopharmaceuticals intended for in vivo administration for diagnostic and monitoring use. It does not apply to radiopharmaceuticals intended for therapeutic purposes. In situations where a particular radiopharmaceutical is proposed for both diagnostic and therapeutic uses, the radiopharmaceutical must be evaluated taking into account each intended use.

Sec. 601.31 Definition.

For purposes of this part, diagnostic radiopharmaceutical means:

(a) An article that is intended for use in the diagnosis or monitoring of a disease or a manifestation of a disease in humans and that exhibits spontaneous disintegration of unstable nuclei with the emission of nuclear particles or photons; or

(b) Any nonradioactive reagent kit or nuclide generator that is intended to be used in the preparation of such article as defined in paragraph (a) of this section.

Sec. 601.32 General factors relevant to safety and effectiveness.

FDA's determination of the safety and effectiveness of a diagnostic radiopharmaceutical includes consideration of the following:

(a) The proposed use of the diagnostic radiopharmaceutical in the practice of medicine;

(b) The pharmacological and toxicological activity of the diagnostic radiopharmaceutical (including any carrier or ligand component of the diagnostic radiopharmaceutical); and

(c) The estimated absorbed radiation dose of the diagnostic radiopharmaceutical.

Sec. 601.33 Indications.

(a) For diagnostic radiopharmaceuticals, the categories of proposed indications for use include, but are not limited to, the following:

(1) Structure delineation;

(2) Functional, physiological, or biochemical assessment;

(3) Disease or pathology detection or assessment; and

(4) Diagnostic or therapeutic patient management.

Part 601

(b) Where a diagnostic radiopharmaceutical is not intended to provide disease-specific information, the proposed indications for use may refer to a biochemical, physiological, anatomical, or pathological process or to more than one disease or condition.

Sec. 601.34 Evaluation of effectiveness.

(a) The effectiveness of a diagnostic radiopharmaceutical is assessed by evaluating its ability to provide useful clinical information related to its proposed indications for use. The method of this evaluation varies depending upon the proposed indication(s) and may use one or more of the following criteria:

(1) The claim of structure delineation is established by demonstrating in a defined clinical setting the ability to locate anatomical structures and to characterize their anatomy.

(2) The claim of functional, physiological, or biochemical assessment is established by demonstrating in a defined clinical setting reliable measurement of function(s) or physiological, biochemical, or molecular process(es).

(3) The claim of disease or pathology detection or assessment is established by demonstrating in a defined clinical setting that the diagnostic radiopharmaceutical has sufficient accuracy in identifying or characterizing the disease or pathology.

(4) The claim of diagnostic or therapeutic patient management is established by demonstrating in a defined clinical setting that the test is useful in diagnostic or therapeutic patient management.

(5) For a claim that does not fall within the indication categories identified in 601.33, the applicant or sponsor should consult FDA on how to establish the effectiveness of the diagnostic radiopharmaceutical for the claim.

(b) The accuracy and usefulness of the diagnostic information is determined by comparison with a reliable assessment of actual clinical status. A reliable assessment of actual clinical status may be provided by a diagnostic standard or standards of demonstrated accuracy. In the absence of such diagnostic standard(s), the actual clinical status must be established in another manner, e.g., patient followup.

Sec. 601.35 Evaluation of safety.

(a) Factors considered in the safety assessment of a diagnostic radiopharmaceutical include, among others, the following:

    (1) The radiation dose;

    (2) The pharmacology and toxicology of the radiopharmaceutical, including any radionuclide, carrier, or ligand;

    (3) The risks of an incorrect diagnostic determination;

    (4) The adverse reaction profile of the drug;

    (5) Results of human experience with the radiopharmaceutical for other uses; and

    (6) Results of any previous human experience with the carrier or ligand of the radiopharmaceutical when the same chemical entity as the carrier or ligand has been used in a previously studied product.

(b) The assessment of the adverse reaction profile includes, but is not limited to, an evaluation of the potential of the diagnostic radiopharmaceutical, including the carrier or ligand, to elicit the following:

    (1) Allergic or hypersensitivity responses,

    (2) Immunologic responses,

    (3) Changes in the physiologic or biochemical function of the target and nontarget tissues, and

    (4) Clinically detectable signs or symptoms.

(c)(1) To establish the safety of a diagnostic radiopharmaceutical, FDA may require, among other information, the following types of data:

    (A) Pharmacology data,

    (B) Toxicology data,

    (C) Clinical adverse event data, and

    (D) Radiation safety assessment.

    (2) The amount of new safety data required will depend on the characteristics of the product and available information regarding the safety of the diagnostic radiopharmaceutical,

Part 601

and its carrier or ligand, obtained from other studies and uses. Such information may include, but is not limited to, the dose, route of administration, frequency of use, half-life of the ligand or carrier, half-life of the radionuclide, and results of clinical and preclinical studies. FDA will establish categories of diagnostic radiopharmaceuticals based on defined characteristics relevant to risk and will specify the amount and type of safety data that are appropriate for each category (e.g., required safety data may be limited for diagnostic radiopharmaceuticals with a well established, low-risk profile). Upon reviewing the relevant product characteristics and safety information, FDA will place each diagnostic radiopharmaceutical into the appropriate safety risk category.

(d) Radiation safety assessment. The radiation safety assessment must establish the radiation dose of a diagnostic radiopharmaceutical by radiation dosimetry evaluations in humans and appropriate animal models. The maximum tolerated dose need not be established.

Subpart E--Accelerated Approval of Biological Products for Serious or Life-Threatening Illnesses

Sec. 601.40 Scope.

This subpart applies to certain biological products that have been studied for their safety and effectiveness in treating serious or life-threatening illnesses and that provide meaningful therapeutic benefit to patients over existing treatments (e.g., ability to treat patients unresponsive to, or intolerant of, available therapy, or improved patient response over available therapy).

Sec. 601.41 Approval based on a surrogate endpoint or on an effect on a clinical endpoint other than survival or irreversible morbidity.

FDA may grant marketing approval for a biological product on the basis of adequate and well-controlled clinical trials establishing that the biological product has an effect on a surrogate endpoint that is reasonably likely, based on epidemiologic, therapeutic, pathophysiologic, or other evidence, to predict clinical benefit or on the basis of an effect on a clinical endpoint other than survival or irreversible morbidity. Approval under this section will be subject to the requirement that the applicant study the biological product further,

to verify and describe its clinical benefit, where there is uncertainty as
to the relation of the surrogate endpoint to clinical benefit, or of the
observed clinical benefit to ultimate outcome. Postmarketing studies
would usually be studies already underway. When required to be
conducted, such studies must also be adequate and well-controlled.
The applicant shall carry out any such studies with due diligence.

Sec. 601.42 Approval with restrictions to assure safe use.

(a) If FDA concludes that a biological product shown to be effective
     can be safely used only if distribution or use is restricted, FDA will
     require such postmarketing restrictions as are needed to assure
     safe use of the biological product, such as:

    (1) Distribution restricted to certain facilities or physicians with
         special training or experience; or

    (2) Distribution conditioned on the performance of specified
         medical procedures.

(b) The limitations imposed will be commensurate with the specific
     safety concerns presented by the biological product.

Sec. 601.43 Withdrawal procedures.

(a) For biological products approved under 601.41 or 601.42, FDA
     may withdraw approval, following a hearing as provided in part 15
     of this chapter, as modified by this section, if:

    (1) A postmarketing clinical study fails to verify clinical benefit;

    (2) The applicant fails to perform the required postmarketing
         study with due diligence;

    (3) Use after marketing demonstrates that postmarketing
         restrictions are inadequate to ensure safe use of the biological
         product;

    (4) The applicant fails to adhere to the postmarketing restrictions
         agreed upon;

    (5) The promotional materials are false or misleading; or

    (6) Other evidence demonstrates that the biological product is
         not shown to be safe or effective under its conditions of use.

(b) Notice of opportunity for a hearing. The Director of the Center
     for Biologics Evaluation and Research or the Director of the

Part 601

Center for Drug Evaluation and Research will give the applicant notice of an opportunity for a hearing on the Center's proposal to withdraw the approval of an application approved under 601.41 or 601.42. The notice, which will ordinarily be a letter, will state generally the reasons for the action and the proposed grounds for the order.

(c) Submission of data and information.

(1) If the applicant fails to file a written request for a hearing within 15 days of receipt of the notice, the applicant waives the opportunity for a hearing.

(2) If the applicant files a timely request for a hearing, the agency will publish a notice of hearing in theFederal Registerin accordance with 12.32(e) and 15.20 of this chapter.

(3) An applicant who requests a hearing under this section must, within 30 days of receipt of the notice of opportunity for a hearing, submit the data and information upon which the applicant intends to rely at the hearing.

(d) Separation of functions. Separation of functions (as specified in 10.55 of this chapter) will not apply at any point in withdrawal proceedings under this section.

(e) Procedures for hearings. Hearings held under this section will be conducted in accordance with the provisions of part 15 of this chapter, with the following modifications:

(1) An advisory committee duly constituted under part 14 of this chapter will be present at the hearing. The committee will be asked to review the issues involved and to provide advice and recommendations to the Commissioner of Food and Drugs.

(2) The presiding officer, the advisory committee members, up to three representatives of the applicant, and up to three representatives of the Center may question any person during or at the conclusion of the person's presentation. No other person attending the hearing may question a person making a presentation. The presiding officer may, as a matter of discretion, permit questions to be submitted to the presiding officer for response by a person making a presentation.

(f) Judicial review. The Commissioner's decision constitutes final agency action from which the applicant may petition for judicial review. Before requesting an order from a court for a stay of action pending review, an applicant must first submit a petition for a stay of action under 10.35 of this chapter.

[57 FR 58959, Dec. 11, 1992, as amended at 68 FR 34797, June 11, 2003; 70 FR 14984, Mar. 24, 2005]

Sec. 601.44 Postmarketing safety reporting.

Biological products approved under this program are subject to the postmarketing recordkeeping and safety reporting applicable to all approved biological products.

Sec. 601.45 Promotional materials.

For biological products being considered for approval under this subpart, unless otherwise informed by the agency, applicants must submit to the agency for consideration during the preapproval review period copies of all promotional materials, including promotional labeling as well as advertisements, intended for dissemination or publication within 120 days following marketing approval. After 120 days following marketing approval, unless otherwise informed by the agency, the applicant must submit promotional materials at least 30 days prior to the intended time of initial dissemination of the labeling or initial publication of the advertisement.

Sec. 601.46 Termination of requirements.

If FDA determines after approval that the requirements established in 601.42, 601.43, or 601.45 are no longer necessary for the safe and effective use of a biological product, it will so notify the applicant. Ordinarily, for biological products approved under 601.41, these requirements will no longer apply when FDA determines that the required postmarketing study verifies and describes the biological product's clinical benefit and the biological product would be appropriate for approval under traditional procedures. For biological products approved under 601.42, the restrictions would no longer apply when FDA determines that safe use of the biological product can be assured through appropriate labeling. FDA also retains the discretion to remove specific postapproval requirements upon review of a petition submitted by the sponsor in accordance with 10.30.

Part 601

Subpart F--Confidentiality of Information

Sec. 601.50 Confidentiality of data and information in an investigational new drug notice for a biological product.

(a) The existence of an IND notice for a biological product will not be disclosed by the Food and Drug Administration unless it has previously been publicly disclosed or acknowledged.

(b) The availability for public disclosure of all data and information in an IND file for a biological product shall be handled in accordance with the provisions established in 601.51.

(c) Notwithstanding the provisions of 601.51, the Food and Drug Administration shall disclose upon request to an individual on whom an investigational biological product has been used a copy of any adverse reaction report relating to such use.

[39 FR 44656, Dec. 24, 1974]

Sec. 601.51 Confidentiality of data and information in applications for biologics licenses.

(a) For purposes of this section the biological product file includes all data and information submitted with or incorporated by reference in any application for a biologics license, IND's incorporated into any such application, master files, and other related submissions. The availability for public disclosure of any record in the biological product file shall be handled in accordance with the provisions of this section.

(b) The existence of a biological product file will not be disclosed by the Food and Drug Administration before a biologics license application has been approved unless it has previously been publicly disclosed or acknowledged. The Food and Drug Administration will maintain a list available for public disclosure of biological products for which a license application has been approved.

(c) If the existence of a biological product file has not been publicly disclosed or acknowledged, no data or information in the biological product file is available for public disclosure.

(d)(1) If the existence of a biological product file has been publicly disclosed or acknowledged before a license has been issued, no data or information contained in the file is available for public disclosure before such license is issued, but the Commissioner may, in his discretion, disclose a summary of such selected portions of the safety and effectiveness data as are appropriate for public consideration of a specific pending issue, e.g., at an open session of a Food and Drug Administration advisory committee or pursuant to an exchange of important regulatory information with a foreign government.

(2) Notwithstanding paragraph (d)(1) of this section, FDA will make available to the public upon request the information in the IND that was required to be filed in Docket Number 95S-0158 in the Division of Dockets Management (HFA-305), Food and Drug Administration, 5630 Fishers Lane, rm. 1061, Rockville, MD 20852, for investigations involving an exception from informed consent under 50.24 of this chapter. Persons wishing to request this information shall submit a request under the Freedom of Information Act.

(e) After a license has been issued, the following data and information in the biological product file are immediately available for public disclosure unless extraordinary circumstances are shown:

(1) All safety and effectiveness data and information.

(2) A protocol for a test or study, unless it is shown to fall within the exemption established for trade secrets and confidential commercial or financial information in 20.61 of this chapter.

(3) Adverse reaction reports, product experience reports, consumer complaints, and other similar data and information, after deletion of:

(i) Names and any information that would identify the person using the product.

(ii) Names and any information that would identify any third party involved with the report, such as a physician or hospital or other institution.

(4) A list of all active ingredients and any inactive ingredients previously disclosed to the public, as defined in 20.81 of this chapter.

Part 601

(5) An assay method or other analytical method, unless it serves no regulatory or compliance purpose and it is shown to fall within the exemption established in 20.61 of this chapter.

(6) All correspondence and written summaries of oral discussions relating to the biological product file, in accordance with the provisions of part 20 of this chapter.

(7) All records showing the manufacturer's testing of a particular lot, after deletion of data or information that would show the volume of the drug produced, manufacturing procedures and controls, yield from raw materials, costs, or other material falling within 20.61 of this chapter.

(8) All records showing the testing of and action on a particular lot by the Food and Drug Administration.

(f) The following data and information in a biological product file are not available for public disclosure unless they have been previously disclosed to the public as defined in 20.81 of this chapter or they relate to a product or ingredient that has been abandoned and they no longer represent a trade secret or confidential commercial or financial information as defined in 20.61 of this chapter:

(1) Manufacturing methods or processes, including quality control procedures.

(2) Production, sales, distribution, and similar data and information, except that any compilation of such data and information aggregated and prepared in a way that does not reveal data or information which is not available for public disclosure under this provision is available for public disclosure.

(3) Quantitative or semiquantitative formulas.

(g) For purposes of this regulation, safety and effectiveness data include all studies and tests of a biological product on animals and humans and all studies and tests on the drug for identity, stability, purity, potency, and bioavailability.

[39 FR 44656, Dec. 24, 1974, as amended at 42 FR 15676, Mar. 22, 1977; 49 FR 23833, June 8, 1984; 55 FR 11013, Mar. 26, 1990; 61 FR 51530, Oct. 2, 1996; 64 FR 56452, Oct. 20, 1999; 68 FR 24879, May 9, 2003; 69 FR 13717, Mar. 24, 2004; 70 FR 14984, Mar. 24, 2005]

Subpart G--Postmarketing Studies

Sec. 601.70 Annual progress reports of postmarketing studies.

(a) General requirements. This section applies to all required postmarketing studies (e.g., accelerated approval clinical benefit studies, pediatric studies) and postmarketing studies that an applicant has committed, in writing, to conduct either at the time of approval of an application or a supplement to an application, or after approval of an application or a supplement. Postmarketing studies within the meaning of this section are those that concern:

    (1) Clinical safety;

    (2) Clinical efficacy;

    (3) Clinical pharmacology; and

    (4) Nonclinical toxicology.

(b) What to report. Each applicant of a licensed biological product shall submit a report to FDA on the status of postmarketing studies for each approved product application. The status of these postmarketing studies shall be reported annually until FDA notifies the applicant, in writing, that the agency concurs with the applicant's determination that the study commitment has been fulfilled, or that the study is either no longer feasible or would no longer provide useful information. Each annual progress report shall be accompanied by a completed transmittal Form FDA-2252, and shall include all the information required under this section that the applicant received or otherwise obtained during the annual reporting interval which ends on the U.S. anniversary date. The report must provide the following information for each postmarketing study:

    (1) Applicant's name.

    (2) Product name. Include the approved product's proper name and the proprietary name, if any.

    (3) Biologics license application (BLA) and supplement number.

    (4) Date of U.S. approval of BLA.

    (5) Date of postmarketing study commitment.

Part 601

(6) Description of postmarketing study commitment. The description must include sufficient information to uniquely describe the study. This information may include the purpose of the study, the type of study, the patient population addressed by the study and the indication(s) and dosage(s) that are to be studied.

(7) Schedule for completion and reporting of the postmarketing study commitment. The schedule should include the actual or projected dates for submission of the study protocol to FDA, completion of patient accrual or initiation of an animal study, completion of the study, submission of the final study report to FDA, and any additional milestones or submissions for which projected dates were specified as part of the commitment. In addition, it should include a revised schedule, as appropriate. If the schedule has been previously revised, provide both the original schedule and the most recent, previously submitted revision.

(8) Current status of the postmarketing study commitment. The status of each postmarketing study should be categorized using one of the following terms that describes the study's status on the anniversary date of U.S. approval of the application or other agreed upon date:

(i) Pending. The study has not been initiated, but does not meet the criterion for delayed.

(ii) Ongoing. The study is proceeding according to or ahead of the original schedule described under paragraph (b)(7) of this section.

(iii) Delayed. The study is behind the original schedule described under paragraph (b)(7) of this section.

(iv) Terminated. The study was ended before completion but a final study report has not been submitted to FDA.

(v) Submitted. The study has been completed or terminated and a final study report has been submitted to FDA.

(9) Explanation of the study's status. Provide a brief description of the status of the study, including the patient accrual rate (expressed by providing the number of patients or subjects enrolled to date, and the total planned enrollment), and an explanation of the study's status identified under paragraph (b)(8) of this section. If the study has been completed, include the date the study was completed and the date the final study

report was submitted to FDA, as applicable. Provide a revised schedule, as well as the reason(s) for the revision, if the schedule under paragraph (b)(7) of this section has changed since the previous report.

(c) *When to report.* Annual progress reports for postmarketing study commitments entered into by applicants shall be reported to FDA within 60 days of the anniversary date of the U.S. approval of the application for the product.

(d) *Where to report.* Submit two copies of the annual progress report of postmarketing studies to the Center for Biologics Evaluation and Research or Center for Drug Evaluation and Research (see mailing addresses in 600.2 of this chapter).

(e) *Public disclosure of information.* Except for the information described in this paragraph, FDA may publicly disclose any information concerning a postmarketing study, within the meaning of this section, if the agency determines that the information is necessary to identify an applicant or to establish the status of the study including the reasons, if any, for failure to conduct, complete, and report the study. Under this section, FDA will not publicly disclose trade secrets, as defined in 20.61 of this chapter, or information, described in 20.63 of this chapter, the disclosure of which would constitute an unwarranted invasion of personal privacy.

[65 FR 64618, Oct. 30, 2000, as amended at 70 FR 14984, Mar. 24, 2005]

Subpart H--Approval of Biological Products When Human Efficacy Studies Are Not Ethical or Feasible

Sec. 601.90 Scope.

This subpart applies to certain biological products that have been studied for their safety and efficacy in ameliorating or preventing serious or life-threatening conditions caused by exposure to lethal or permanently disabling toxic biological, chemical, radiological, or nuclear substances. This subpart applies only to those biological products for which: Definitive human efficacy studies cannot be conducted because it would be unethical to deliberately expose healthy human volunteers to a lethal or permanently disabling toxic biological,

Part 601

chemical, radiological, or nuclear substance; and field trials to study the product's efficacy after an accidental or hostile exposure have not been feasible. This subpart does not apply to products that can be approved based on efficacy standards described elsewhere in FDA's regulations (e.g., accelerated approval based on surrogate markers or clinical endpoints other than survival or irreversible morbidity), nor does it address the safety evaluation for the products to which it does apply.

Sec. 601.91 Approval based on evidence of effectiveness from studies in animals.

(a) FDA may grant marketing approval for a biological product for which safety has been established and for which the requirements of 601.90 are met based on adequate and well-controlled animal studies when the results of those animal studies establish that the biological product is reasonably likely to produce clinical benefit in humans. In assessing the sufficiency of animal data, the agency may take into account other data, including human data, available to the agency. FDA will rely on the evidence from studies in animals to provide substantial evidence of the effectiveness of these products only when:

(1) There is a reasonably well-understood pathophysiological mechanism of the toxicity of the substance and its prevention or substantial reduction by the product;

(2) The effect is demonstrated in more than one animal species expected to react with a response predictive for humans, unless the effect is demonstrated in a single animal species that represents a sufficiently well-characterized animal model for predicting the response in humans;

(3) The animal study endpoint is clearly related to the desired benefit in humans, generally the enhancement of survival or prevention of major morbidity; and

(4) The data or information on the kinetics and pharmacodynamics of the product or other relevant data or information, in animals and humans, allows selection of an effective dose in humans.

(b) Approval under this subpart will be subject to three requirements:

(1) Postmarketing studies. The applicant must conduct postmarketing studies, such as field studies, to verify and

describe the biological product's clinical benefit and to assess its safety when used as indicated when such studies are feasible and ethical. Such postmarketing studies would not be feasible until an exigency arises. When such studies are feasible, the applicant must conduct such studies with due diligence. Applicants must include as part of their application a plan or approach to postmarketing study commitments in the event such studies become ethical and feasible.

(2) Approval with restrictions to ensure safe use. If FDA concludes that a biological product shown to be effective under this subpart can be safely used only if distribution or use is restricted, FDA will require such postmarketing restrictions as are needed to ensure safe use of the biological product, commensurate with the specific safety concerns presented by the biological product, such as:

    (i) Distribution restricted to certain facilities or health care practitioners with special training or experience;

    (ii) Distribution conditioned on the performance of specified medical procedures, including medical followup; and

    (iii) Distribution conditioned on specified recordkeeping requirements.

(3) Information to be provided to patient recipients. For biological products or specific indications approved under this subpart, applicants must prepare, as part of their proposed labeling, labeling to be provided to patient recipients. The patient labeling must explain that, for ethical or feasibility reasons, the biological product's approval was based on efficacy studies conducted in animals alone and must give the biological product's indication(s), directions for use (dosage and administration), contraindications, a description of any reasonably foreseeable risks, adverse reactions, anticipated benefits, drug interactions, and any other relevant information required by FDA at the time of approval. The patient labeling must be available with the product to be provided to patients prior to administration or dispensing of the biological product for the use approved under this subpart, if possible.

Sec. 601.92 Withdrawal procedures.

(a) Reasons to withdraw approval. For biological products approved under this subpart, FDA may withdraw approval, following a hearing as provided in part 15 of this chapter, as modified by this section, if:

Part 601

(1) A postmarketing clinical study fails to verify clinical benefit;

(2) The applicant fails to perform the postmarketing study with due diligence;

(3) Use after marketing demonstrates that postmarketing restrictions are inadequate to ensure safe use of the biological product;

(4) The applicant fails to adhere to the postmarketing restrictions applied at the time of approval under this subpart;

(5) The promotional materials are false or misleading; or

(6) Other evidence demonstrates that the biological product is not shown to be safe or effective under its conditions of use.

(b) Notice of opportunity for a hearing. The Director of the Center for Biologics Evaluation and Research or the Director of the Center for Drug Evaluation and Research will give the applicant notice of an opportunity for a hearing on the proposal to withdraw the approval of an application approved under this subpart. The notice, which will ordinarily be a letter, will state generally the reasons for the action and the proposed grounds for the order.

(c) Submission of data and information.

(1) If the applicant fails to file a written request for a hearing within 15 days of receipt of the notice, the applicant waives the opportunity for a hearing.

(2) If the applicant files a timely request for a hearing, the agency will publish a notice of hearing in theFederal Registerin accordance with 12.32(e) and 15.20 of this chapter.

(3) An applicant who requests a hearing under this section must, within 30 days of receipt of the notice of opportunity for a hearing, submit the data and information upon which the applicant intends to rely at the hearing.

(d) Separation of functions. Separation of functions (as specified in 10.55 of this chapter) will not apply at any point in withdrawal proceedings under this section.

(e) Procedures for hearings. Hearings held under this section will be conducted in accordance with the provisions of part 15 of this chapter, with the following modifications:

(1) An advisory committee duly constituted under part 14 of this chapter will be present at the hearing. The committee will be asked to review the issues involved and to provide advice and recommendations to the Commissioner of Food and Drugs.

(2) The presiding officer, the advisory committee members, up to three representatives of the applicant, and up to three representatives of CBER may question any person during or at the conclusion of the person's presentation. No other person attending the hearing may question a person making a presentation. The presiding officer may, as a matter of discretion, permit questions to be submitted to the presiding officer for response by a person making a presentation.

(f) Judicial review. The Commissioner of Food and Drugs' decision constitutes final agency action from which the applicant may petition for judicial review. Before requesting an order from a court for a stay of action pending review, an applicant must first submit a petition for a stay of action under 10.35 of this chapter.

[67 FR 37996, May 31, 2002, as amended at 70 FR 14984, Mar. 24, 2005]

Sec. 601.93 Postmarketing safety reporting.

Biological products approved under this subpart are subject to the postmarketing recordkeeping and safety reporting applicable to all approved biological products.

Sec. 601.94 Promotional materials.

For biological products being considered for approval under this subpart, unless otherwise informed by the agency, applicants must submit to the agency for consideration during the preapproval review period copies of all promotional materials, including promotional labeling as well as advertisements, intended for dissemination or publication within 120 days following marketing approval. After 120 days following marketing approval, unless otherwise informed by the agency, the applicant must submit promotional materials at least 30 days prior to the intended time of initial dissemination of the labeling or initial publication of the advertisement.

Sec. 601.95 Termination of requirements.

If FDA determines after approval under this subpart that the requirements established in 601.91(b)(2), 601.92, and 601.93 are no longer necessary for the safe and effective use of a biological product,

Part 601

FDA will so notify the applicant. Ordinarily, for biological products approved under 601.91, these requirements will no longer apply when FDA determines that the postmarketing study verifies and describes the biological product's clinical benefit. For biological products approved under 601.91, the restrictions would no longer apply when FDA determines that safe use of the biological product can be ensured through appropriate labeling. FDA also retains the discretion to remove specific postapproval requirements upon review of a petition submitted by the sponsor in accordance with 10.30 of this chapter.

Authority: 15 U.S.C. 1451-1561; 21 U.S.C. 321, 351, 352, 353, 355, 356b, 360, 360c-360f, 360h-360j, 371, 374, 379e, 381; 42 U.S.C. 216, 241, 262, 263, 264; sec 122, Pub. L. 105-115, 111 Stat. 2322 (21 U.S.C. 355 note).

Source: 38 FR 32052, Nov. 20, 1973, unless otherwise noted.

Part 812: Investigational Device Exemptions

[Code of Federal Regulations]

[Title 21, Volume 8]

[Revised as of April 1, 2009]

[CITE: 21CFR812]

Title 21--Food and Drugs

Chapter I--Food and Drug Administration

Department of Health and Human Services

Subchapter H--Medical Devices

Part 812 Investigational Device Exemptions[1]

Subpart A--General Provisions

Sec. 812.1 Scope.

(a) The purpose of this part is to encourage, to the extent consistent with the protection of public health and safety and with ethical standards, the discovery and development of useful devices intended for human use, and to that end to maintain optimum freedom for scientific investigators in their pursuit of this purpose. This part provides procedures for the conduct of clinical investigations of devices. An approved investigational device exemption (IDE) permits a device that otherwise would be required to comply with a performance standard or to have premarket approval to be shipped lawfully for the purpose of conducting investigations of that device. An IDE approved under

---

[1] Available on the FDA website at http://www.accessdata.fda.gov/scripts/cdrh/cfdocs/cfCFR/CFRSearch.cfm?CFRPart=812&showFR=1

812.30 or considered approved under 812.2(b) exempts a device from the requirements of the following sections of the Federal Food, Drug, and Cosmetic Act (the act) and regulations issued thereunder: Misbranding under section 502 of the act, registration, listing, and premarket notification under section 510, performance standards under section 514, premarket approval under section 515, a banned device regulation under section 516, records and reports under section 519, restricted device requirements under section 520(e), good manufacturing practice requirements under section 520(f) except for the requirements found in 820.30, if applicable (unless the sponsor states an intention to comply with these requirements under 812.20(b)(3) or 812.140(b)(4)(v)) and color additive requirements under section 721.

(b) References in this part to regulatory sections of the Code of Federal Regulations are to chapter I of title 21, unless otherwise noted.

[45 FR 3751, Jan. 18, 1980, as amended at 59 FR 14366, Mar. 28, 1994; 61 FR 52654, Oct. 7, 1996]

Sec. 812.2 Applicability.

(a) General. This part applies to all clinical investigations of devices to determine safety and effectiveness, except as provided in paragraph (c) of this section.

(b) Abbreviated requirements. The following categories of investigations are considered to have approved applications for IDE's, unless FDA has notified a sponsor under 812.20(a) that approval of an application is required:

(1) An investigation of a device other than a significant risk device, if the device is not a banned device and the sponsor:

(i) Labels the device in accordance with 812.5;

(ii) Obtains IRB approval of the investigation after presenting the reviewing IRB with a brief explanation of why the device is not a significant risk device, and maintains such approval;

(iii) Ensures that each investigator participating in an investigation of the device obtains from each subject under the investigator's care, informed consent under part 50 and documents it, unless documentation is waived by an IRB under 56.109(c).

(iv) Complies with the requirements of 812.46 with respect to monitoring investigations;

(v) Maintains the records required under 812.140(b) (4) and (5) and makes the reports required under 812.150(b) (1) through (3) and (5) through (10);

(vi) Ensures that participating investigators maintain the records required by 812.140(a)(3)(i) and make the reports required under 812.150(a) (1), (2), (5), and (7); and

(vii) Complies with the prohibitions in 812.7 against promotion and other practices.

(2) An investigation of a device other than one subject to paragraph (e) of this section, if the investigation was begun on or before July 16, 1980, and to be completed, and is completed, on or before January 19, 1981.

(c) Exempted investigations. This part, with the exception of 812.119, does not apply to investigations of the following categories of devices:

(1) A device, other than a transitional device, in commercial distribution immediately before May 28, 1976, when used or investigated in accordance with the indications in labeling in effect at that time.

(2) A device, other than a transitional device, introduced into commercial distribution on or after May 28, 1976, that FDA has determined to be substantially equivalent to a device in commercial distribution immediately before May 28, 1976, and that is used or investigated in accordance with the indications in the labeling FDA reviewed under subpart E of part 807 in determining substantial equivalence.

(3) A diagnostic device, if the sponsor complies with applicable requirements in 809.10(c) and if the testing:

(i) Is noninvasive,

(ii) Does not require an invasive sampling procedure that presents significant risk,

(iii) Does not by design or intention introduce energy into a subject, and

   (iv) Is not used as a diagnostic procedure without confirmation of the diagnosis by another, medically established diagnostic product or procedure.

  (4) A device undergoing consumer preference testing, testing of a modification, or testing of a combination of two or more devices in commercial distribution, if the testing is not for the purpose of determining safety or effectiveness and does not put subjects at risk.

  (5) A device intended solely for veterinary use.

  (6) A device shipped solely for research on or with laboratory animals and labeled in accordance with 812.5(c).

  (7) A custom device as defined in 812.3(b), unless the device is being used to determine safety or effectiveness for commercial distribution.

 (d) Limit on certain exemptions. In the case of class II or class III device described in paragraph (c)(1) or (2) of this section, this part applies beginning on the date stipulated in an FDA regulation or order that calls for the submission of premarket approval applications for an unapproved class III device, or establishes a performance standard for a class II device.

 (e) Investigations subject to IND's. A sponsor that, on July 16, 1980, has an effective investigational new drug application (IND) for an investigation of a device shall continue to comply with the requirements of part 312 until 90 days after that date. To continue the investigation after that date, a sponsor shall comply with paragraph (b)(1) of this section, if the device is not a significant risk device, or shall have obtained FDA approval under 812.30 of an IDE application for the investigation of the device.

[45 FR 3751, Jan. 18, 1980, as amended at 46 FR 8956, Jan. 27, 1981; 46 FR 14340, Feb. 27, 1981; 53 FR 11252, Apr. 6, 1988; 62 FR 4165, Jan, 29, 1997; 62 FR 12096, Mar. 14, 1997]

Sec. 812.3 Definitions.

 (a) *Act* means the Federal Food, Drug, and Cosmetic Act (sections 201-901, 52 Stat. 1040 et seq., as amended (21 U.S.C. 301-392)).

 (b) *Custom device* means a device that:

(1) Necessarily deviates from devices generally available or from an applicable performance standard or premarket approval requirement in order to comply with the order of an individual physician or dentist;

(2) Is not generally available to, or generally used by, other physicians or dentists;

(3) Is not generally available in finished form for purchase or for dispensing upon prescription;

(4) Is not offered for commercial distribution through labeling or advertising; and

(5) Is intended for use by an individual patient named in the order of a physician or dentist, and is to be made in a specific form for that patient, or is intended to meet the special needs of the physician or dentist in the course of professional practice.

(c) **FDA** means the Food and Drug Administration.

(d) **Implant** means a device that is placed into a surgically or naturally formed cavity of the human body if it is intended to remain there for a period of 30 days or more. FDA may, in order to protect public health, determine that devices placed in subjects for shorter periods are also "implants" for purposes of this part.

(e) **Institution** means a person, other than an individual, who engages in the conduct of research on subjects or in the delivery of medical services to individuals as a primary activity or as an adjunct to providing residential or custodial care to humans. The term includes, for example, a hospital, retirement home, confinement facility, academic establishment, and device manufacturer. The term has the same meaning as "facility" in section 520(g) of the act.

(f) **Institutional review board (IRB)** means any board, committee, or other group formally designated by an institution to review biomedical research involving subjects and established, operated, and functioning in conformance with part 56. The term has the same meaning as "institutional review committee" in section 520(g) of the act.

(g) **Investigational device** means a device, including a transitional device, that is the object of an investigation.

(h) **Investigation** means a clinical investigation or research involving one or more subjects to determine the safety or effectiveness of a device.

(i) **Investigator** means an individual who actually conducts a clinical investigation, i.e., under whose immediate direction the test article is administered or dispensed to, or used involving, a subject, or, in the event of an investigation conducted by a team of individuals, is the responsible leader of that team.

(j) **Monitor**, when used as a noun, means an individual designated by a sponsor or contract research organization to oversee the progress of an investigation. The monitor may be an employee of a sponsor or a consultant to the sponsor, or an employee of or consultant to a contract research organization.Monitor, when used as a verb, means to oversee an investigation.

(k) **Noninvasive**, when applied to a diagnostic device or procedure, means one that does not by design or intention: (1) Penetrate or pierce the skin or mucous membranes of the body, the ocular cavity, or the urethra, or (2) enter the ear beyond the external auditory canal, the nose beyond the nares, the mouth beyond the pharynx, the anal canal beyond the rectum, or the vagina beyond the cervical os. For purposes of this part, blood sampling that involves simple venipuncture is considered noninvasive, and the use of surplus samples of body fluids or tissues that are left over from samples taken for noninvestigational purposes is also considered noninvasive.

(l) **Person** includes any individual, partnership, corporation, association, scientific or academic establishment, Government agency or organizational unit of a Government agency, and any other legal entity.

(m) **Significant risk device** means an investigational device that:

(1) Is intended as an implant and presents a potential for serious risk to the health, safety, or welfare of a subject;

(2) Is purported or represented to be for a use in supporting or sustaining human life and presents a potential for serious risk to the health, safety, or welfare of a subject;

(3) Is for a use of substantial importance in diagnosing, curing, mitigating, or treating disease, or otherwise preventing

impairment of human health and presents a potential for serious risk to the health, safety, or welfare of a subject; or

(4) Otherwise presents a potential for serious risk to the health, safety, or welfare of a subject.

(n) **Sponsor** means a person who initiates, but who does not actually conduct, the investigation, that is, the investigational device is administered, dispensed, or used under the immediate direction of another individual. A person other than an individual that uses one or more of its own employees to conduct an investigation that it has initiated is a sponsor, not a sponsor-investigator, and the employees are investigators.

(o) **Sponsor-investigator** means an individual who both initiates and actually conducts, alone or with others, an investigation, that is, under whose immediate direction the investigational device is administered, dispensed, or used. The term does not include any person other than an individual. The obligations of a sponsor-investigator under this part include those of an investigator and those of a sponsor.

(p) **Subject** means a human who participates in an investigation, either as an individual on whom or on whose specimen an investigational device is used or as a control. A subject may be in normal health or may have a medical condition or disease.

(q) **Termination** means a discontinuance, by sponsor or by withdrawal of IRB or FDA approval, of an investigation before completion.

(r) **Transitional device** means a device subject to section 520(l) of the act, that is, a device that FDA considered to be a new drug or an antibiotic drug before May 28, 1976.

(s) **Unanticipated adverse device effect** means any serious adverse effect on health or safety or any life-threatening problem or death caused by, or associated with, a device, if that effect, problem, or death was not previously identified in nature, severity, or degree of incidence in the investigational plan or application (including a supplementary plan or application), or any other unanticipated serious problem associated with a device that relates to the rights, safety, or welfare of subjects.

[45 FR 3751, Jan. 18, 1980, as amended at 46 FR 8956, Jan. 27, 1981; 48 FR 15622, Apr. 12, 1983]

Sec. 812.5 Labeling of investigational devices.

(a) Contents. An investigational device or its immediate package shall bear a label with the following information: the name and place of business of the manufacturer, packer, or distributor (in accordance with 801.1), the quantity of contents, if appropriate, and the following statement: "CAUTION--Investigational device. Limited by Federal (or United States) law to investigational use." The label or other labeling shall describe all relevant contraindications, hazards, adverse effects, interfering substances or devices, warnings, and precautions.

(b) Prohibitions. The labeling of an investigational device shall not bear any statement that is false or misleading in any particular and shall not represent that the device is safe or effective for the purposes for which it is being investigated.

(c) Animal research. An investigational device shipped solely for research on or with laboratory animals shall bear on its label the following statement: "CAUTION--Device for investigational use in laboratory animals or other tests that do not involve human subjects."

(d) The appropriate FDA Center Director, according to the procedures set forth in 801.128 or 809.11 of this chapter, may grant an exception or alternative to the provisions in paragraphs (a) and (c) of this section, to the extent that these provisions are not explicitly required by statute, for specified lots, batches, or other units of a device that are or will be included in the Strategic National Stockpile.

[45 FR 3751, Jan. 18, 1980, as amended at 45 FR 58842, Sept. 5, 1980; 72 FR 73602, Dec. 28, 2007]

Sec. 812.7 Prohibition of promotion and other practices.

A sponsor, investigator, or any person acting for or on behalf of a sponsor or investigator shall not:

(a) Promote or test market an investigational device, until after FDA has approved the device for commercial distribution.

(b) Commercialize an investigational device by charging the subjects or investigators for a device a price larger than that necessary to recover costs of manufacture, research, development, and handling.

(c) Unduly prolong an investigation. If data developed by the investigation indicate in the case of a class III device that premarket approval cannot be justified or in the case of a class II device that it will not comply with an applicable performance standard or an amendment to that standard, the sponsor shall promptly terminate the investigation.

(d) Represent that an investigational device is safe or effective for the purposes for which it is being investigated.

Sec. 812.10 Waivers.

(a) Request. A sponsor may request FDA to waive any requirement of this part. A waiver request, with supporting documentation, may be submitted separately or as part of an application to the address in 812.19.

(b) FDA action. FDA may by letter grant a waiver of any requirement that FDA finds is not required by the act and is unnecessary to protect the rights, safety, or welfare of human subjects.

(c) Effect of request. Any requirement shall continue to apply unless and until FDA waives it.

Sec. 812.18 Import and export requirements.

(a) Imports. In addition to complying with other requirements of this part, a person who imports or offers for importation an investigational device subject to this part shall be the agent of the foreign exporter with respect to investigations of the device and shall act as the sponsor of the clinical investigation, or ensure that another person acts as the agent of the foreign exporter and the sponsor of the investigation.

(b) Exports. A person exporting an investigational device subject to this part shall obtain FDA's prior approval, as required by section 801(e) of the act or comply with section 802 of the act.

[45 FR 3751, Jan. 18, 1980, as amended at 62 FR 26229, May 13, 1997]

Sec. 812.19 Address for IDE correspondence.

(a) If you are sending an application, supplemental application, report, request for waiver, request for import or export approval, or other correspondence relating to matters covered by this part, you must send the submission to the appropriate address as follows:

> (1) For devices regulated by the Center for Devices and Radiological Health, send it to Food and Drug Administration, Center for Devices and Radiological Health, Document Mail Center, 10903 New Hampshire Ave., Bldg. 66, rm. G609, Silver Spring, MD 20993-0002.

> (2) For devices regulated by the Center for Biologics Evaluation and Research, send it to the Document Control Center (HFM-99), Center for Biologics Evaluation and Research, Food and Drug Administration, 1401 Rockville Pike, suite 200N, Rockville, MD 20852-1448.

> (3) For devices regulated by the Center for Drug Evaluation and Research, send it to Central Document Control Room, Center for Drug Evaluation and Research, Food and Drug Administration, 5901-B Ammendale Rd., Beltsville, MD 20705-1266.

(b) You must state on the outside wrapper of each submission what the submission is, for example, an "IDE application," a "supplemental IDE application," or a "correspondence concerning an IDE (or an IDE application)."

[71 FR 42048, July 25, 2006, as amended at 75 FR 20915, Apr. 22, 2010]

Subpart B--Application and Administrative Action

Sec. 812.20 Application.

(a) Submission.

> (1) A sponsor shall submit an application to FDA if the sponsor intends to use a significant risk device in an investigation, intends to conduct an investigation that involves an exception from informed consent under 50.24 of this chapter, or if FDA notifies the sponsor that an application is required for an investigation.

(2) A sponsor shall not begin an investigation for which FDA's approval of an application is required until FDA has approved the application.

(3) A sponsor shall submit three copies of a signed "Application for an Investigational Device Exemption" (IDE application), together with accompanying materials, by registered mail or by hand to the address in 812.19. Subsequent correspondence concerning an application or a supplemental application shall be submitted by registered mail or by hand.

(4)(i) A sponsor shall submit a separate IDE for any clinical investigation involving an exception from informed consent under 50.24 of this chapter. Such a clinical investigation is not permitted to proceed without the prior written authorization of FDA. FDA shall provide a written determination 30 days after FDA receives the IDE or earlier.

   (ii) If the investigation involves an exception from informed consent under 50.24 of this chapter, the sponsor shall prominently identify on the cover sheet that the investigation is subject to the requirements in 50.24 of this chapter.

(b) Contents. An IDE application shall include, in the following order:

(1) The name and address of the sponsor.

(2) A complete report of prior investigations of the device and an accurate summary of those sections of the investigational plan described in 812.25(a) through (e) or, in lieu of the summary, the complete plan. The sponsor shall submit to FDA a complete investigational plan and a complete report of prior investigations of the device if no IRB has reviewed them, if FDA has found an IRB's review inadequate, or if FDA requests them.

(3) A description of the methods, facilities, and controls used for the manufacture, processing, packing, storage, and, where appropriate, installation of the device, in sufficient detail so that a person generally familiar with good manufacturing practices can make a knowledgeable judgment about the quality control used in the manufacture of the device.

(4) An example of the agreements to be entered into by all investigators to comply with investigator obligations under

this part, and a list of the names and addresses of all investigators who have signed the agreement.

(5) A certification that all investigators who will participate in the investigation have signed the agreement, that the list of investigators includes all the investigators participating in the investigation, and that no investigators will be added to the investigation until they have signed the agreement.

(6) A list of the name, address, and chairperson of each IRB that has been or will be asked to review the investigation and a certification of the action concerning the investigation taken by each such IRB.

(7) The name and address of any institution at which a part of the investigation may be conducted that has not been identified in accordance with paragraph (b)(6) of this section.

(8) If the device is to be sold, the amount to be charged and an explanation of why sale does not constitute commercialization of the device.

(9) A claim for categorical exclusion under 25.30 or 25.34 or an environmental assessment under 25.40.

(10) Copies of all labeling for the device.

(11) Copies of all forms and informational materials to be provided to subjects to obtain informed consent.

(12) Any other relevant information FDA requests for review of the application.

(c) Additional information. FDA may request additional information concerning an investigation or revision in the investigational plan. The sponsor may treat such a request as a disapproval of the application for purposes of requesting a hearing under part 16.

(d) Information previously submitted. Information previously submitted to the Center for Devices and Radiological Health, the Center for Biologics Evaluation and Research, or the Center for Drug Evaluation and Research, as applicable, in accordance with this chapter ordinarily need not be resubmitted, but may be incorporated by reference.

[45 FR 3751, Jan. 18, 1980, as amended at 46 FR 8956, Jan. 27, 1981; 50 FR 16669, Apr. 26, 1985; 53 FR 11252, Apr. 6, 1988; 61 FR 51530, Oct. 2, 1996; 62 FR 40600, July 29, 1997; 64 FR 10942, Mar. 8, 1999; 73 FR 49942, Aug. 25, 2008]

Sec. 812.25 Investigational plan.

The investigational plan shall include, in the following order:

(a) Purpose. The name and intended use of the device and the objectives and duration of the investigation.

(b) Protocol. A written protocol describing the methodology to be used and an analysis of the protocol demonstrating that the investigation is scientifically sound.

(c) Risk analysis. A description and analysis of all increased risks to which subjects will be exposed by the investigation; the manner in which these risks will be minimized; a justification for the investigation; and a description of the patient population, including the number, age, sex, and condition.

(d) Description of device. A description of each important component, ingredient, property, and principle of operation of the device and of each anticipated change in the device during the course of the investigation.

(e) Monitoring procedures. The sponsor's written procedures for monitoring the investigation and the name and address of any monitor.

(f) Labeling. Copies of all labeling for the device.

(g) Consent materials. Copies of all forms and informational materials to be provided to subjects to obtain informed consent.

(h) IRB information. A list of the names, locations, and chairpersons of all IRB's that have been or will be asked to review the investigation, and a certification of any action taken by any of those IRB's with respect to the investigation.

(i) Other institutions. The name and address of each institution at which a part of the investigation may be conducted that has not been identified in paragraph (h) of this section.

(j) Additional records and reports. A description of records and reports that will be maintained on the investigation in addition to those prescribed in subpart G.

Sec. 812.27 Report of prior investigations.

(a) General. The report of prior investigations shall include reports of all prior clinical, animal, and laboratory testing of the device and shall be comprehensive and adequate to justify the proposed investigation.

(b) Specific contents. The report also shall include:

(1) A bibliography of all publications, whether adverse or supportive, that are relevant to an evaluation of the safety or effectiveness of the device, copies of all published and unpublished adverse information, and, if requested by an IRB or FDA, copies of other significant publications.

(2) A summary of all other unpublished information (whether adverse or supportive) in the possession of, or reasonably obtainable by, the sponsor that is relevant to an evaluation of the safety or effectiveness of the device.

(3) If information on nonclinical laboratory studies is provided, a statement that all such studies have been conducted in compliance with applicable requirements in the good laboratory practice regulations in part 58, or if any such study was not conducted in compliance with such regulations, a brief statement of the reason for the noncompliance. Failure or inability to comply with this requirement does not justify failure to provide information on a relevant nonclinical test study.

[45 FR 3751, Jan. 18, 1980, as amended at 50 FR 7518, Feb. 22, 1985]

Sec. 812.30 FDA action on applications.

(a) Approval or disapproval. FDA will notify the sponsor in writing of the date it receives an application. FDA may approve an investigation as proposed, approve it with modifications, or disapprove it. An investigation may not begin until:

(1) Thirty days after FDA receives the application at the address in 812.19 for the investigation of a device other than a banned device, unless FDA notifies the sponsor that the investigation may not begin; or

(2) FDA approves, by order, an IDE for the investigation.

(b) Grounds for disapproval or withdrawal. FDA may disapprove or withdraw approval of an application if FDA finds that:

(1) There has been a failure to comply with any requirement of this part or the act, any other applicable regulation or statute, or any condition of approval imposed by an IRB or FDA.

(2) The application or a report contains an untrue statement of a material fact, or omits material information required by this part.

(3) The sponsor fails to respond to a request for additional information within the time prescribed by FDA.

(4) There is reason to believe that the risks to the subjects are not outweighed by the anticipated benefits to the subjects and the importance of the knowledge to be gained, or informed consent is inadquate, or the investigation is scientifically unsound, or there is reason to believe that the device as used is ineffective.

(5) It is otherwise unreasonable to begin or to continue the investigation owing to the way in which the device is used or the inadequacy of:

(i) The report of prior investigations or the investigational plan;

(ii) The methods, facilities, and controls used for the manufacturing, processing, packaging, storage, and, where appropriate, installation of the device; or

(iii) Monitoring and review of the investigation.

(c) Notice of disapproval or withdrawal. If FDA disapproves an application or proposes to withdraw approval of an application, FDA will notify the sponsor in writing.

(1) A disapproval order will contain a complete statement of the reasons for disapproval and a statement that the sponsor has an opportunity to request a hearing under part 16.

(2) A notice of a proposed withdrawal of approval will contain a complete statement of the reasons for withdrawal and a statement that the sponsor has an opportunity to request a hearing under part 16. FDA will provide the opportunity for hearing before withdrawal of approval, unless FDA determines in the notice that continuation of testing under

Part 812

the exemption will result in an unreasonble risk to the public health and orders withdrawal of approval before any hearing.

[45 FR 3751, Jan. 18, 1980, as amended at 45 FR 58842, Sept. 5, 1980]

Sec. 812.35 Supplemental applications.

(a) Changes in investigational plan –

(1) Changes requiring prior approval. Except as described in paragraphs (a)(2) through (a)(4) of this section, a sponsor must obtain approval of a supplemental application under 812.30(a), and IRB approval when appropriate (see 56.110 and 56.111 of this chapter), prior to implementing a change to an investigational plan. If a sponsor intends to conduct an investigation that involves an exception to informed consent under 50.24 of this chapter, the sponsor shall submit a separate investigational device exemption (IDE) application in accordance with 812.20(a).

(2) Changes effected for emergency use. The requirements of paragraph (a)(1) of this section regarding FDA approval of a supplement do not apply in the case of a deviation from the investigational plan to protect the life or physical well-being of a subject in an emergency. Such deviation shall be reported to FDA within 5-working days after the sponsor learns of it (see 812.150(a)(4)).

(3) Changes effected with notice to FDA within 5 days. A sponsor may make certain changes without prior approval of a supplemental application under paragraph (a)(1) of this section if the sponsor determines that these changes meet the criteria described in paragraphs (a)(3)(i) and (a)(3)(ii) of this section, on the basis of credible information defined in paragraph (a)(3)(iii) of this section, and the sponsor provides notice to FDA within 5-working days of making these changes.

(i) Developmental changes. The requirements in paragraph (a)(1) of this section regarding FDA approval of a supplement do not apply to developmental changes in the device (including manufacturing changes) that do not constitute a significant change in design or basic principles of operation and that are made in response to information gathered during the course of an investigation.

(ii) Changes to clinical protocol. The requirements in paragraph (a)(1) of this section regarding FDA approval of a supplement do not apply to changes to clinical protocols that do not affect:

(A) The validity of the data or information resulting from the completion of the approved protocol, or the relationship of likely patient risk to benefit relied upon to approve the protocol;

(B) The scientific soundness of the investigational plan; or

(C) The rights, safety, or welfare of the human subjects involved in the investigation.

(iii) Definition of credible information.

(A) Credible information to support developmental changes in the device (including manufacturing changes) includes data generated under the design control procedures of 820.30, preclinical/animal testing, peer reviewed published literature, or other reliable information such as clinical information gathered during a trial or marketing.

(B) Credible information to support changes to clinical protocols is defined as the sponsor's documentation supporting the conclusion that a change does not have a significant impact on the study design or planned statistical analysis, and that the change does not affect the rights, safety, or welfare of the subjects. Documentation shall include information such as peer reviewed published literature, the recommendation of the clinical investigator(s), and/or the data gathered during the clinical trial or marketing.

(iv) Notice of IDE change. Changes meeting the criteria in paragraphs (a)(3)(i) and (a)(3)(ii) of this section that are supported by credible information as defined in paragraph (a)(3)(iii) of this section may be made without prior FDA approval if the sponsor submits a notice of the change to the IDE not later than 5-working days after making the change. Changes to devices are deemed to occur on the date the device, manufactured incorporating the design or manufacturing change, is distributed to the investigator(s). Changes to a clinical protocol are deemed to occur when a clinical investigator is notified by the sponsor that the change should be implemented in the protocol or, for sponsor-investigator studies, when a sponsor-investigator incorporates the change in the protocol. Such notices shall be identified as a "notice of IDE change."

(A) For a developmental or manufacturing change to the device, the notice shall include a summary of the relevant information gathered during the course of the investigation upon which the change was based; a description of the change to the device or manufacturing process (cross-referenced to the appropriate sections of the original device description or manufacturing process); and, if design controls were used to assess the change, a statement that no new risks were identified by appropriate risk analysis and that the verification and validation testing, as appropriate, demonstrated that the design outputs met the design input requirements. If another method of assessment was used, the notice shall include a summary of the information which served as the credible information supporting the change.

(B) For a protocol change, the notice shall include a description of the change (cross-referenced to the appropriate sections of the original protocol); an assessment supporting the conclusion that the change does not have a significant impact on the study design or planned statistical analysis; and a summary of the information that served as the credible information supporting the sponsor's determination that the change does not affect the rights, safety, or welfare of the subjects.

(4) Changes submitted in annual report. The requirements of paragraph (a)(1) of this section do not apply to minor changes to the purpose of the study, risk analysis, monitoring procedures, labeling, informed consent materials, and IRB information that do not affect:

(i) The validity of the data or information resulting from the completion of the approved protocol, or the relationship of likely patient risk to benefit relied upon to approve the protocol;

(ii) The scientific soundness of the investigational plan; or

(iii) The rights, safety, or welfare of the human subjects involved in the investigation. Such changes shall be reported in the annual progress report for the IDE, under 812.150(b)(5).

(b) IRB approval for new facilities. A sponsor shall submit to FDA a certification of any IRB approval of an investigation or a part of an investigation not included in the IDE application. If the investigation is otherwise unchanged, the supplemental application shall consist of an updating of the information required by 812.20(b) and (c) and a description of any modifications in the investigational plan required by the IRB as a condition of approval. A certification of IRB approval need not be included in the initial submission of the supplemental application, and such certification is not a precondition for agency consideration of the application. Nevertheless, a sponsor may not begin a part of an investigation at a facility until the IRB has approved the investigation, FDA has received the certification of IRB approval, and FDA, under 812.30(a), has approved the supplemental application relating to that part of the investigation (see 56.103(a)).

[50 FR 25909, June 24, 1985; 50 FR 28932, July 17, 1985, as amended at 61 FR 51531, Oct. 2, 1996; 63 FR 64625, Nov. 23, 1998]

Sec. 812.36 Treatment use of an investigational device.

(a) General. A device that is not approved for marketing may be under clinical investigation for a serious or immediately life-threatening disease or condition in patients for whom no comparable or satisfactory alternative device or other therapy is available. During the clinical trial or prior to final action on the marketing application, it may be appropriate to use the device in the treatment of patients not in the trial under the provisions of a treatment investigational device exemption (IDE). The purpose of this section is to facilitate the availability of promising new devices to desperately ill patients as early in the device development process as possible, before general marketing begins, and to obtain additional data on the device's safety and effectiveness. In the case of a serious disease, a device ordinarily may be made available for treatment use under this section after all clinical trials have been completed. In the case of an immediately life-threatening disease, a device may be made available for treatment use under this section prior to the completion of all clinical trials. For the purpose of this section, an "immediately life-threatening" disease means a stage of a disease in which there is a reasonable likelihood that death will occur within a matter of months or in which premature death is likely without early treatment. For purposes of this section, "treatment use" of a device includes the use of a device for diagnostic purposes.

(b) Criteria. FDA shall consider the use of an investigational device under a treatment IDE if:

(1) The device is intended to treat or diagnose a serious or immediately life-threatening disease or condition;

(2) There is no comparable or satisfactory alternative device or other therapy available to treat or diagnose that stage of the disease or condition in the intended patient population;

(3) The device is under investigation in a controlled clinical trial for the same use under an approved IDE, or such clinical trials have been completed; and

(4) The sponsor of the investigation is actively pursuing marketing approval/clearance of the investigational device with due diligence.

(c) Applications for treatment use. (1) A treatment IDE application shall include, in the following order:

(i) The name, address, and telephone number of the sponsor of the treatment IDE;

(ii) The intended use of the device, the criteria for patient selection, and a written protocol describing the treatment use;

(iii) An explanation of the rationale for use of the device, including, as appropriate, either a list of the available regimens that ordinarily should be tried before using the investigational device or an explanation of why the use of the investigational device is preferable to the use of available marketed treatments;

(iv) A description of clinical procedures, laboratory tests, or other measures that will be used to evaluate the effects of the device and to minimize risk;

(v) Written procedures for monitoring the treatment use and the name and address of the monitor;

(vi) Instructions for use for the device and all other labeling as required under 812.5(a) and (b);

(vii) Information that is relevant to the safety and effectiveness of the device for the intended treatment use. Information from other IDE's may be incorporated by reference to support the treatment use;

(viii) A statement of the sponsor's commitment to meet all applicable responsibilities under this part and part 56 of this chapter and to ensure compliance of all participating investigators with the informed consent requirements of part 50 of this chapter;

(ix) An example of the agreement to be signed by all investigators participating in the treatment IDE and certification that no investigator will be added to the treatment IDE before the agreement is signed; and

(x) If the device is to be sold, the price to be charged and a statement indicating that the price is based on manufacturing and handling costs only.

(2) A licensed practitioner who receives an investigational device for treatment use under a treatment IDE is an "investigator" under the IDE and is responsible for meeting all applicable investigator responsibilities under this part and parts 50 and 56 of this chapter.

(d) FDA action on treatment IDE applications –

(1) Approval of treatment IDE's. Treatment use may begin 30 days after FDA receives the treatment IDE submission at the address specified in 812.19, unless FDA notifies the sponsor in writing earlier than the 30 days that the treatment use may or may not begin. FDA may approve the treatment use as proposed or approve it with modifications.

(2) Disapproval or withdrawal of approval of treatment IDE's. FDA may disapprove or withdraw approval of a treatment IDE if:

(i) The criteria specified in 812.36(b) are not met or the treatment IDE does not contain the information required in 812.36(c);

(ii) FDA determines that any of the grounds for disapproval or withdrawal of approval listed in 812.30(b)(1) through (b)(5) apply;

(iii) The device is intended for a serious disease or condition and there is insufficient evidence of safety and effectiveness to support such use;

(iv) The device is intended for an immediately life-threatening disease or condition and the available scientific evidence, taken as a whole, fails to provide a reasonable basis for concluding that the device:

(A) May be effective for its intended use in its intended population; or

(B) Would not expose the patients to whom the device is to be administered to an unreasonable and significant additional risk of illness or injury;

(v) There is reasonable evidence that the treatment use is impeding enrollment in, or otherwise interfering with the conduct or completion of, a controlled investigation of the same or another investigational device;

(vi) The device has received marketing approval/clearance or a comparable device or therapy becomes available to treat or diagnose the same indication in the same patient population for which the investigational device is being used;

(vii) The sponsor of the controlled clinical trial is not pursuing marketing approval/clearance with due diligence;

(viii) Approval of the IDE for the controlled clinical investigation of the device has been withdrawn; or

(ix) The clinical investigator(s) named in the treatment IDE are not qualified by reason of their scientific training and/or experience to use the investigational device for the intended treatment use.

(3) Notice of disapproval or withdrawal. If FDA disapproves or proposes to withdraw approval of a treatment IDE, FDA will follow the procedures set forth in 812.30(c).

(e) Safeguards. Treatment use of an investigational device is conditioned upon the sponsor and investigators complying with the safeguards of the IDE process and the regulations governing informed consent (part 50 of this chapter) and institutional review boards (part 56 of this chapter).

(f) Reporting requirements. The sponsor of a treatment IDE shall submit progress reports on a semi-annual basis to all reviewing IRB's and FDA until the filing of a marketing application. These reports shall be based on the period of time since initial approval of the treatment IDE and shall include the number of patients treated with the device under the treatment IDE, the names of the investigators participating in the treatment IDE, and a brief description of the sponsor's efforts to pursue marketing approval/clearance of the device. Upon filing of a marketing application, progress reports shall be submitted annually in accordance with 812.150(b)(5). The sponsor of a treatment IDE is responsible for submitting all other reports required under 812.150.

[62 FR 48947, Sept. 18, 1997]

Sec. 812.38 Confidentiality of data and information.

(a) Existence of IDE. FDA will not disclose the existence of an IDE unless its existence has previously been publicly disclosed or acknowledged, until FDA approves an application for premarket approval of the device subject to the IDE; or a notice of completion of a product development protocol for the device has become effective.

(b) Availability of summaries or data.

(1) FDA will make publicly available, upon request, a detailed summary of information concerning the safety and effectiveness of the device that was the basis for an order approving, disapproving, or withdrawing approval of an application for an IDE for a banned device. The summary shall include information on any adverse effect on health caused by the device.

(2) If a device is a banned device or if the existence of an IDE has been publicly disclosed or acknowledged, data or information contained in the file is not available for public disclosure before approval of an application for premarket approval or the effective date of a notice of completion of a product development protocol except as provided in this section. FDA may, in its discretion, disclose a summary of selected portions of the safety and effectiveness data, that is, clinical, animal, or laboratory studies and tests of the device, for public consideration of a specific pending issue.

(3) If the existence of an IDE file has not been publicly disclosed or acknowledged, no data or information in the file are available for public disclosure except as provided in paragraphs (b)(1) and (c) of this section.

(4) Notwithstanding paragraph (b)(2) of this section, FDA will make available to the public, upon request, the information in the IDE that was required to be filed in Docket Number 95S-0158 in the Division of Dockets Management (HFA-305), Food and Drug Administration, 5630 Fishers Lane, rm. 1061, Rockville, MD 20852, for investigations involving an exception from informed consent under 50.24 of this chapter. Persons wishing to request this information shall submit a request under the Freedom of Information Act.

(c) Reports of adverse effects. Upon request or on its own initiative, FDA shall disclose to an individual on whom an investigational device has been used a copy of a report of adverse device effects relating to that use.

(d) Other rules. Except as otherwise provided in this section, the availability for public disclosure of data and information in an IDE file shall be handled in accordance with 814.9.

[45 FR 3751, Jan. 18, 1980, as amended at 53 FR 11253, Apr. 6, 1988; 61 FR 51531, Oct. 2, 1996]

Subpart C--Responsibilities of Sponsors

Sec. 812.40 General responsibilities of sponsors.

Sponsors are responsible for selecting qualified investigators and providing them with the information they need to conduct the investigation properly, ensuring proper monitoring of the investigation, ensuring that IRB review and approval are obtained, submitting an IDE application to FDA, and ensuring that any reviewing IRB and FDA are promptly informed of significant new information about an investigation. Additional responsibilities of sponsors are described in subparts B and G.

Sec. 812.42 FDA and IRB approval.

A sponsor shall not begin an investigation or part of an investigation until an IRB and FDA have both approved the application or supplemental application relating to the investigation or part of an investigation.

[46 FR 8957, Jan. 27, 1981]

Sec. 812.43 Selecting investigators and monitors.

(a) Selecting investigators. A sponsor shall select investigators qualified by training and experience to investigate the device.

(b) Control of device. A sponsor shall ship investigational devices only to qualified investigators participating in the investigation.

(c) Obtaining agreements. A sponsor shall obtain from each participating investigator a signed agreement that includes:

    (1) The investigator's curriculum vitae.

    (2) Where applicable, a statement of the investigator's relevant experience, including the dates, location, extent, and type of experience.

    (3) If the investigator was involved in an investigation or other research that was terminated, an explanation of the circumstances that led to termination.

    (4) A statement of the investigator's commitment to:

        (i) Conduct the investigation in accordance with the agreement, the investigational plan, this part and other applicable FDA regulations, and conditions of approval imposed by the reviewing IRB or FDA;

        (ii) Supervise all testing of the device involving human subjects; and

        (iii) Ensure that the requirements for obtaining informed consent are met.

Part 812

(5) Sufficient accurate financial disclosure information to allow the sponsor to submit a complete and accurate certification or disclosure statement as required under part 54 of this chapter. The sponsor shall obtain a commitment from the clinical investigator to promptly update this information if any relevant changes occur during the course of the investigation and for 1 year following completion of the study. This information shall not be submitted in an investigational device exemption application, but shall be submitted in any marketing application involving the device.

(d) Selecting monitors. A sponsor shall select monitors qualified by training and experience to monitor the investigational study in accordance with this part and other applicable FDA regulations.

[45 FR 3751, Jan. 18, 1980, as amended at 63 FR 5253, Feb. 2, 1998]

Sec. 812.45 Informing investigators.

A sponsor shall supply all investigators participating in the investigation with copies of the investigational plan and the report of prior investigations of the device.

Sec. 812.46 Monitoring investigations.

(a) Securing compliance. A sponsor who discovers that an investigator is not complying with the signed agreement, the investigational plan, the requirements of this part or other applicable FDA regulations, or any conditions of approval imposed by the reviewing IRB or FDA shall promptly either secure compliance, or discontinue shipments of the device to the investigator and terminate the investigator's participation in the investigation. A sponsor shall also require such an investigator to dispose of or return the device, unless this action would jeopardize the rights, safety, or welfare of a subject.

(b) Unanticipated adverse device effects.

(1) A sponsor shall immediately conduct an evaluation of any unanticipated adverse device effect.

(2) A sponsor who determines that an unanticipated adverse device effect presents an unreasonable risk to subjects shall terminate all investigations or parts of investigations presenting that risk as soon as possible. Termination shall

occur not later than 5 working days after the sponsor makes this determination and not later than 15 working days after the sponsor first received notice of the effect.

(c) Resumption of terminated studies. If the device is a significant risk device, a sponsor may not resume a terminated investigation without IRB and FDA approval. If the device is not a significant risk device, a sponsor may not resume a terminated investigation without IRB approval and, if the investigation was terminated under paragraph (b)(2) of this section, FDA approval.

Sec. 812.47 Emergency research under 50.24 of this chapter.

(a) The sponsor shall monitor the progress of all investigations involving an exception from informed consent under 50.24 of this chapter. When the sponsor receives from the IRB information concerning the public disclosures under 50.24(a)(7)(ii) and (a)(7)(iii) of this chapter, the sponsor shall promptly submit to the IDE file and to Docket Number 95S-0158 in the Division of Dockets Management (HFA-305), Food and Drug Administration, 5630 Fishers Lane, rm. 1061, Rockville, MD 20852, copies of the information that was disclosed, identified by the IDE number.

(b) The sponsor also shall monitor such investigations to determine when an IRB determines that it cannot approve the research because it does not meet the criteria in the exception in 50.24(a) of this chapter or because of other relevant ethical concerns. The sponsor promptly shall provide this information in writing to FDA, investigators who are asked to participate in this or a substantially equivalent clinical investigation, and other IRB's that are asked to review this or a substantially equivalent investigation.

[61 FR 51531, Oct. 2, 1996, as amended at 64 FR 10943, Mar. 8, 1999]

Subpart D--IRB Review and Approval

Sec. 812.60 IRB composition, duties, and functions.

An IRB reviewing and approving investigations under this part shall comply with the requirements of part 56 in all respects, including its composition, duties, and functions.

[46 FR 8957, Jan. 27, 1981]

Sec. 812.62 IRB approval.

(a) An IRB shall review and have authority to approve, require modifications in (to secure approval), or disapprove all investigations covered by this part.

(b) If no IRB exists or if FDA finds that an IRB's review is inadequate, a sponsor may submit an application to FDA.

[46 FR 8957, Jan. 27, 1981]

Sec. 812.64 IRB's continuing review.

The IRB shall conduct its continuing review of an investigation in accordance with part 56.

[46 FR 8957, Jan. 27, 1981]

Sec. 812.65 [Reserved]

Sec. 812.66 Significant risk device determinations.

If an IRB determines that an investigation, presented for approval under 812.2(b)(1)(ii), involves a significant risk device, it shall so notify the investigator and, where appropriate, the sponsor. A sponsor may not begin the investigation except as provided in 812.30(a).

[46 FR 8957, Jan. 27, 1981]

Subpart E--Responsibilities of Investigators

Sec. 812.100 General responsibilities of investigators.

An investigator is responsible for ensuring that an investigation is conducted according to the signed agreement, the investigational plan and applicable FDA regulations, for protecting the rights, safety, and welfare of subjects under the investigator's care, and for the control of devices under investigation. An investigator also is responsible for ensuring that informed consent is obtained in accordance with part 50 of this chapter. Additional responsibilities of investigators are described in subpart G.

[45 FR 3751, Jan. 18, 1980, as amended at 46 FR 8957, Jan. 27, 1981]

Sec. 812.110 Specific responsibilities of investigators.

(a) Awaiting approval. An investigator may determine whether potential subjects would be interested in participating in an investigation, but shall not request the written informed consent of any subject to participate, and shall not allow any subject to participate before obtaining IRB and FDA approval.

(b) Compliance. An investigator shall conduct an investigation in accordance with the signed agreement with the sponsor, the investigational plan, this part and other applicable FDA regulations, and any conditions of approval imposed by an IRB or FDA.

(c) Supervising device use. An investigator shall permit an investigational device to be used only with subjects under the investigator's supervision. An investigator shall not supply an investigational device to any person not authorized under this part to receive it.

(d) Financial disclosure. A clinical investigator shall disclose to the sponsor sufficient accurate financial information to allow the applicant to submit complete and accurate certification or disclosure statements required under part 54 of this chapter. The investigator shall promptly update this information if any relevant changes occur during the course of the investigation and for 1 year following completion of the study.

(e) Disposing of device. Upon completion or termination of a clinical investigation or the investigator's part of an investigation, or at the sponsor's request, an investigator shall return to the sponsor any remaining supply of the device or otherwise dispose of the device as the sponsor directs.

[45 FR 3751, Jan. 18, 1980, as amended at 63 FR 5253, Feb. 2, 1998]

Sec. 812.119 Disqualification of a clinical investigator.

(a) If FDA has information indicating that an investigator has repeatedly or deliberately failed to comply with the requirements of this part, part 50, or part 56 of this chapter, or has repeatedly or deliberately submitted false information either to the sponsor of the investigation or in any required report, the Center for Devices and Radiological Health, the Center for Biologics Evaluation and

Research, or the Center for Drug Evaluation and Research will furnish the investigator written notice of the matter under complaint and offer the investigator an opportunity to explain the matter in writing, or, at the option of the investigator, in an informal conference. If an explanation is offered and accepted by the applicable Center, the disqualification process will be terminated. If an explanation is offered but not accepted by the Center, the investigator will be given an opportunity for a regulatory hearing under part 16 of this chapter on the question of whether the investigator is entitled to receive investigational devices.

(b) After evaluating all available information, including any explanation presented by the investigator, if the Commissioner determines that the investigator has repeatedly or deliberately failed to comply with the requirements of this part, part 50, or part 56 of this chapter, or has deliberately or repeatedly submitted false information either to the sponsor of the investigation or in any required report, the Commissioner will notify the investigator, the sponsor of any investigation in which the investigator has been named as a participant, and the reviewing IRB that the investigator is not entitled to receive investigational devices. The notification will provide a statement of basis for such determination.

(c) Each investigational device exemption (IDE) and each cleared or approved application submitted under this part, subpart E of part 807 of this chapter, or part 814 of this chapter containing data reported by an investigator who has been determined to be ineligible to receive investigational devices will be examined to determine whether the investigator has submitted unreliable data that are essential to the continuation of the investigation or essential to the approval or clearance of any marketing application.

(d) If the Commissioner determines, after the unreliable data submitted by the investigator are eliminated from consideration, that the data remaining are inadequate to support a conclusion that it is reasonably safe to continue the investigation, the Commissioner will notify the sponsor who shall have an opportunity for a regulatory hearing under part 16 of this chapter. If a danger to the public health exists, however, the Commissioner shall terminate the IDE immediately and notify the sponsor and the reviewing IRB of the determination. In such case, the sponsor shall have an opportunity for a regulatory hearing before FDA under part 16 of this chapter on the question of whether the IDE should be reinstated.

(e) If the Commissioner determines, after the unreliable data submitted by the investigator are eliminated from consideration, that the continued clearance or approval of the marketing application for which the data were submitted cannot be justified, the Commissioner will proceed to withdraw approval or rescind clearance of the medical device in accordance with the applicable provisions of the act.

(f) An investigator who has been determined to be ineligible to receive investigational devices may be reinstated as eligible when the Commissioner determines that the investigator has presented adequate assurances that the investigator will employ investigational devices solely in compliance with the provisions of this part and of parts 50 and 56 of this chapter.

[62 FR 12096, Mar. 14, 1997, as amended at 71 FR 76902, Dec. 22, 2006]

Subpart F [Reserved]

Subpart G--Records and Reports

Sec. 812.140 Records.

(a) Investigator records. A participating investigator shall maintain the following accurate, complete, and current records relating to the investigator's participation in an investigation:

   (1) All correspondence with another investigator, an IRB, the sponsor, a monitor, or FDA, including required reports.

   (2) Records of receipt, use or disposition of a device that relate to:

      (i) The type and quantity of the device, the dates of its receipt, and the batch number or code mark.

      (ii) The names of all persons who received, used, or disposed of each device.

      (iii) Why and how many units of the device have been returned to the sponsor, repaired, or otherwise disposed of.

(3) Records of each subject's case history and exposure to the device. Case histories include the case report forms and supporting data including, for example, signed and dated consent forms and medical records including, for example, progress notes of the physician, the individual's hospital chart(s), and the nurses' notes. Such records shall include:

    (i) Documents evidencing informed consent and, for any use of a device by the investigator without informed consent, any written concurrence of a licensed physician and a brief description of the circumstances justifying the failure to obtain informed consent. The case history for each individual shall document that informed consent was obtained prior to participation in the study.

    (ii) All relevant observations, including records concerning adverse device effects (whether anticipated or unanticipated), information and data on the condition of each subject upon entering, and during the course of, the investigation, including information about relevant previous medical history and the results of all diagnostic tests.

    (iii) A record of the exposure of each subject to the investigational device, including the date and time of each use, and any other therapy.

(4) The protocol, with documents showing the dates of and reasons for each deviation from the protocol.

(5) Any other records that FDA requires to be maintained by regulation or by specific requirement for a category of investigations or a particular investigation.

(b) Sponsor records. A sponsor shall maintain the following accurate, complete, and current records relating to an investigation:

(1) All correspondence with another sponsor, a monitor, an investigator, an IRB, or FDA, including required reports.

(2) Records of shipment and disposition. Records of shipment shall include the name and address of the consignee, type and quantity of device, date of shipment, and batch number or code mark. Records of disposition shall describe the batch number or code marks of any devices returned to the sponsor, repaired, or disposed of in other ways by the

investigator or another person, and the reasons for and method of disposal.

(3) Signed investigator agreements including the financial disclosure information required to be collected under 812.43(c)(5) in accordance with part 54 of this chapter.

(4) For each investigation subject to 812.2(b)(1) of a device other than a significant risk device, the records described in paragraph (b)(5) of this section and the following records, consolidated in one location and available for FDA inspection and copying:

(i) The name and intended use of the device and the objectives of the investigation;

(ii) A brief explanation of why the device is not a significant risk device:

(iii) The name and address of each investigator:

(iv) The name and address of each IRB that has reviewed the investigation:

(v) A statement of the extent to which the good manufacturing practice regulation in part 820 will be followed in manufacturing the device; and

(vi) Any other information required by FDA.

(5) Records concerning adverse device effects (whether anticipated or unanticipated) and complaints and

(6) Any other records that FDA requires to be maintained by regulation or by specific requirement for a category of investigation or a particular investigation.

(c) IRB records. An IRB shall maintain records in accordance with part 56 of this chapter.

(d) Retention period. An investigator or sponsor shall maintain the records required by this subpart during the investigation and for a period of 2 years after the latter of the following two dates: The date on which the investigation is terminated or completed, or the date that the records are no longer required for purposes of supporting a premarket approval application or a notice of completion of a product development protocol.

(e) Records custody. An investigator or sponsor may withdraw from the responsibility to maintain records for the period required in paragraph (d) of this section and transfer custody of the records to any other person who will accept responsibility for them under this part, including the requirements of 812.145. Notice of a transfer shall be given to FDA not later than 10 working days after transfer occurs.

[45 FR 3751, Jan. 18, 1980, as amended at 45 FR 58843, Sept. 5, 1980; 46 FR 8957, Jan. 27, 1981; 61 FR 57280, Nov. 5, 1996; 63 FR 5253, Feb. 2, 1998]

Sec. 812.145 Inspections.

(a) Entry and inspection. A sponsor or an investigator who has authority to grant access shall permit authorized FDA employees, at reasonable times and in a reasonable manner, to enter and inspect any establishment where devices are held (including any establishment where devices are manufactured, processed, packed, installed, used, or implanted or where records of results from use of devices are kept).

(b) Records inspection. A sponsor, IRB, or investigator, or any other person acting on behalf of such a person with respect to an investigation, shall permit authorized FDA employees, at reasonable times and in a reasonable manner, to inspect and copy all records relating to an investigation.

(c) Records identifying subjects. An investigator shall permit authorized FDA employees to inspect and copy records that identify subjects, upon notice that FDA has reason to suspect that adequate informed consent was not obtained, or that reports required to be submitted by the investigator to the sponsor or IRB have not been submitted or are incomplete, inaccurate, false, or misleading.

Sec. 812.150 Reports.

(a) Investigator reports. An investigator shall prepare and submit the following complete, accurate, and timely reports:

(1) Unanticipated adverse device effects. An investigator shall submit to the sponsor and to the reviewing IRB a report of any unanticipated adverse device effect occurring during an

investigation as soon as possible, but in no event later than 10 working days after the investigator first learns of the effect.

(2) Withdrawal of IRB approval. An investigator shall report to the sponsor, within 5 working days, a withdrawal of approval by the reviewing IRB of the investigator's part of an investigation.

(3) Progress. An investigator shall submit progress reports on the investigation to the sponsor, the monitor, and the reviewing IRB at regular intervals, but in no event less often than yearly.

(4) Deviations from the investigational plan. An investigator shall notify the sponsor and the reviewing IRB (see 56.108(a) (3) and (4)) of any deviation from the investigational plan to protect the life or physical well-being of a subject in an emergency. Such notice shall be given as soon as possible, but in no event later than 5 working days after the emergency occurred. Except in such an emergency, prior approval by the sponsor is required for changes in or deviations from a plan, and if these changes or deviations may affect the scientific soundness of the plan or the rights, safety, or welfare of human subjects, FDA and IRB in accordance with 812.35(a) also is required.

(5) Informed consent. If an investigator uses a device without obtaining informed consent, the investigator shall report such use to the sponsor and the reviewing IRB within 5 working days after the use occurs.

(6) Final report. An investigator shall, within 3 months after termination or completion of the investigation or the investigator's part of the investigation, submit a final report to the sponsor and the reviewing IRB.

(7) Other. An investigator shall, upon request by a reviewing IRB or FDA, provide accurate, complete, and current information about any aspect of the investigation.

(b) Sponsor reports. A sponsor shall prepare and submit the following complete, accurate, and timely reports:

(1) Unanticipated adverse device effects. A sponsor who conducts an evaluation of an unanticipated adverse device effect under 812.46(b) shall report the results of such evaluation to FDA and to all reviewing IRB's and participating investigators within 10 working days after the

sponsor first receives notice of the effect. Thereafter the sponsor shall submit such additional reports concerning the effect as FDA requests.

(2) Withdrawal of IRB approval. A sponsor shall notify FDA and all reviewing IRB's and participating investigators of any withdrawal of approval of an investigation or a part of an investigation by a reviewing IRB within 5 working days after receipt of the withdrawal of approval.

(3) Withdrawal of FDA approval. A sponsor shall notify all reviewing IRB's and participating investigators of any withdrawal of FDA approval of the investigation, and shall do so within 5 working days after receipt of notice of the withdrawal of approval.

(4) Current investigator list. A sponsor shall submit to FDA, at 6-month intervals, a current list of the names and addresses of all investigators participating in the investigation. The sponsor shall submit the first such list 6 months after FDA approval.

(5) Progress reports. At regular intervals, and at least yearly, a sponsor shall submit progress reports to all reviewing IRB's. In the case of a significant risk device, a sponsor shall also submit progress reports to FDA. A sponsor of a treatment IDE shall submit semi-annual progress reports to all reviewing IRB's and FDA in accordance with 812.36(f) and annual reports in accordance with this section.

(6) Recall and device disposition. A sponsor shall notify FDA and all reviewing IRB's of any request that an investigator return, repair, or otherwise dispose of any units of a device. Such notice shall occur within 30 working days after the request is made and shall state why the request was made.

(7) Final report. In the case of a significant risk device, the sponsor shall notify FDA within 30 working days of the completion or termination of the investigation and shall submit a final report to FDA and all reviewing the IRB's and participating investigators within 6 months after completion or termination. In the case of a device that is not a significant risk device, the sponsor shall submit a final report to all reviewing IRB's within 6 months after termination or completion.

(8) Informed consent. A sponsor shall submit to FDA a copy of any report by an investigator under paragraph (a)(5) of this section of use of a device without obtaining informed consent, within 5 working days of receipt of notice of such use.

(9) Significant risk device determinations. If an IRB determines that a device is a significant risk device, and the sponsor had proposed that the IRB consider the device not to be a significant risk device, the sponsor shall submit to FDA a report of the IRB's determination within 5 working days after the sponsor first learns of the IRB's determination.

(10) Other. A sponsor shall, upon request by a reviewing IRB or FDA, provide accurate, complete, and current information about any aspect of the investigation.

[45 FR 3751, Jan. 18, 1980, as amended at 45 FR 58843, Sept. 5, 1980; 48 FR 15622, Apr. 12, 1983; 62 FR 48948, Sept. 18, 1997]

Authority: 21 U.S.C. 331, 351, 352, 353, 355, 360, 360c-360f, 360h-360j, 371, 372, 374, 379e, 381, 382, 383; 42 U.S.C. 216, 241, 262, 263b-263n.

Source: 45 FR 3751, Jan. 18, 1980, unless otherwise noted.

Part 814: Premarket Approval of Medical Devices

[Code of Federal Regulations]

[Title 21, Volume 8]

[Revised as of April 1, 2009]

[CITE: 21CFR814]

Title 21--Food and Drugs

Chapter I--Food and Drug Administration

Department of Health and Human Services

Subchapter H--Medical Devices

Part 814 Premarket Approval of Medical Devices[1]

Subpart A--General

Sec. 814.1 Scope.

(a) This part implements section 515 of the act by providing procedures for the premarket approval of medical devices intended for human use.

(b) References in this part to regulatory sections of the Code of Federal Regulations are to chapter I of title 21, unless otherwise noted.

(c) This part applies to any class III medical device, unless exempt under section 520(g) of the act, that:

---

[1] Available on the FDA website at http://www.accessdata.fda.gov/scripts/cdrh/cfdocs/cfCFR/CFRSearch.cfm?CFRPart=814&showFR=1

(1) Was not on the market (introduced or delivered for introduction into commerce for commercial distribution) before May 28, 1976, and is not substantially equivalent to a device on the market before May 28, 1976, or to a device first marketed on, or after that date, which has been classified into class I or class II; or

(2) Is required to have an approved premarket approval application (PMA) or a declared completed product development protocol under a regulation issued under section 515(b) of the act; or

(3) Was regulated by FDA as a new drug or antibiotic drug before May 28, 1976, and therefore is governed by section 520(1) of the act.

(d) This part amends the conditions to approval for any PMA approved before the effective date of this part. Any condition to approval for an approved PMA that is inconsistent with this part is revoked. Any condition to approval for an approved PMA that is consistent with this part remains in effect.

Sec. 814.2 Purpose.

The purpose of this part is to establish an efficient and thorough device review process--

(a) To facilitate the approval of PMA's for devices that have been shown to be safe and effective and that otherwise meet the statutory criteria for approval; and

(b) To ensure the disapproval of PMA's for devices that have not been shown to be safe and effective or that do not otherwise meet the statutory criteria for approval. This part shall be construed in light of these objectives.

Sec. 814.3 Definitions.

For the purposes of this part:

(a) *Act* means the Federal Food, Drug, and Cosmetic Act (sections 201-902, 52 Stat. 1040 et seq., as amended (21 U.S.C. 321-392)).

(b) *FDA* means the Food and Drug Administration.

(c) **IDE** means an approved or considered approved investigational device exemption under section 520(g) of the act and parts 812 and 813.

(d) **Master file** means a reference source that a person submits to FDA. A master file may contain detailed information on a specific manufacturing facility, process, methodology, or component used in the manufacture, processing, or packaging of a medical device.

(e) **PMA** means any premarket approval application for a class III medical device, including all information submitted with or incorporated by reference therein. "PMA" includes a new drug application for a device under section 520(1) of the act.

(f) **PMA amendment** means information an applicant submits to FDA to modify a pending PMA or a pending PMA supplement.

(g) **PMA supplement** means a supplemental application to an approved PMA for approval of a change or modification in a class III medical device, including all information submitted with or incorporated by reference therein.

(h) **Person** includes any individual, partnership, corporation, association, scientific or academic establishment, Government agency, or organizational unit thereof, or any other legal entity.

(i) **Statement of material fact** means a representation that tends to show that the safety or effectiveness of a device is more probable than it would be in the absence of such a representation. A false affirmation or silence or an omission that would lead a reasonable person to draw a particular conclusion as to the safety or effectiveness of a device also may be a false statement of material fact, even if the statement was not intended by the person making it to be misleading or to have any probative effect.

(j) **30-day PMA supplement** means a supplemental application to an approved PMA in accordance with 814.39(e).

(k) **Reasonable probability** means that it is more likely than not that an event will occur.

(l) **Serious, adverse health consequences** means any significant adverse experience, including those which may be either life-threatening or involve permanent or long term injuries, but

Part 814

excluding injuries that are nonlife-threatening and that are temporary and reasonably reversible.

(m) *HDE* means a premarket approval application submitted pursuant to this subpart seeking a humanitarian device exemption from the effectiveness requirements of sections 514 and 515 of the act as authorized by section 520(m)(2) of the act.

(n) *HUD (humanitarian use device)* means a medical device intended to benefit patients in the treatment or diagnosis of a disease or condition that affects or is manifested in fewer than 4,000 individuals in the United States per year.

(o) *Newly acquired information* means data, analyses, or other information not previously submitted to the agency, which may include (but are not limited to) data derived from new clinical studies, reports of adverse events, or new analyses of previously submitted data (e.g., meta-analyses) if the studies, events or analyses reveal risks of a different type or greater severity or frequency than previously included in submissions to FDA.

[51 FR 26364, July 22, 1986, as amended at 61 FR 15190, Apr. 5, 1996; 61 FR 33244, June 26, 1996; 73 FR 49610, Aug. 22, 2008]

Sec. 814.9 Confidentiality of data and information in a premarket approval application (PMA) file.

(a) A "PMA file" includes all data and information submitted with or incorporated by reference in the PMA, any IDE incorporated into the PMA, any PMA supplement, any report under 814.82, any master file, or any other related submission. Any record in the PMA file will be available for public disclosure in accordance with the provisions of this section and part 20. The confidentiality of information in a color additive petition submitted as part of a PMA is governed by 71.15.

(b) The existence of a PMA file may not be disclosed by FDA before an approval order is issued to the applicant unless it previously has been publicly disclosed or acknowledged.

(c) If the existence of a PMA file has not been publicly disclosed or acknowledged, data or information in the PMA file are not available for public disclosure.

(d)(1) If the existence of a PMA file has been publicly disclosed or acknowledged before an order approving, or an order denying approval of the PMA is issued, data or information contained in the file are not available for public disclosure before such order issues. FDA may, however, disclose a summary of portions of the safety and effectiveness data before an approval order or an order denying approval of the PMA issues if disclosure is relevant to public consideration of a specific pending issue.

(2) Notwithstanding paragraph (d)(1) of this section, FDA will make available to the public upon request the information in the IDE that was required to be filed in Docket Number 95S-0158 in the Division of Dockets Management (HFA-305), Food and Drug Administration, 12420 Parklawn Dr., rm. 1-23, Rockville, MD 20857, for investigations involving an exception from informed consent under 50.24 of this chapter. Persons wishing to request this information shall submit a request under the Freedom of Information Act.

(e) Upon issuance of an order approving, or an order denying approval of any PMA, FDA will make available to the public the fact of the existence of the PMA and a detailed summary of information submitted to FDA respecting the safety and effectiveness of the device that is the subject of the PMA and that is the basis for the order.

(f) After FDA issues an order approving, or an order denying approval of any PMA, the following data and information in the PMA file are immediately available for public disclosure:

(1) All safety and effectiveness data and information previously disclosed to the public, as such disclosure is defined in 20.81.

(2) Any protocol for a test or study unless the protocol is shown to constitute trade secret or confidential commercial or financial information under 20.61.

(3) Any adverse reaction report, product experience report, consumer complaint, and other similar data and information, after deletion of:

(i) Any information that constitutes trade secret or confidential commercial or financial information under 20.61; and

Part 814

(ii) Any personnel, medical, and similar information disclosure of which would constitute a clearly unwarranted invasion of personal privacy under 20.63; provided, however, that except for the information that constitutes trade secret or confidential commercial or financial information under 20.61, FDA will disclose to a patient who requests a report all the information in the report concerning that patient.

(4) A list of components previously disclosed to the public, as such disclosure is defined in 20.81.

(5) An assay method or other analytical method, unless it does not serve any regulatory purpose and is shown to fall within the exemption in 20.61 for trade secret or confidential commercial or financial information.

(6) All correspondence and written summaries of oral discussions relating to the PMA file, in accordance with the provisions of 20.103 and 20.104.

(g) All safety and effectiveness data and other information not previously disclosed to the public are available for public disclosure if any one of the following events occurs and the data and information do not constitute trade secret or confidential commercial or financial information under 20.61:

(1) The PMA has been abandoned. FDA will consider a PMA abandoned if:

(i)(A) The applicant fails to respond to a request for additional information within 180 days after the date FDA issues the request or

(B) Other circumstances indicate that further work is not being undertaken with respect to it, and

(ii) The applicant fails to communicate with FDA within 7 days after the date on which FDA notifies the applicant that the PMA appears to have been abandoned.

(2) An order denying approval of the PMA has issued, and all legal appeals have been exhausted.

(3) An order withdrawing approval of the PMA has issued, and all legal appeals have been exhausted.

(4) The device has been reclassified.

(5) The device has been found to be substantially equivalent to a class I or class II device.

(6) The PMA is considered voluntarily withdrawn under 814.44(g).

(h) The following data and information in a PMA file are not available for public disclosure unless they have been previously disclosed to the public, as such disclosure is defined in 20.81, or they relate to a device for which a PMA has been abandoned and they no longer represent a trade secret or confidential commercial or financial information as defined in 20.61:

(1) Manufacturing methods or processes, including quality control procedures.

(2) Production, sales, distribution, and similar data and information, except that any compilation of such data and information aggregated and prepared in a way that does not reveal data or information which are not available for public disclosure under this provision is available for public disclosure.

(3) Quantitative or semiquantitative formulas.

[51 FR 26364, July 22, 1986, as amended at 61 FR 51531, Oct. 2, 1996]

Sec. 814.15 Research conducted outside the United States.

(a) A study conducted outside the United States submitted in support of a PMA and conducted under an IDE shall comply with part 812. A study conducted outside the United States submitted in support of a PMA and not conducted under an IDE shall comply with the provisions in paragraph (b) or (c) of this section, as applicable.

(b) Research begun on or after effective date. FDA will accept studies submitted in support of a PMA which have been conducted outside the United States and begun on or after November 19, 1986, if the data are valid and the investigator has conducted the studies in conformance with the "Declaration of Helsinki" or the laws and regulations of the country in which the research is conducted, whichever accords greater protection to the human subjects. If the standards of the country are used, the applicant shall state in detail any differences between those standards and the "Declaration of Helsinki" and explain why they offer greater protection to the human subjects.

(c) Research begun before effective date. FDA will accept studies submitted in support of a PMA which have been conducted outside the United States and begun before November 19, 1986, if FDA is satisfied that the data are scientifically valid and that the rights, safety, and welfare of human subjects have not been violated.

(d) As sole basis for marketing approval. A PMA based solely on foreign clinical data and otherwise meeting the criteria for approval under this part may be approved if:

(1) The foreign data are applicable to the U.S. population and U.S. medical practice;

(2) The studies have been performed by clinical investigators of recognized competence; and

(3) The data may be considered valid without the need for an on-site inspection by FDA or, if FDA considers such an inspection to be necessary, FDA can validate the data through an on-site inspection or other appropriate means.

(e) Consultation between FDA and applicants. Applicants are encouraged to meet with FDA officials in a "presubmission" meeting when approval based solely on foreign data will be sought.

[51 FR 26364, July 22, 1986; 51 FR 40415, Nov. 7, 1986, as amended at 51 FR 43344, Dec. 2, 1986]

Sec. 814.17 Service of orders.

Orders issued under this part will be served in person by a designated officer or employee of FDA on, or by registered mail to, the applicant or the designated agent at the applicant's or designated agent's last known address in FDA's records.

Sec. 814.19 Product development protocol (PDP).

A class III device for which a product development protocol has been declared completed by FDA under this chapter will be considered to have an approved PMA.

Subpart B--Premarket Approval Application (PMA)

Sec. 814.20 Application.

(a) The applicant or an authorized representative shall sign the PMA. If the applicant does not reside or have a place of business within the United States, the PMA shall be countersigned by an authorized representative residing or maintaining a place of business in the United States and shall identify the representative's name and address.

(b) Unless the applicant justifies an omission in accordance with paragraph (d) of this section, a PMA shall include:

(1) The name and address of the applicant.

(2) A table of contents that specifies the volume and page number for each item referred to in the table. A PMA shall include separate sections on nonclinical laboratory studies and on clinical investigations involving human subjects. A PMA shall be submitted in six copies each bound in one or more numbered volumes of reasonable size. The applicant shall include information that it believes to be trade secret or confidential commercial or financial information in all copies of the PMA and identify in at least one copy the information that it believes to be trade secret or confidential commercial or financial information.

(3) A summary in sufficient detail that the reader may gain a general understanding of the data and information in the application. The summary shall contain the following information:

(i) Indications for use. A general description of the disease or condition the device will diagnose, treat, prevent, cure, or mitigate, including a description of the patient population for which the device is intended.

(ii) Device description. An explanation of how the device functions, the basic scientific concepts that form the basis for the device, and the significant physical and performance characteristics of the device. A brief description of the manufacturing process should be included if it will significantly enhance the reader's

Part 814

understanding of the device. The generic name of the device as well as any proprietary name or trade name should be included.

(iii) Alternative practices and procedures. A description of existing alternative practices or procedures for diagnosing, treating, preventing, curing, or mitigating the disease or condition for which the device is intended.

(iv) Marketing history. A brief description of the foreign and U.S. marketing history, if any, of the device, including a list of all countries in which the device has been marketed and a list of all countries in which the device has been withdrawn from marketing for any reason related to the safety or effectiveness of the device. The description shall include the history of the marketing of the device by the applicant and, if known, the history of the marketing of the device by any other person.

(v) Summary of studies. An abstract of any information or report described in the PMA under paragraph (b)(8)(ii) of this section and a summary of the results of technical data submitted under paragraph (b)(6) of this section. Such summary shall include a description of the objective of the study, a description of the experimental design of the study, a brief description of how the data were collected and analyzed, and a brief description of the results, whether positive, negative, or inconclusive. This section shall include the following:

(A) A summary of the nonclinical laboratory studies submitted in the application;

(B) A summary of the clinical investigations involving human subjects submitted in the application including a discussion of subject selection and exclusion criteria, study population, study period, safety and effectiveness data, adverse reactions and complications, patient discontinuation, patient complaints, device failures and replacements, results of statistical analyses of the clinical investigations, contraindications and precautions for use of the device, and other information from the clinical investigations as appropriate (any investigation conducted under an IDE shall be identified as such).

(vi) Conclusions drawn from the studies. A discussion demonstrating that the data and information in the application constitute valid scientific evidence within the meaning of 860.7 and provide reasonable assurance that the device is safe and effective for its intended use. A concluding discussion shall present benefit and risk considerations related to the device including a discussion of any adverse effects of the device on health and any proposed additional studies or surveillance the applicant intends to conduct following approval of the PMA.

(4) A complete description of:

(i) The device, including pictorial representations;

(ii) Each of the functional components or ingredients of the device if the device consists of more than one physical component or ingredient;

(iii) The properties of the device relevant to the diagnosis, treatment, prevention, cure, or mitigation of a disease or condition;

(iv) The principles of operation of the device; and

(v) The methods used in, and the facilities and controls used for, the manufacture, processing, packing, storage, and, where appropriate, installation of the device, in sufficient detail so that a person generally familiar with current good manufacturing practice can make a knowledgeable judgment about the quality control used in the manufacture of the device.

(5) Reference to any performance standard under section 514 of the act or under section 534 of Subchapter C--Electronic Product Radiation Control of the Federal Food, Drug, and Cosmetic Act (formerly the Radiation Control for Health and Safety Act of 1968) in effect or proposed at the time of the submission and to any voluntary standard that is relevant to any aspect of the safety or effectiveness of the device and that is known to or that should reasonably be known to the applicant. The applicant shall--

(i) Provide adequate information to demonstrate how the device meets, or justify any deviation from, any performance standard established under section 514 of the act or under section 534 of Subchapter C--Electronic Product Radiation Control of the Federal Food, Drug,

Part 814

and Cosmetic Act (formerly the Radiation Control for Health and Safety Act of 1968), and

(ii) Explain any deviation from a voluntary standard.

(6) The following technical sections which shall contain data and information in sufficient detail to permit FDA to determine whether to approve or deny approval of the application:

(i) A section containing results of the nonclinical laboratory studies with the device including microbiological, toxicological, immunological, biocompatibility, stress, wear, shelf life, and other laboratory or animal tests as appropriate. Information on nonclinical laboratory studies shall include a statement that each such study was conducted in compliance with part 58, or, if the study was not conducted in compliance with such regulations, a brief statement of the reason for the noncompliance.

(ii) A section containing results of the clinical investigations involving human subjects with the device including clinical protocols, number of investigators and subjects per investigator, subject selection and exclusion criteria, study population, study period, safety and effectiveness data, adverse reactions and complications, patient discontinuation, patient complaints, device failures and replacements, tabulations of data from all individual subject report forms and copies of such forms for each subject who died during a clinical investigation or who did not complete the investigation, results of statistical analyses of the clinical investigations, device failures and replacements, contraindications and precautions for use of the device, and any other appropriate information from the clinical investigations. Any investigation conducted under an IDE shall be identified as such. Information on clinical investigations involving human subjects shall include the following:

(A) A statement with respect to each study that it either was conducted in compliance with the institutional review board regulations in part 56, or was not subject to the regulations under 56.104 or 56.105, and that it was conducted in compliance with the informed consent regulations in part 50; or if the study was not conducted in compliance with those regulations, a brief statement of the reason for the noncompliance.

(B) A statement that each study was conducted in compliance with part 812 or part 813 concerning sponsors of clinical investigations and clinical investigators, or if the study was not conducted in compliance with those regulations, a brief statement of the reason for the noncompliance.

(7) For a PMA supported solely by data from one investigation, a justification showing that data and other information from a single investigator are sufficient to demonstrate the safety and effectiveness of the device and to ensure reproducibility of test results.

(8)(i) A bibliography of all published reports not submitted under paragraph (b)(6) of this section, whether adverse or supportive, known to or that should reasonably be known to the applicant and that concern the safety or effectiveness of the device.

(ii) An identification, discussion, and analysis of any other data, information, or report relevant to an evaluation of the safety and effectiveness of the device known to or that should reasonably be known to the applicant from any source, foreign or domestic, including information derived from investigations other than those proposed in the application and from commercial marketing experience.

(iii) Copies of such published reports or unpublished information in the possession of or reasonably obtainable by the applicant if an FDA advisory committee or FDA requests.

(9) One or more samples of the device and its components, if requested by FDA. If it is impractical to submit a requested sample of the device, the applicant shall name the location at which FDA may examine and test one or more devices.

(10) Copies of all proposed labeling for the device. Such labeling may include, e.g., instructions for installation and any information, literature, or advertising that constitutes labeling under section 201(m) of the act.

(11) An environmental assessment under 25.20(n) prepared in the applicable format in 25.40, unless the action qualifies for

exclusion under 25.30 or 25.34. If the applicant believes that the action qualifies for exclusion, the PMA shall under 25.15(a) and (d) provide information that establishes to FDA's satisfaction that the action requested is included within the excluded category and meets the criteria for the applicable exclusion.

(12) A financial certification or disclosure statement or both as required by part 54 of this chapter.

(13) Such other information as FDA may request. If necessary, FDA will obtain the concurrence of the appropriate FDA advisory committee before requesting additional information.

(c) Pertinent information in FDA files specifically referred to by an applicant may be incorporated into a PMA by reference. Information in a master file or other information submitted to FDA by a person other than the applicant will not be considered part of a PMA unless such reference is authorized in writing by the person who submitted the information or the master file. If a master file is not referenced within 5 years after the date that it is submitted to FDA, FDA will return the master file to the person who submitted it.

(d) If the applicant believes that certain information required under paragraph (b) of this section to be in a PMA is not applicable to the device that is the subject of the PMA, and omits any such information from its PMA, the applicant shall submit a statement that identifies the omitted information and justifies the omission. The statement shall be submitted as a separate section in the PMA and identified in the table of contents. If the justification for the omission is not accepted by the agency, FDA will so notify the applicant.

(e) The applicant shall periodically update its pending application with new safety and effectiveness information learned about the device from ongoing or completed studies that may reasonably affect an evaluation of the safety or effectiveness of the device or that may reasonably affect the statement of contraindications, warnings, precautions, and adverse reactions in the draft labeling. The update report shall be consistent with the data reporting provisions of the protocol. The applicant shall submit three copies of any update report and shall include in the report the number assigned by FDA to the PMA. These updates are considered to be amendments to the PMA. The time frame for review of a PMA will not be extended due to the submission of an update report unless the update is a major amendment under 814.37(c)(1). The applicant shall submit these reports--

(1) 3 months after the filing date,

(2) Following receipt of an approvable letter, and

(3) At any other time as requested by FDA.

(f) If a color additive subject to section 721 of the act is used in or on the device and has not previously been listed for such use, then, in lieu of submitting a color additive petition under part 71, at the option of the applicant, the information required to be submitted under part 71 may be submitted as part of the PMA. When submitted as part of the PMA, the information shall be submitted in three copies each bound in one or more numbered volumes of reasonable size. A PMA for a device that contains a color additive that is subject to section 721 of the act will not be approved until the color additive is listed for use in or on the device.

(g) Additional information on FDA policies and procedures, as well as links to PMA guidance documents, is available on the Internet athttp://www.fda.gov/cdrh/devadvice/pma/.

(h) If you are sending a PMA, PMA amendment, PMA supplement, or correspondence with respect to a PMA, you must send the submission to the appropriate address as follows:

(1) For devices regulated by the Center for Devices and Radiological Health, Food and Drug Administration, Center for Devices and Radiological Health, Document Mail Center, 10903 New Hampshire Ave., Bldg. 66, rm. G609, Silver Spring, MD 20993-0002.

(2) For devices regulated by the Center for Biologics Evaluation and Research, send it to: Document Control Center (HFM-99), Center for Biologics Evaluation and Research, Food and Drug Administration, 1401 Rockville Pike, suite 200N, Rockville, MD 20852-1448.

(3) For devices regulated by the Center for Drug Evaluation and Research, send it to: Central Document Control Room, Center for Drug Evaluation and Research, Food and Drug Administration, 5901-B Ammendale Rd., Beltsville, MD 20705-1266.

Part 814

[51 FR 26364, July 22, 1986; 51 FR 40415, Nov. 7, 1986, as amended at 51 FR 43344, Dec. 2, 1986; 55 FR 11169, Mar. 27, 1990; 62 FR 40600, July 29, 1997; 63 FR 5253, Feb. 2, 1998; 65 FR 17137, Mar. 31, 2000; 65 FR 56480, Sept. 19, 2000; 67 FR 9587, Mar. 4, 2002; 71 FR 42048, July 25, 2006; 72 FR 17399, Apr. 9, 2007; 73 FR 34859, June 19, 2008; 74 FR 14478, Mar. 31, 2009; 75 FR 20915, Apr. 22, 2010]

Sec. 814.37 PMA amendments and resubmitted PMA's.

(a) An applicant may amend a pending PMA or PMA supplement to revise existing information or provide additional information.

(b) FDA may request the applicant to amend a PMA or PMA supplement with any information regarding the device that is necessary for FDA or the appropriate advisory committee to complete the review of the PMA or PMA supplement.

(c) A PMA amendment submitted to FDA shall include the PMA or PMA supplement number assigned to the original submission and, if submitted on the applicant's own initiative, the reason for submitting the amendment. FDA may extend the time required for its review of the PMA, or PMA supplement, as follows:

   (1) If the applicant on its own initiative or at FDA's request submits a major PMA amendment (e.g., an amendment that contains significant new data from a previously unreported study, significant updated data from a previously reported study, detailed new analyses of previously submitted data, or significant required information previously omitted), the review period may be extended up to 180 days.

   (2) If an applicant declines to submit a major amendment requested by FDA, the review period may be extended for the number of days that elapse between the date of such request and the date that FDA receives the written response declining to submit the requested amendment.

(d) An applicant may on its own initiative withdraw a PMA or PMA supplement. If FDA requests an applicant to submit a PMA amendment and a written response to FDA's request is not received within 180 days of the date of the request, FDA will consider the pending PMA or PMA supplement to be withdrawn voluntarily by the applicant.

(e) An applicant may resubmit a PMA or PMA supplement after withdrawing it or after it is considered withdrawn under paragraph

(d) of this section, or after FDA has refused to accept it for filing, or has denied approval of the PMA or PMA supplement. A resubmitted PMA or PMA supplement shall comply with the requirements of 814.20 or 814.39, respectively, and shall include the PMA number assigned to the original submission and the applicant's reasons for resubmission of the PMA or PMA supplement.

Sec. 814.39 PMA supplements.

(a) After FDA's approval of a PMA, an applicant shall submit a PMA supplement for review and approval by FDA before making a change affecting the safety or effectiveness of the device for which the applicant has an approved PMA, unless the change is of a type for which FDA, under paragraph (e) of this section, has advised that an alternate submission is permitted or is of a type which, under section 515(d)(6)(A) of the act and paragraph (f) of this section, does not require a PMA supplement under this paragraph. While the burden for determining whether a supplement is required is primarily on the PMA holder, changes for which an applicant shall submit a PMA supplement include, but are not limited to, the following types of changes if they affect the safety or effectiveness of the device:

(1) New indications for use of the device.

(2) Labeling changes.

(3) The use of a different facility or establishment to manufacture, process, or package the device.

(4) Changes in sterilization procedures.

(5) Changes in packaging.

(6) Changes in the performance or design specifications, circuits, components, ingredients, principle of operation, or physical layout of the device.

(7) Extension of the expiration date of the device based on data obtained under a new or revised stability or sterility testing protocol that has not been approved by FDA. If the protocol has been approved, the change shall be reported to FDA under paragraph (b) of this section.

(b) An applicant may make a change in a device after FDA's approval of a PMA for the device without submitting a PMA supplement if the change does not affect the device's safety or effectiveness and

Part 814

the change is reported to FDA in postapproval periodic reports required as a condition to approval of the device, e.g., an editorial change in labeling which does not affect the safety or effectiveness of the device.

(c) All procedures and actions that apply to an application under 814.20 also apply to PMA supplements except that the information required in a supplement is limited to that needed to support the change. A summary under 814.20(b)(3) is required for only a supplement submitted for new indications for use of the device, significant changes in the performance or design specifications, circuits, components, ingredients, principles of operation, or physical layout of the device, or when otherwise required by FDA. The applicant shall submit three copies of a PMA supplement and shall include information relevant to the proposed changes in the device. A PMA supplement shall include a separate section that identifies each change for which approval is being requested and explains the reason for each such change. The applicant shall submit additional copies and additional information if requested by FDA. The time frames for review of, and FDA action on, a PMA supplement are the same as those provided in 814.40 for a PMA.

(d)(1) After FDA approves a PMA, any change described in paragraph (d)(2) of this section to reflect newly acquired information that enhances the safety of the device or the safety in the use of the device may be placed into effect by the applicant prior to the receipt under 814.17 of a written FDA order approving the PMA supplement provided that:

  (i)   The PMA supplement and its mailing cover are plainly marked "Special PMA Supplement--Changes Being Effected";

  (ii) The PMA supplement provides a full explanation of the basis for the changes;

  (iii) The applicant has received acknowledgement from FDA of receipt of the supplement; and

  (iv) The PMA supplement specifically identifies the date that such changes are being effected.

  (2)   The following changes are permitted by paragraph (d)(1) of this section:

(i) Labeling changes that add or strengthen a contraindication, warning, precaution, or information about an adverse reaction for which there is reasonable evidence of a causal association.

(ii) Labeling changes that add or strengthen an instruction that is intended to enhance the safe use of the device.

(iii) Labeling changes that delete misleading, false, or unsupported indications.

(iv) Changes in quality controls or manufacturing process that add a new specification or test method, or otherwise provide additional assurance of purity, identity, strength, or reliability of the device.

(e)(1) FDA will identify a change to a device for which an applicant has an approved PMA and for which a PMA supplement under paragraph (a) is not required. FDA will identify such a change in an advisory opinion under 10.85, if the change applies to a generic type of device, or in correspondence to the applicant, if the change applies only to the applicant's device. FDA will require that a change for which a PMA supplement under paragraph (a) is not required be reported to FDA in:

(i) A periodic report under 814.84 or

(ii) A 30-day PMA supplement under this paragraph.

(2) FDA will identify, in the advisory opinion or correspondence, the type of information that is to be included in the report or 30-day PMA supplement. If the change is required to be reported to FDA in a periodic report, the change may be made before it is reported to FDA. If the change is required to be reported in a 30-day PMA supplement, the change may be made 30 days after FDA files the 30-day PMA supplement unless FDA requires the PMA holder to provide additional information, informs the PMA holder that the supplement is not approvable, or disapproves the supplement. The 30-day PMA supplement shall follow the instructions in the correspondence or advisory opinion. Any 30-day PMA supplement that does not meet the requirements of the correspondence or advisory opinion will not be filed and, therefore, will not be deemed approved 30 days after receipt.

(f) Under section 515(d) of the act, modifications to manufacturing procedures or methods of manufacture that affect the safety and effectiveness of a device subject to an approved PMA do not require submission of a PMA supplement under paragraph (a) of this section and are eligible to be the subject of a 30-day notice. A 30-day notice shall describe in detail the change, summarize the data or information supporting the change, and state that the change has been made in accordance with the requirements of part 820 of this chapter. The manufacturer may distribute the device 30 days after the date on which FDA receives the 30-day notice, unless FDA notifies the applicant within 30 days from receipt of the notice that the notice is not adequate. If the notice is not adequate, FDA shall inform the applicant in writing that a 135-day PMA supplement is needed and shall describe what further information or action is required for acceptance of such change. The number of days under review as a 30-day notice shall be deducted from the 135-day PMA supplement review period if the notice meets appropriate content requirements for a PMA supplement.

(g) The submission and grant of a written request for an exception or alternative under 801.128 or 809.11 of this chapter satisfies the requirement in paragraph (a) of this section.

[51 FR 26364, July 22, 1986, as amended at 51 FR 43344, Dec. 2, 1986; 63 FR 54044, Oct. 8, 1998; 67 FR 9587, Mar. 4, 2002; 69 FR 11313, Mar. 10, 2004; 72 FR 73602, Dec. 28, 2007; 73 FR 49610, Aug. 22, 2008]

Subpart C--FDA Action on a PMA

Sec. 814.40 Time frames for reviewing a PMA.

Within 180 days after receipt of an application that is accepted for filing and to which the applicant does not submit a major amendment, FDA will review the PMA and, after receiving the report and recommendation of the appropriate FDA advisory committee, send the applicant an approval order under 814.44(d), an approvable letter under 814.44(e), a not approvable letter under 814.44(f), or an order denying approval under 814.45. The approvable letter and the not approvable letter will provide an opportunity for the applicant to amend or withdraw the application, or to consider the letter to be a denial of approval of the PMA under 814.45 and to request administrative review under section 515 (d)(3) and (g) of the act.

Sec. 814.42 Filing a PMA.

(a) The filing of an application means that FDA has made a threshold determination that the application is sufficiently complete to permit a substantive review. Within 45 days after a PMA is received by FDA, the agency will notify the applicant whether the application has been filed.

(b) If FDA does not find that any of the reasons in paragraph (e) of this section for refusing to file the PMA applies, the agency will file the PMA and will notify the applicant in writing of the filing. The notice will include the PMA reference number and the date FDA filed the PMA. The date of filing is the date that a PMA accepted for filing was received by the agency. The 180-day period for review of a PMA starts on the date of filing.

(c) If FDA refuses to file a PMA, the agency will notify the applicant of the reasons for the refusal. This notice will identify the deficiencies in the application that prevent filing and will include the PMA reference number.

(d) If FDA refuses to file the PMA, the applicant may:

(1) Resubmit the PMA with additional information necessary to comply with the requirements of section 515(c)(1) (A)-(G) of the act and 814.20. A resubmitted PMA shall include the PMA reference number of the original submission. If the resubmitted PMA is accepted for filing, the date of filing is the date FDA receives the resubmission;

(2) Request in writing within 10 working days of the date of receipt of the notice refusing to file the PMA, an informal conference with the Director of the Office of Device Evaluation to review FDA's decision not to file the PMA. FDA will hold the informal conference within 10 working days of its receipt of the request and will render its decision on filing within 5 working days after the informal conference. If, after the informal conference, FDA accepts the PMA for filing, the date of filing will be the date of the decision to accept the PMA for filing. If FDA does not reverse its decision not to file the PMA, the applicant may request reconsideration of the decision from the Director of the Center for Devices and Radiological Health, the Director of the Center for Biologics Evaluation and Research, or the Director of the Center for Drug Evaluation and Research, as

applicable. The Director's decision will constitute final administrative action for the purpose of judicial review.

(e) FDA may refuse to file a PMA if any of the following applies:

(1) The application is incomplete because it does not on its face contain all the information required under section 515(c)(1)(A)-(G) of the act;

(2) The PMA does not contain each of the items required under 814.20 and justification for omission of any item is inadequate;

(3) The applicant has a pending premarket notification under section 510(k) of the act with respect to the same device, and FDA has not determined whether the device falls within the scope of 814.1(c).

(4) The PMA contains a false statement of material fact.

(5) The PMA is not accompanied by a statement of either certification or disclosure as required by part 54 of this chapter.

[51 FR 26364, July 22, 1986, as amended at 63 FR 5254, Feb. 2, 1998; 73 FR 49942, Aug. 25, 2008]

Sec. 814.44 Procedures for review of a PMA.

(a) FDA will begin substantive review of a PMA after the PMA is accepted for filing under 814.42. FDA may refer the PMA to a panel on its own initiative, and will do so upon request of an applicant, unless FDA determines that the application substantially duplicates information previously reviewed by a panel. If FDA refers an application to a panel, FDA will forward the PMA, or relevant portions thereof, to each member of the appropriate FDA panel for review. During the review process, FDA may communicate with the applicant as set forth under 814.37(b), or with a panel to respond to questions that may be posed by panel members or to provide additional information to the panel. FDA will maintain a record of all communications with the applicant and with the panel.

(b) The advisory committee shall submit a report to FDA which includes the committee's recommendation and the basis for such recommendation on the PMA. Before submission of this report, the committee shall hold a public meeting to review the PMA in accordance with part 14. This meeting may be held by a telephone conference under 14.22(g). The advisory committee report and recommendation may be in the form of a meeting transcript signed by the chairperson of the committee.

(c) FDA will complete its review of the PMA and the advisory committee report and recommendation and, within the later of 180 days from the date of filing of the PMA under 814.42 or the number of days after the date of filing as determined under 814.37(c), issue an approval order under paragraph (d) of this section, an approvable letter under paragraph (e) of this section, a not approvable letter under paragraph (f) of this section, or an order denying approval of the application under 814.45(a).

(d)(1) FDA will issue to the applicant an order approving a PMA if none of the reasons in 814.45 for denying approval of the application applies. FDA will approve an application on the basis of draft final labeling if the only deficiencies in the application concern editorial or similar minor deficiencies in the draft final labeling. Such approval will be conditioned upon the applicant incorporating the specified labeling changes exactly as directed and upon the applicant submitting to FDA a copy of the final printed labeling before marketing. FDA will also give the public notice of the order, including notice of and opportunity for any interested persons to request review under section 515(d)(3) of the act. The notice of approval will be placed on FDA's home page on the Internet (http://www.fda.gov), and it will state that a detailed summary of information respecting the safety and effectiveness of the device, which was the basis for the order approving the PMA, including information about any adverse effects of the device on health, is available on the Internet and has been placed on public display, and that copies are available upon request. FDA will publish in theFederal Registerafter each quarter a list of the approvals announced in that quarter. When a notice of approval is published, data and information in the PMA file will be available for public disclosure in accordance with 814.9.

(2) A request for copies of the current PMA approvals and denials document and for copies of summaries of safety and effectiveness shall be sent in writing to the Division of Dockets Management (HFA-305), Food and Drug Administration, 5630 Fishers Lane, rm. 1061, Rockville, MD 20852.

(e) FDA will send the applicant an approvable letter if the application substantially meets the requirements of this part and the agency believes it can approve the application if specific additional information is submitted or specific conditions are agreed to by the applicant.

(1) The approvable letter will describe the information FDA requires to be provided by the applicant or the conditions the applicant is required to meet to obtain approval. For example, FDA may require, as a condition to approval:

(i) The submission of certain information identified in the approvable letter, e.g., final labeling;

(ii) An FDA inspection that finds the manufacturing facilities, methods, and controls in compliance with part 820 and, if applicable, that verifies records pertinent to the PMA;

(iii) Restrictions imposed on the device under section 515(d)(1)(B)(ii) or 520(e) of the act;

(iv) Postapproval requirements as described in subpart E of this part.

(2) In response to an approvable letter the applicant may:

(i) Amend the PMA as requested in the approvable letter; or

(ii) Consider the approvable letter to be a denial of approval of the PMA under 814.45 and request administrative review under section 515(d)(3) of the act by filing a petition in the form of a petition for reconsideration under 10.33; or

(iii) Withdraw the PMA.

(f) FDA will send the applicant a not approvable letter if the agency believes that the application may not be approved for one or more of the reasons given in 814.45(a). The not approvable letter will describe the deficiencies in the application, including each applicable ground for denial under section 515(d)(2) (A)-(E) of the act, and, where practical, will identify measures required to place the PMA in approvable form. In response to a not approvable letter, the applicant may:

(1) Amend the PMA as requested in the not approvable letter (such an amendment will be considered a major amendment under 814.37(c)(1)); or

(2) Consider the not approvable letter to be a denial of approval of the PMA under 814.45 and request administrative review under section 515(d)(3) of the act by filing a petition in the form of a petition for reconsideration under 10.33; or

(3) Withdraw the PMA.

(g) FDA will consider a PMA to have been withdrawn voluntarily if:

(1) The applicant fails to respond in writing to a written request for an amendment within 180 days after the date FDA issues such request;

(2) The applicant fails to respond in writing to an approvable or not approvable letter within 180 days after the date FDA issues such letter; or

(3) The applicant submits a written notice to FDA that the PMA has been withdrawn.

[51 FR 26364, July 22, 1986, as amended at 57 FR 58403, Dec. 10, 1992; 63 FR 4572, Jan. 30, 1998]

Sec. 814.45 Denial of approval of a PMA.

(a) FDA may issue an order denying approval of a PMA if the applicant fails to follow the requirements of this part or if, upon the basis of the information submitted in the PMA or any other information before the agency, FDA determines that any of the grounds for denying approval of a PMA specified in section 515(d)(2) (A)-(E) of the act applies. In addition, FDA may deny approval of a PMA for any of the following reasons:

(1) The PMA contains a false statement of material fact;

(2) The device's proposed labeling does not comply with the requirements in part 801 or part 809;

(3) The applicant does not permit an authorized FDA employee an opportunity to inspect at a reasonable time and in a reasonable manner the facilities, controls, and to have access to and to copy and verify all records pertinent to the application;

(4) A nonclinical laboratory study that is described in the PMA and that is essential to show that the device is safe for use under the conditions prescribed, recommended, or suggested in its proposed labeling, was not conducted in compliance with the good laboratory practice regulations in part 58 and no reason for the noncompliance is provided or, if it is, the differences between the practices used in conducting the study and the good laboratory practice regulations do not support the validity of the study; or

(5) Any clinical investigation involving human subjects described in the PMA, subject to the institutional review board regulations in part 56 or informed consent regulations in part 50, was not conducted in compliance with those regulations such that the rights or safety of human subjects were not adequately protected.

(b) FDA will issue any order denying approval of the PMA in accordance with 814.17. The order will inform the applicant of the deficiencies in the PMA, including each applicable ground for denial under section 515(d)(2) of the act and the regulations under this part, and, where practical, will identify measures required to place the PMA in approvable form. The order will include a notice of an opportunity to request review under section 515(d)(4) of the act.

(c) FDA will use the criteria specified in 860.7 to determine the safety and effectiveness of a device in deciding whether to approve or deny approval of a PMA. FDA may use information other than that submitted by the applicant in making such determination.

(d)(1) FDA will give the public notice of an order denying approval of the PMA. The notice will be placed on the FDA's home page on the Internet (http://www.fda.gov), and it will state that a detailed summary of information respecting the safety and effectiveness of the device, including information about any adverse effects of the device on health, is available on the Internet and has been placed on public display and that copies are available upon request. FDA will publish in theFederal Registerafter each quarter a list of the denials announced in that quarter. When a notice of denial of approval is made publicly available, data and information in the PMA file will be available for public disclosure in accordance with 814.9.

(2) A request for copies of the current PMA approvals and denials document and copies of summaries of safety and effectiveness shall be sent in writing to the Freedom of Information Staff (HFI-35), Food and Drug Administration, 5600 Fishers Lane, Rockville, MD 20857.

(e) FDA will issue an order denying approval of a PMA after an approvable or not approvable letter has been sent and the applicant:

(1) Submits a requested amendment but any ground for denying approval of the application under section 515(d)(2) of the act still applies; or

(2) Notifies FDA in writing that the requested amendment will not be submitted; or

(3) Petitions for review under section 515(d)(3) of the act by filing a petition in the form of a petition for reconsideration under 10.33.

[51 FR 26364, July 22, 1986, as amended at 63 FR 4572, Jan. 30, 1998; 73 FR 34859, June 19, 2008]

Sec. 814.46 Withdrawal of approval of a PMA.

(a) FDA may issue an order withdrawing approval of a PMA if, from any information available to the agency, FDA determines that:

(1) Any of the grounds under section 515(e)(1) (A)-(G) of the act applies.

(2) Any postapproval requirement imposed by the PMA approval order or by regulation has not been met.

(3) A nonclinical laboratory study that is described in the PMA and that is essential to show that the device is safe for use under the conditions prescribed, recommended, or suggested in its proposed labeling, was not conducted in compliance with the good laboratory practice regulations in part 58 and no reason for the noncompliance is provided or, if it is, the differences between the practices used in conducting the study and the good laboratory practice regulations do not support the validity of the study.

(4) Any clinical investigation involving human subjects described in the PMA, subject to the institutional review board

regulations in part 56 or informed consent regulations in part 50, was not conducted in compliance with those regulations such that the rights or safety of human subjects were not adequately protected.

(b)(1) FDA may seek advice on scientific matters from any appropriate FDA advisory committee in deciding whether to withdraw approval of a PMA.

(2) FDA may use information other than that submitted by the applicant in deciding whether to withdraw approval of a PMA.

(c) Before issuing an order withdrawing approval of a PMA, FDA will issue the holder of the approved application a notice of opportunity for an informal hearing under part 16.

(d) If the applicant does not request a hearing or if after the part 16 hearing is held the agency decides to proceed with the withdrawal, FDA will issue to the holder of the approved application an order withdrawing approval of the application. The order will be issued under 814.17, will state each ground for withdrawing approval, and will include a notice of an opportunity for administrative review under section 515(e)(2) of the act.

(e) FDA will give the public notice of an order withdrawing approval of a PMA. The notice will be published in theFederal Registerand will state that a detailed summary of information respecting the safety and effectiveness of the device, including information about any adverse effects of the device on health, has been placed on public display and that copies are available upon request. When a notice of withdrawal of approval is published, data and information in the PMA file will be available for public disclosure in accordance with 814.9.

Sec. 814.47 Temporary suspension of approval of a PMA.

(a) Scope.

(1) This section describes the procedures that FDA will follow in exercising its authority under section 515(e)(3) of the act (21 U.S.C. 360e(e)(3)). This authority applies to the original PMA, as well as any PMA supplement(s), for a medical device.

(2) FDA will issue an order temporarily suspending approval of a PMA if FDA determines that there is a reasonable probability that continued distribution of the device would cause serious, adverse health consequences or death.

(b) Regulatory hearing.

(1) If FDA believes that there is a reasonable probability that the continued distribution of a device subject to an approved PMA would cause serious, adverse health consequences or death, FDA may initiate and conduct a regulatory hearing to determine whether to issue an order temporarily suspending approval of the PMA.

(2) Any regulatory hearing to determine whether to issue an order temporarily suspending approval of a PMA shall be initiated and conducted by FDA pursuant to part 16 of this chapter. If FDA believes that immediate action to remove a dangerous device from the market is necessary to protect the public health, the agency may, in accordance with 16.60(h) of this chapter, waive, suspend, or modify any part 16 procedure pursuant to 10.19 of this chapter.

(3) FDA shall deem the PMA holder's failure to request a hearing within the timeframe specified by FDA in the notice of opportunity for hearing to be a waiver.

(c) Temporary suspension order. If the PMA holder does not request a regulatory hearing or if, after the hearing, and after consideration of the administrative record of the hearing, FDA determines that there is a reasonable probability that the continued distribution of a device under an approved PMA would cause serious, adverse health consequences or death, the agency shall, under the authority of section 515(e)(3) of the act, issue an order to the PMA holder temporarily suspending approval of the PMA.

(d) Permanent withdrawal of approval of the PMA. If FDA issues an order temporarily suspending approval of a PMA, the agency shall proceed expeditiously, but within 60 days, to hold a hearing on whether to permanently withdraw approval of the PMA in accordance with section 515(e)(1) of the act and the procedures set out in 814.46.

[61 FR 15190, Apr. 5, 1996]

Part 814

Subpart D--Administrative Review [Reserved]

Subpart E--Postapproval Requirements

Sec. 814.80 General.

A device may not be manufactured, packaged, stored, labeled, distributed, or advertised in a manner that is inconsistent with any conditions to approval specified in the PMA approval order for the device.

Sec. 814.82 Postapproval requirements.

(a) FDA may impose postapproval requirements in a PMA approval order or by regulation at the time of approval of the PMA or by regulation subsequent to approval. Postapproval requirements may include as a condition to approval of the device:

  (1) Restriction of the sale, distribution, or use of the device as provided by section 515(d)(1)(B)(ii) or 520(e) of the act.

  (2) Continuing evaluation and periodic reporting on the safety, effectiveness, and reliability of the device for its intended use. FDA will state in the PMA approval order the reason or purpose for such requirement and the number of patients to be evaluated and the reports required to be submitted.

  (3) Prominent display in the labeling of a device and in the advertising of any restricted device of warnings, hazards, or precautions important for the device's safe and effective use, including patient information, e.g., information provided to the patient on alternative modes of therapy and on risks and benefits associated with the use of the device.

  (4) Inclusion of identification codes on the device or its labeling, or in the case of an implant, on cards given to patients if necessary to protect the public health.

  (5) Maintenance of records that will enable the applicant to submit to FDA information needed to trace patients if such information is necessary to protect the public health. Under section 519(a)(4) of the act, FDA will require that the identity of any patient be disclosed in records maintained under this paragraph only to the extent required for the medical welfare of the individual, to determine the safety or effectiveness of

the device, or to verify a record, report, or information submitted to the agency.

(6) Maintenance of records for specified periods of time and organization and indexing of records into identifiable files to enable FDA to determine whether there is reasonable assurance of the continued safety and effectiveness of the device.

(7) Submission to FDA at intervals specified in the approval order of periodic reports containing the information required by 814.84(b).

(8) Batch testing of the device.

(9) Such other requirements as FDA determines are necessary to provide reasonable assurance, or continued reasonable assurance, of the safety and effectiveness of the device.

(b) An applicant shall grant to FDA access to any records and reports required under the provisions of this part, and shall permit authorized FDA employees to copy and verify such records and reports and to inspect at a reasonable time and in a reasonable manner all manufacturing facilities to verify that the device is being manufactured, stored, labeled, and shipped under approved conditions.

(c) Failure to comply with any postapproval requirement constitutes a ground for withdrawal of approval of a PMA.

[51 FR 26364, July 22, 1986, as amended at 51 FR 43344, Dec. 2, 1986]

Sec. 814.84 Reports.

(a) The holder of an approved PMA shall comply with the requirements of part 803 and with any other requirements applicable to the device by other regulations in this subchapter or by order approving the device.

(b) Unless FDA specifies otherwise, any periodic report shall:

(1) Identify changes described in 814.39(a) and changes required to be reported to FDA under 814.39(b).

(2) Contain a summary and bibliography of the following information not previously submitted as part of the PMA:

(i) Unpublished reports of data from any clinical investigations or nonclinical laboratory studies involving the device or related devices and known to or that reasonably should be known to the applicant.

(ii) Reports in the scientific literature concerning the device and known to or that reasonably should be known to the applicant. If, after reviewing the summary and bibliography, FDA concludes that the agency needs a copy of the unpublished or published reports, FDA will notify the applicant that copies of such reports shall be submitted.

(3) Identify changes made pursuant to an exception or alternative granted under 801.128 or 809.11 of this chapter.

[51 FR 26364, July 22, 1986, as amended at 51 FR 43344, Dec. 2, 1986; 67 FR 9587, Mar. 4, 2002; 72 FR 73602, Dec. 28, 2007]

Subparts F-G [Reserved]

Subpart H--Humanitarian Use Devices

Sec. 814.100 Purpose and scope.

(a) This subpart H implements section 520(m) of the act. The purpose of section 520(m) is, to the extent consistent with the protection of the public health and safety and with ethical standards, to encourage the discovery and use of devices intended to benefit patients in the treatment or diagnosis of diseases or conditions that affect or are manifested in fewer than 4,000 individuals in the United States per year. This subpart provides procedures for obtaining:

(1) HUD designation of a medical device; and

(2) Marketing approval for the HUD notwithstanding the absence of reasonable assurance of effectiveness that would otherwise be required under sections 514 and 515 of the act.

(b) Although a HUD may also have uses that differ from the humanitarian use, applicants seeking approval of any non-HUD use shall submit a PMA as required under 814.20, or a premarket notification as required under part 807 of this chapter.

(c) Obtaining marketing approval for a HUD involves two steps:

(1) Obtaining designation of the device as a HUD from FDA's Office of Orphan Products Development, and

(2) Submitting an HDE to the Office of Device Evaluation (ODE), Center for Devices and Radiological Health (CDRH), the Center for Biologics Evaluation and Research (CBER), or the Center for Drug Evaluation and Research (CDER), as applicable.

(d) A person granted an exemption under section 520(m) of the act shall submit periodic reports as described in 814.126(b).

(e) FDA may suspend or withdraw approval of an HDE after providing notice and an opportunity for an informal hearing.

[61 FR 33244, June 26, 1996, as amended at 63 FR 59220, Nov. 3, 1998; 73 FR 49942, Aug. 25, 2008]

Sec. 814.102 Designation of HUD status.

(a) Request for designation. Prior to submitting an HDE application, the applicant shall submit a request for HUD designation to FDA's Office of Orphan Products Development. The request shall contain the following:

(1) A statement that the applicant requests HUD designation for a rare disease or condition or a valid subset of a disease or condition which shall be identified with specificity;

(2) The name and address of the applicant, the name of the applicant's primary contact person and/or resident agent, including title, address, and telephone number;

(3) A description of the rare disease or condition for which the device is to be used, the proposed indication or indications for use of the device, and the reasons why such therapy is needed. If the device is proposed for an indication that represents a subset of a common disease or condition, a demonstration that the subset is medically plausible should be included;

(4) A description of the device and a discussion of the scientific rationale for the use of the device for the rare disease or condition; and

(5) Documentation, with appended authoritative references, to demonstrate that the device is designed to treat or diagnose a

disease or condition that affects or is manifested in fewer than 4,000 people in the United States per year. If the device is for diagnostic purposes, the documentation must demonstrate that fewer than 4,000 patients per year would be subjected to diagnosis by the device in the United States. Authoritative references include literature citations in specialized medical journals, textbooks, specialized medical society proceedings, or governmental statistics publications. When no such studies or literature citations exist, the applicant may be able to demonstrate the prevalence of the disease or condition in the United States by providing credible conclusions from appropriate research or surveys.

(b) FDA action. Within 45 days of receipt of a request for HUD designation, FDA will take one of the following actions:

(1) Approve the request and notify the applicant that the device has been designated as a HUD based on the information submitted;

(2) Return the request to the applicant pending further review upon submission of additional information. This action will ensue if the request is incomplete because it does not on its face contain all of the information required under 814.102(a). Upon receipt of this additional information, the review period may be extended up to 45 days; or

(3) Disapprove the request for HUD designation based on a substantive review of the information submitted. FDA may disapprove a request for HUD designation if:

(i) There is insufficient evidence to support the estimate that the disease or condition for which the device is designed to treat or diagnose affects or is manifested in fewer than 4,000 people in the United States per year;

(ii) FDA determines that, for a diagnostic device, 4,000 or more patients in the United States would be subjected to diagnosis using the device per year; or

(iii) FDA determines that the patient population defined in the request is not a medically plausible subset of a larger population.

(c) Revocation of designation. FDA may revoke a HUD designation if the agency finds that:

(1) The request for designation contained an untrue statement of material fact or omitted material information; or

(2) Based on the evidence available, the device is not eligible for HUD designation.

(d) Submission. The applicant shall submit two copies of a completed, dated, and signed request for HUD designation to: Office of Orphan Products Development (HF-35), Food and Drug Administration, 5600 Fishers Lane, Rockville, MD 20857.

Sec. 814.104 Original applications.

(a) United States applicant or representative. The applicant or an authorized representative shall sign the HDE. If the applicant does not reside or have a place of business within the United States, the HDE shall be countersigned by an authorized representative residing or maintaining a place of business in the United States and shall identify the representative's name and address.

(b) Contents. Unless the applicant justifies an omission in accordance with paragraph (d) of this section, an HDE shall include:

(1) A copy of or reference to the determination made by FDA's Office of Orphan Products Development (in accordance with 814.102) that the device qualifies as a HUD;

(2) An explanation of why the device would not be available unless an HDE were granted and a statement that no comparable device (other than another HUD approved under this subpart or a device under an approved IDE) is available to treat or diagnose the disease or condition. The application also shall contain a discussion of the risks and benefits of currently available devices or alternative forms of treatment in the United States;

(3) An explanation of why the probable benefit to health from the use of the device outweighs the risk of injury or illness from its use, taking into account the probable risks and benefits of currently available devices or alternative forms of treatment. Such explanation shall include a description, explanation, or theory of the underlying disease process or condition, and known or postulated mechanism(s) of action of the device in relation to the disease process or condition;

(4) All of the information required to be submitted under 814.20(b), except that:

   (i) In lieu of the summaries, conclusions, and results from clinical investigations required under 814.20(b)(3)(v)(B), (b)(3)(vi), and (b)(6)(ii), the applicant shall include the summaries, conclusions, and results of all clinical experience or investigations (whether adverse or supportive) reasonably obtainable by the applicant that are relevant to an assessment of the risks and probable benefits of the device; and

   (ii) In addition to the proposed labeling requirement set forth in 814.20(b)(10), the labeling shall bear the following statement: Humanitarian Device. Authorized by Federal law for use in the [treatment or diagnosis] of [specify disease or condition]. The effectiveness of this device for this use has not been demonstrated; and

(5) The amount to be charged for the device and, if the amount is more than $250, a report by an independent certified public accountant, made in accordance with the Statement on Standards for Attestation established by the American Institute of Certified Public Accountants, or in lieu of such a report, an attestation by a responsible individual of the organization, verifying that the amount charged does not exceed the costs of the device's research, development, fabrication, and distribution. If the amount charged is $250 or less, the requirement for a report by an independent certified public accountant or an attestation by a responsible individual of the organization is waived.

(c) Omission of information. If the applicant believes that certain information required under paragraph (b) of this section is not applicable to the device that is the subject of the HDE, and omits any such information from its HDE, the applicant shall submit a statement that identifies and justifies the omission. The statement shall be submitted as a separate section in the HDE and identified in the table of contents. If the justification for the omission is not accepted by the agency, FDA will so notify the applicant.

(d) Address for submissions and correspondence. Copies of all original HDEs amendments and supplements, as well as any correspondence relating to an HDE, must be sent or delivered to the following:

(1) For devices regulated by the Center for Devices and Radiological Health, send to Document Mail Center, 10903 New Hampshire Ave., Bldg. 66, rm. G609, Silver Spring, MD 20993-0002.

(2) For devices regulated by the Center for Biologics Evaluation and Research, send this information to the Document Control Center (HFM-99), Center for Biologics Evaluation and Research, Food and Drug Administration, 1401 Rockville Pike, suite 200N, Rockville, MD 20852-1448.

(3) For devices regulated by the Center for Drug Evaluation and Research, send this information to the Central Document Control Room, Center for Drug Evaluation and Research, Food and Drug Administration, 5901-B Ammendale Rd., Beltsville, MD 20705-1266.

[61 FR 33244, June 26, 1996, as amended at 63 FR 59220, Nov. 3, 1998; 73 FR 49942, Aug. 25, 2008; 75 FR 20915, Apr. 22, 2010]

Part 814

Sec. 814.106 HDE amendments and resubmitted HDE's.

An HDE or HDE supplement may be amended or resubmitted upon an applicant's own initiative, or at the request of FDA, for the same reasons and in the same manner as prescribed for PMA's in 814.37, except that the timeframes set forth in 814.37(c)(1) and (d) do not apply. If FDA requests an HDE applicant to submit an HDE amendment, and a written response to FDA's request is not received within 75 days of the date of the request, FDA will consider the pending HDE or HDE supplement to be withdrawn voluntarily by the applicant. Furthermore, if the HDE applicant, on its own initiative or at FDA's request, submits a major amendment as described in 814.37(c)(1), the review period may be extended up to 75 days.

[63 FR 59220, Nov. 3, 1998]

Sec. 814.108 Supplemental applications.

After FDA approval of an original HDE, an applicant shall submit supplements in accordance with the requirements for PMA's under 814.39, except that a request for a new indication for use of a HUD shall comply with requirements set forth in 814.110. The timeframes for review of, and FDA action on, an HDE supplement are the same as those provided in 814.114 for an HDE.

[63 FR 59220, Nov. 3, 1998]

Sec. 814.110 New indications for use.

(a) An applicant seeking a new indication for use of a HUD approved under this subpart H shall obtain a new designation of HUD status in accordance with 814.102 and shall submit an original HDE in accordance with 814.104.

(b) An application for a new indication for use made under 814.104 may incorporate by reference any information or data previously submitted to the agency under an HDE.

Sec. 814.112 Filing an HDE.

(a) The filing of an HDE means that FDA has made a threshold determination that the application is sufficiently complete to permit substantive review. Within 30 days from the date an HDE is received by FDA, the agency will notify the applicant whether the application has been filed. FDA may refuse to file an HDE if any of the following applies:

    (1) The application is incomplete because it does not on its face contain all the information required under 814.104(b);

    (2) FDA determines that there is a comparable device available (other than another HUD approved under this subpart or a device under an approved IDE) to treat or diagnose the disease or condition for which approval of the HUD is being sought; or

    (3) The application contains an untrue statement of material fact or omits material information.

    (4) The HDE is not accompanied by a statement of either certification or disclosure, or both, as required by part 54 of this chapter.

(b) The provisions contained in 814.42(b), (c), and (d) regarding notification of filing decisions, filing dates, the start of the 75-day review period, and applicant's options in response to FDA refuse to file decisions shall apply to HDE's.

[61 FR 33244, June 26, 1996, as amended at 63 FR 5254, Feb. 2, 1998; 63 FR 59221, Nov. 3, 1998]

Sec. 814.114 Timeframes for reviewing an HDE.

Within 75 days after receipt of an HDE that is accepted for filing and to which the applicant does not submit a major amendment, FDA shall send the applicant an approval order, an approvable letter, a not approvable letter (under 814.116), or an order denying approval (under 814.118).

[63 FR 59221, Nov. 3, 1998]

Sec. 814.116 Procedures for review of an HDE.

(a) Substantive review. FDA will begin substantive review of an HDE after the HDE is accepted for filing under 814.112. FDA may refer an original HDE application to a panel on its own initiative, and shall do so upon the request of an applicant, unless FDA determines that the application substantially duplicates information previously reviewed by a panel. If the HDE is referred to a panel, the agency shall follow the procedures set forth under 814.44, with the exception that FDA will complete its review of the HDE and the advisory committee report and recommendations within 75 days from receipt of an HDE that is accepted for filing under 814.112 or the date of filing as determined under 814.106, whichever is later. Within the later of these two timeframes, FDA will issue an approval order under paragraph (b) of this section, an approvable letter under paragraph (c) of this section, a not approvable letter under paragraph (d) of this section, or an order denying approval of the application under 814.118(a).

(b) Approval order. FDA will issue to the applicant an order approving an HDE if none of the reasons in 814.118 for denying approval of the application applies. FDA will approve an application on the basis of draft final labeling if the only deficiencies in the application concern editorial or similar minor deficiencies in the draft final labeling. Such approval will be conditioned upon the applicant incorporating the specified labeling changes exactly as directed and upon the applicant submitting to FDA a copy of the final printed labeling before marketing. The notice of approval of an HDE will be published in theFederal Registerin accordance with the rules and policies applicable to PMA's submitted under 814.20. Following the issuance of an approval order, data and information in the HDE file will be available for public disclosure in accordance with 814.9(b) through (h), as applicable.

(c) Approvable letter. FDA will send the applicant an approvable letter if the application substantially meets the requirements of this subpart and the agency believes it can approve the application if specific additional information is submitted or specific conditions are agreed to by the applicant. The approvable letter will describe the information FDA requires to be provided by the applicant or the conditions the applicant is required to meet to obtain approval. For example, FDA may require as a condition to approval:

(1) The submission of certain information identified in the approvable letter, e.g., final labeling;

(2) Restrictions imposed on the device under section 520(e) of the act;

(3) Postapproval requirements as described in subpart E of this part; and

(4) An FDA inspection that finds the manufacturing facilities, methods, and controls in compliance with part 820 of this chapter and, if applicable, that verifies records pertinent to the HDE.

(d) Not approvable letter. FDA will send the applicant a not approvable letter if the agency believes that the application may not be approved for one or more of the reasons given in 814.118. The not approvable letter will describe the deficiencies in the application and, where practical, will identify measures required to place the HDE in approvable form. The applicant may respond to the not approvable letter in the same manner as permitted for not approvable letters for PMA's under 814.44(f), with the exception that if a major HDE amendment is submitted, the review period may be extended up to 75 days.

(e) FDA will consider an HDE to have been withdrawn voluntarily if:

(1) The applicant fails to respond in writing to a written request for an amendment within 75 days after the date FDA issues such request;

(2) The applicant fails to respond in writing to an approvable or not approvable letter within 75 days after the date FDA issues such letter; or

(3) The applicant submits a written notice to FDA that the HDE has been withdrawn.

[61 FR 33244, June 26, 1996, as amended at 63 FR 59221, Nov. 3, 1998]

Sec. 814.118 Denial of approval or withdrawal of approval of an HDE.

(a) FDA may deny approval or withdraw approval of an application if the applicant fails to meet the requirements of section 520(m) of the act or of this part, or of any condition of approval imposed by an IRB or by FDA, or any postapproval requirements imposed under 814.126. In addition, FDA may deny approval or withdraw approval of an application if, upon the basis of the information submitted in the HDE or any other information before the agency, FDA determines that:

(1) There is a lack of a showing of reasonable assurance that the device is safe under the conditions of use prescribed, recommended, or suggested in the labeling thereof;

(2) The device is ineffective under the conditions of use prescribed, recommended, or suggested in the labeling thereof;

(3) The applicant has not demonstrated that there is a reasonable basis from which to conclude that the probable benefit to health from the use of the device outweighs the risk of injury or illness, taking into account the probable risks and benefits of currently available devices or alternative forms of treatment;

(4) The application or a report submitted by or on behalf of the applicant contains an untrue statement of material fact, or omits material information;

(5) The device's labeling does not comply with the requirements in part 801 or part 809 of this chapter;

(6) A nonclinical laboratory study that is described in the HDE and that is essential to show that the device is safe for use under the conditions prescribed, recommended, or suggested in its proposed labeling, was not conducted in compliance with the good laboratory practice regulations in part 58 of this chapter and no reason for the noncompliance is provided or, if it is, the differences between the practices used in conducting the study and the good laboratory practice regulations do not support the validity of the study;

Part 814

(7) Any clinical investigation involving human subjects described in the HDE, subject to the institutional review board regulations in part 56 of this chapter or the informed consent regulations in part 50 of this chapter, was not conducted in compliance with those regulations such that the rights or safety of human subjects were not adequately protected;

(8) The applicant does not permit an authorized FDA employee an opportunity to inspect at a reasonable time and in a reasonable manner the facilities and controls, and to have access to and to copy and verify all records pertinent to the application; or

(9) The device's HUD designation should be revoked in accordance with 814.102(c).

(b) If FDA issues an order denying approval of an application, the agency will comply with the same notice and disclosure provisions required for PMA's under 814.45(b) and (d), as applicable.

(c) FDA will issue an order denying approval of an HDE after an approvable or not approvable letter has been sent and the applicant:

(1) Submits a requested amendment but any ground for denying approval of the application under 814.118(a) still applies;

(2) Notifies FDA in writing that the requested amendment will not be submitted; or

(3) Petitions for review under section 515(d)(3) of the act by filing a petition in the form of a petition for reconsideration under 10.33 of this chapter.

(d) Before issuing an order withdrawing approval of an HDE, FDA will provide the applicant with notice and an opportunity for a hearing as required for PMA's under 814.46(c) and (d), and will provide the public with notice in accordance with 814.46(e), as applicable.

[61 FR 33244, June 26, 1996, as amended at 63 FR 59221, Nov. 3, 1998]

Sec. 814.120 Temporary suspension of approval of an HDE.

An HDE or HDE supplement may be temporarily suspended for the same reasons and in the same manner as prescribed for PMA's in 814.47.

[63 FR 59221, Nov. 3, 1998]

Sec. 814.122 Confidentiality of data and information.

(a) Requirement for disclosure. The "HDE file" includes all data and information submitted with or referenced in the HDE, any IDE incorporated into the HDE, any HDE amendment or supplement, any report submitted under 814.126, any master file, or any other related submission. Any record in the HDE file will be available for public disclosure in accordance with the provisions of this section and part 20 of this chapter.

(b) Extent of disclosure. Disclosure by FDA of the existence and contents of an HDE file shall be subject to the same rules that pertain to PMA's under 814.9(b) through (h), as applicable.

Sec. 814.124 Institutional Review Board requirements.

(a) IRB approval. The HDE holder is responsible for ensuring that a HUD approved under this subpart is administered only in facilities having an Institutional Review Board (IRB) constituted and acting pursuant to part 56 of this chapter, including continuing review of use of the device. In addition, a HUD may be administered only if such use has been approved by the IRB located at the facility or by a similarly constituted IRB that has agreed to oversee such use and to which the local IRB has deferred in a letter to the HDE holder, signed by the IRB chair or an authorized designee. If, however, a physician in an emergency situation determines that approval from an IRB cannot be obtained in time to prevent serious harm or death to a patient, a HUD may be administered without prior approval by the IRB located at the facility or by a similarly constituted IRB that has agreed to oversee such use. In such an emergency situation, the physician shall, within 5 days after the use of the device, provide written notification to the chairman of the IRB of such use. Such written notification shall include the identification of the patient involved, the date on which the device was used, and the reason for the use.

(b) Withdrawal of IRB approval. A holder of an approved HDE shall notify FDA of any withdrawal of approval for the use of a HUD by a reviewing IRB within 5 working days after being notified of the withdrawal of approval.

[61 FR 33244, June 26, 1996, as amended at 63 FR 59221, Nov. 3, 1998]

Sec. 814.126 Postapproval requirements and reports.

(a) An HDE approved under this subpart H shall be subject to the postapproval requirements and reports set forth under subpart E of this part, as applicable, with the exception of 814.82(a)(7). In addition, medical device reports submitted to FDA in compliance with the requirements of part 803 of this chapter shall also be submitted to the IRB of record.

(b) In addition to the reports identified in paragraph (a) of this section, the holder of an approved HDE shall prepare and submit the following complete, accurate, and timely reports:

    (1) Periodic reports. An HDE applicant is required to submit reports in accordance with the approval order. Unless FDA specifies otherwise, any periodic report shall include:

        (i) An update of the information required under 814.102(a) in a separately bound volume;

        (ii) An update of the information required under 814.104(b)(2), (b)(3), and (b)(5);

        (iii) The number of devices that have been shipped or sold since initial marketing approval under this subpart H and, if the number shipped or sold exceeds 4,000, an explanation and estimate of the number of devices used per patient. If a single device is used on multiple patients, the applicant shall submit an estimate of the number of patients treated or diagnosed using the device together with an explanation of the basis for the estimate;

        (iv) Information describing the applicant's clinical experience with the device since the HDE was initially approved. This information shall include safety information that is known or reasonably should be known to the applicant, medical device reports made under part 803 of this chapter, any data generated from the postmarketing studies, and information (whether published or unpublished) that is known or reasonably expected to be known by the applicant that may affect an evaluation of the safety of the device or that may affect the statement of contraindications, warnings, precautions, and adverse reactions in the device's labeling; and

        (v) A summary of any changes made to the device in accordance with supplements submitted under 814.108.

If information provided in the periodic reports, or any other information in the possession of FDA, gives the agency reason to believe that a device raises public health concerns or that the criteria for exemption are no longer met, the agency may require the HDE holder to submit additional information to demonstrate continued compliance with the HDE requirements.

(2) Other. An HDE holder shall maintain records of the names and addresses of the facilities to which the HUD has been shipped, correspondence with reviewing IRB's, as well as any other information requested by a reviewing IRB or FDA. Such records shall be maintained in accordance with the HDE approval order.

[61 FR 33244, June 26, 1996, as amended at 63 FR 59221, Nov. 3, 1998, 71 FR 16228, Mar. 31, 2006]

Authority: 21 U.S.C. 351, 352, 353, 360, 360c-360j, 371, 372, 373, 374, 375, 379, 379e, 381.

Source: 51 FR 26364, July 22, 1986, unless otherwise noted.

Part 814

Part II

Combined Glossary and Index

Combined Glossary

505(b)(2) Application means an application submitted under section 505(b)(1) of the act for a drug for which the investigations described in section 505(b)(1)(A) of the act and relied upon by the applicant for approval of the application were not conducted by or for the applicant and for which the applicant has not obtained a right of reference or use from the person by or for whom the investigations were conducted. [21 CFR § 314]

A

Abbreviated application means the application described under 314.94, including all amendments and supplements to the application. "Abbreviated application" applies to both an abbreviated new drug application and an abbreviated antibiotic application. [21 CFR § 314]

Acceptance criteria means the product specifications and acceptance/rejection criteria, such as acceptable quality level and unacceptable quality level, with an associated sampling plan, that are necessary for making a decision to accept or reject a lot or batch (or any other convenient subgroups of manufactured units). [21 CFR § 210]

Act means the Federal Food, Drug, and Cosmetic Act (secs. 201-903 (21 U.S.C. 321-393)). [21 CFR § 11]

> ***Act*** means the Federal Food, Drug, and Cosmetic Act, as amended (secs. 201-902, 52 Stat. 1040et seq. as amended (21 U.S.C. 321-392)). [21 CFR § 50, § 56, § 58, § 312, § 812]

> ***Act*** means the Federal Food, Drug, and Cosmetic Act, as amended (21 U.S.C. 301et seq.). [21 CFR § 210]

> ***Act*** means the Federal Food, Drug, and Cosmetic Act (sections 201-901 (21 U.S.C. 301-392)). [21 CFR § 314]

Act means the Federal Food, Drug, and Cosmetic Act (sections 201-902, 52 Stat. 1040 et seq., as amended (21 U.S.C. 321-392)). [21 CFR § 814]

Active ingredient means any component that is intended to furnish pharmacological activity or other direct effect in the diagnosis, cure, mitigation, treatment, or prevention of disease, or to affect the structure or any function of the body of man or other animals. The term includes those components that may undergo chemical change in the manufacture of the drug product and be present in the drug product in a modified form intended to furnish the specified activity or effect. [21 CFR § 210]

Actual yield means the quantity that is actually produced at any appropriate phase of manufacture, processing, or packing of a particular drug product.

Adverse drug experience is any adverse event associated with the use of a new animal drug, whether or not considered to be drug related, and whether or not the new animal drug was used in accordance with the approved labeling (i.e., used according to label directions or used in an extralabel manner, including but not limited to different route of administration, different species, different indications, or other than labeled dosage). Adverse drug experience includes, but is not limited to: [21 CFR § 514]

(1) An adverse event occurring in animals in the course of the use of an animal drug product by a veterinarian or by a livestock producer or other animal owner or caretaker.

(2) Failure of a new animal drug to produce its expected pharmacological or clinical effect (lack of expected effectiveness).

(3) An adverse event occurring in humans from exposure during manufacture, testing, handling, or use of a new animal drug.

Agency means the Food and Drug Administration. [21 CFR § 11]

ANADA is an abbreviated new animal drug application including all amendments and supplements. [21 CFR § 514]

Applicant means the party who submits a marketing application to FDA for approval of a drug, device, or biologic product. The applicant is responsible for submitting the appropriate certification and disclosure statements required in this part. [21 CFR § 54]

Applicant means any person who submits an application or abbreviated application or an amendment or supplement to them under this part to obtain FDA approval of a new drug or an antibiotic drug and any person who owns an approved application or abbreviated application. [21 CFR § 314]

Applicant is a person or entity who owns or holds on behalf of the owner the approval for an NADA or an ANADA, and is responsible for compliance with applicable provisions of the act and regulations. [21 CFR § 514]

Application means the application described under 314.50, including all amendements and supplements to the application. [21 CFR § 314]

Application for research or marketing permit includes: [21 CFR § 50]

(1) A color additive petition, described in part 71.

(2) A food additive petition, described in parts 171 and 571.

(3) Data and information about a substance submitted as part of the procedures for establishing that the substance is generally recognized as safe for use that results or may reasonably be expected to result, directly or indirectly, in its becoming a component or otherwise affecting the characteristics of any food, described in 170.30 and 570.30.

(4) Data and information about a food additive submitted as part of the procedures for food additives permitted to be used on an interim basis pending additional study, described in 180.1.

(5) Data and information about a substance submitted as part of the procedures for establishing a tolerance for unavoidable contaminants in food and food-packaging materials, described in section 406 of the act.

(6) An investigational new drug application, described in part 312 of this chapter.

(7) A new drug application, described in part 314.

(8) Data and information about the bioavailability or bioequivalence of drugs for human use submitted as part of the procedures for issuing, amending, or repealing a bioequivalence requirement, described in part 320.

(9) Data and information about an over-the-counter drug for human use submitted as part of the procedures for classifying these drugs as generally recognized as safe and effective and not misbranded, described in part 330.

(10) Data and information about a prescription drug for human use submitted as part of the procedures for classifying these drugs as generally recognized as safe and effective and not misbranded, described in this chapter.

(11) [Reserved]

(12) An application for a biologics license, described in part 601 of this chapter.

(13) Data and information about a biological product submitted as part of the procedures for determining that licensed biological products are safe and effective and not misbranded, described in part 601.

(14) Data and information about an in vitro diagnostic product submitted as part of the procedures for establishing, amending, or repealing a standard for these products, described in part 809.

(15) An Application for an Investigational Device Exemption, described in part 812.

(16) Data and information about a medical device submitted as part of the procedures for classifying these devices, described in section 513.

(17) Data and information about a medical device submitted as part of the procedures for establishing, amending, or repealing a standard for these devices, described in section 514.

(18) An application for premarket approval of a medical device, described in section 515.

(19) A product development protocol for a medical device, described in section 515.

(20) Data and information about an electronic product submitted as part of the procedures for establishing, amending, or repealing a standard for these products, described in section 358 of the Public Health Service Act.

(21) Data and information about an electronic product submitted as part of the procedures for obtaining a variance from any

electronic product performance standard, as described in 1010.4.

(22) Data and information about an electronic product submitted as part of the procedures for granting, amending, or extending an exemption from a radiation safety performance standard, as described in 1010.5.

(23) Data and information about a clinical study of an infant formula when submitted as part of an infant formula notification under section 412(c) of the Federal Food, Drug, and Cosmetic Act.

(24) Data and information submitted in a petition for a nutrient content claim, described in 101.69 of this chapter, or for a health claim, described in 101.70 of this chapter.

(25) Data and information from investigations involving children submitted in a new dietary ingredient notification, described in 190.6 of this chapter.

Application for research or marketing permit includes: [21 CFR § 56]

(1) A color additive petition, described in part 71.

(2) Data and information regarding a substance submitted as part of the procedures for establishing that a substance is generally recognized as safe for a use which results or may reasonably be expected to result, directly or indirectly, in its becoming a component or otherwise affecting the characteristics of any food, described in 170.35.

(3) A food additive petition, described in part 171.

(4) Data and information regarding a food additive submitted as part of the procedures regarding food additives permitted to be used on an interim basis pending additional study, described in 180.1.

(5) Data and information regarding a substance submitted as part of the procedures for establishing a tolerance for unavoidable contaminants in food and food-packaging materials, described in section 406 of the act.

(6) An investigational new drug application, described in part 312 of this chapter.

(7) A new drug application, described in part 314.

(8) Data and information regarding the bioavailability or bioequivalence of drugs for human use submitted as part of the procedures for issuing, amending, or repealing a bioequivalence requirement, described in part 320.

(9) Data and information regarding an over-the-counter drug for human use submitted as part of the procedures for classifying such drugs as generally recognized as safe and effective and not misbranded, described in part 330.

(10) An application for a biologics license, described in part 601 of this chapter.

(11) Data and information regarding a biological product submitted as part of the procedures for determining that licensed biological products are safe and effective and not misbranded, as described in part 601 of this chapter.

(12) An Application for an Investigational Device Exemption, described in part 812.

(13) Data and information regarding a medical device for human use submitted as part of the procedures for classifying such devices, described in part 860.

(14) Data and information regarding a medical device for human use submitted as part of the procedures for establishing, amending, or repealing a standard for such device, described in part 861.

(15) An application for premarket approval of a medical device for human use, described in section 515 of the act.

(16) A product development protocol for a medical device for human use, described in section 515 of the act.

(17) Data and information regarding an electronic product submitted as part of the procedures for establishing, amending, or repealing a standard for such products, described in section 358 of the Public Health Service Act.

(18) Data and information regarding an electronic product submitted as part of the procedures for obtaining a variance from any electronic product performance standard, as described in 1010.4.

(19) Data and information regarding an electronic product submitted as part of the procedures for granting, amending, or extending an exemption from a radiation safety performance standard, as described in 1010.5.

(20) Data and information regarding an electronic product submitted as part of the procedures for obtaining an exemption from notification of a radiation safety defect or failure of compliance with a radiation safety performance standard, described in subpart D of part 1003.

(21) Data and information about a clinical study of an infant formula when submitted as part of an infant formula notification under section 412(c) of the Federal Food, Drug, and Cosmetic Act.

(22) Data and information submitted in a petition for a nutrient content claim, described in 101.69 of this chapter, and for a health claim, described in 101.70 of this chapter.

(23) Data and information from investigations involving children submitted in a new dietary ingredient notification, described in 190.6 of this chapter.

Application for research or marketing permit includes: [21 CFR § 58]

(1) A color additive petition, described in part 71.

(2) A food additive petition, described in parts 171 and 571.

(3) Data and information regarding a substance submitted as part of the procedures for establishing that a substance is generally recognized as safe for use, which use results or may reasonably be expected to result, directly or indirectly, in its becoming a component or otherwise affecting the characteristics of any food, described in 170.35 and 570.35.

(4) Data and information regarding a food additive submitted as part of the procedures regarding food additives permitted to be used on an interim basis pending additional study, described in 180.1.

(5) Aninvestigational new drug application, described in part 312 of this chapter.

(6) Anew drug application, described in part 314.

(7) Data and information regarding an over-the-counter drug for human use, submitted as part of the procedures for classifying such drugs as generally recognized as safe and effective and not misbranded, described in part 330.

(8) Data and information about a substance submitted as part of the procedures for establishing a tolerance for unavoidable contaminants in food and food-packaging materials, described in parts 109 and 509.

(9) [Reserved]

(10) A Notice of Claimed Investigational Exemption for a New Animal Drug, described in part 511.

(11) A new animal drug application, described in part 514.

(12) [Reserved]

(13) An application for a biologics license, described in part 601 of this chapter.

(14) An application for an investigational device exemption, described in part 812.

(15) An Application for Premarket Approval of a Medical Device, described in section 515 of the act.

(16) A Product Development Protocol for a Medical Device, described in section 515 of the act.

(17) Data and information regarding a medical device submitted as part of the procedures for classifying such devices, described in part 860.

(18) Data and information regarding a medical device submitted as part of the procedures for establishing, amending, or repealing a performance standard for such devices, described in part 861.

(19) Data and information regarding an electronic product submitted as part of the procedures for obtaining an exemption from notification of a radiation safety defect or failure of compliance with a radiation safety performance standard, described in subpart D of part 1003.

(20) Data and information regarding an electronic product submitted as part of the procedures for establishing, amending, or repealing a standard for such product, described in section 358 of the Public Health Service Act.

(21) Data and information regarding an electronic product submitted as part of the procedures for obtaining a variance from any electronic product performance standard as described in 1010.4.

(22) Data and information regarding an electronic product submitted as part of the procedures for granting, amending, or extending an exemption from any electronic product performance standard, as described in 1010.5.

(23) A premarket notification for a food contact substance, described in part 170, subpart D, of this chapter.

Approval letter means a written communication to an applicant from FDA approving an application or an abbreviated application. [21 CFR § 314]

Assent means a child's affirmative agreement to participate in a clinical investigation. Mere failure to object may not, absent affirmative agreement, be construed as assent. [21 CFR § 50]

Assess the effects of the change means to evaluate the effects of a manufacturing change on the identity, strength, quality, purity, and potency of a drug product as these factors may relate to the safety or effectiveness of the drug product. [21 CFR § 314]

Authorized generic drug means a listed drug, as defined in this section, that has been approved under section 505(c) of the act and is marketed, sold, or distributed directly or indirectly to retail class of trade with labeling, packaging (other than repackaging as the listed drug in blister packs, unit doses, or similar packaging for use in institutions), product code, labeler code, trade name, or trademark that differs from that of the listed drug. [21 CFR § 314]

B

Batch means a specific quantity or lot of a test or control article that has been characterized according to 58.105(a). [21 CFR § 58]

> ***Batch*** means a specific quantity of a drug or other material that is intended to have uniform character and quality, within specified limits, and is produced according to a single manufacturing order during the same cycle of manufacture. [21 CFR § 210]

Bioavailability means the rate and extent to which the active ingredient or active moiety is absorbed from a drug product and becomes available at the site of action. For drug products that are not intended to be absorbed into the bloodstream, bioavailability may be assessed by measurements intended to reflect the rate and extent to which the active ingredient or active moiety becomes available at the site of action. [21 CFR § 320]

Bioequivalence means the absence of a significant difference in the rate and extent to which the active ingredient or active moiety in pharmaceutical equivalents or pharmaceutical alternatives becomes available at the site of drug action when administered at the same molar dose under similar conditions in an appropriately designed study. Where there is an intentional difference in rate (e.g., in certain extended release dosage forms), certain pharmaceutical equivalents or alternatives may be considered bioequivalent if there is no significant difference in the extent to which the active ingredient or moiety from each product becomes available at the site of drug action. This applies only if the difference in the rate at which the active ingredient or moiety becomes available at the site of drug action is intentional and is reflected in the proposed labeling, is not essential to the attainment of effective body drug concentrations on chronic use, and is considered medically insignificant for the drug. [21 CFR § 320]

Bioequivalence requirement means a requirement imposed by the Food and Drug Administration for in vitro and/or in vivo testing of specified drug products which must be satisfied as a condition of marketing. [21 CFR § 320]

Biometrics means a method of verifying an individual's identity based on measurement of the individual's physical feature(s) or repeatable action(s) where those features and/or actions are both unique to that individual and measurable. [21 CFR § 11]

C

Children means persons who have not attained the legal age for consent to treatments or procedures involved in clinical investigations, under the applicable law of the jurisdiction in which the clinical investigation will be conducted. [21 CFR § 50]

Class 1 resubmission means the resubmission of an application or efficacy supplement, following receipt of a complete response letter, that contains one or more of the following: Final printed labeling, draft labeling, certain safety updates, stability updates to support provisional or final dating periods, commitments to perform postmarketing studies (including proposals for such studies), assay validation data, final release testing on the last lots used to support approval, minor reanalyses of previously submitted data, and other comparatively minor information. [21 CFR § 314]

Class 2 resubmission means the resubmission of an application or efficacy supplement, following receipt of a complete response letter, that includes any item not specified in the definition of "Class 1 resubmission," including any item that would require presentation to an advisory committee. [21 CFR § 314]

Closed system means an environment in which system access is controlled by persons who are responsible for the content of electronic records that are on the system. [21 CFR § 11]

Clinical investigation means any experiment that involves a test article and one or more human subjects and that either is subject to requirements for prior submission to the Food and Drug Administration under section 505(i) or 520(g) of the act, or is not subject to requirements for prior submission to the Food and Drug Administration under these sections of the act, but the results of which are intended to be submitted later to, or held for inspection by, the Food and Drug Administration as part of an application for a research or marketing permit. The term does not include experiments that are subject to the provisions of part 58 of this chapter, regarding nonclinical laboratory studies. [21 CFR § 50]

Clinical investigation means any experiment that involves a test article and one or more human subjects, and that either must meet the requirements for prior submission to the Food and Drug Administration under section 505(i) or 520(g) of the act, or need not meet the requirements for prior submission to the Food and Drug Administration under these sections of the act, but the results of which are intended to be later submitted to, or held for inspection by, the Food and Drug Administration as part of an application for a research or marketing permit. The term does not include experiments that must meet the provisions of part 58, regarding nonclinical laboratory studies. The termsresearch, clinical research, clinical study, study, andclinical investigation are deemed to be synonymous for purposes of this part. [21 CFR § 56]

Clinical investigation means any experiment in which a drug is administered or dispensed to, or used involving, one or more human subjects. For the purposes of this part, an experiment is any use of a drug except for the use of a marketed drug in the course of medical practice. [21 CFR § 312]

Clinical investigator means only a listed or identified investigator or subinvestigator who is directly involved in the treatment or evaluation of research subjects. The term also includes the spouse and each dependent child of the investigator. [21 CFR § 54]

Compensation affected by the outcome of clinical studies means compensation that could be higher for a favorable outcome than for an unfavorable outcome, such as compensation that is explicitly greater for a favorable result or compensation to the investigator in the form of an equity interest in the sponsor of a covered study or in the form of compensation tied to sales of the product, such as a royalty interest. [21 CFR § 54]

Complete response letter means a written communication to an applicant from FDA usually describing all of the deficiencies that the agency has identified in an application or abbreviated application that must be satisfactorily addressed before it can be approved. [21 CFR § 314]

Component means any ingredient intended for use in the manufacture of a drug product, including those that may not appear in such drug product. [21 CFR § 210]

Contract research organization means a person that assumes, as an independent contractor with the sponsor, one or more of the obligations of a sponsor, e.g., design of a protocol, selection or monitoring of investigations, evaluation of reports, and preparation of materials to be submitted to the Food and Drug Administration. [21 CFR § 312]

Control article means any food additive, color additive, drug, biological product, electronic product, medical device for human use, or any article other than a test article, feed, or water that is administered to the test system in the course of a nonclinical laboratory study for the purpose of establishing a basis for comparison with the test article. [21 CFR § 58]

Covered clinical study means any study of a drug or device in humans submitted in a marketing application or reclassification petition subject to this part that the applicant or FDA relies on to establish that the product is effective (including studies that show equivalence to an effective product) or any study in which a single investigator makes a significant contribution to the demonstration of safety. This would, in general, not include phase 1 tolerance studies or pharmacokinetic studies, most clinical pharmacology studies (unless they are critical to an efficacy determination), large open safety studies conducted at multiple sites, treatment protocols, and parallel track protocols. An applicant may consult with FDA as to which clinical studies constitute "covered clinical studies" for purposes of complying with financial disclosure requirements. [21 CFR § 54]

Custom device means a device that: [21 CFR § 812]

(1) Necessarily deviates from devices generally available or from an applicable performance standard or premarket approval requirement in order to comply with the order of an individual physician or dentist;

(2) Is not generally available to, or generally used by, other physicians or dentists;

(3) Is not generally available in finished form for purchase or for dispensing upon prescription;

(4) Is not offered for commercial distribution through labeling or advertising; and

(5) Is intended for use by an individual patient named in the order of a physician or dentist, and is to be made in a specific form for that patient, or is intended to meet the special needs of the physician or dentist in the course of professional practice.

D

Digital signature means an electronic signature based upon cryptographic methods of originator authentication, computed by using a set of rules and a set of parameters such that the identity of the signer and the integrity of the data can be verified. [21 CFR § 11]

Drug product means a finished dosage form, for example, tablet, capsule, solution, etc., that contains an active drug ingredient generally, but not necessarily, in association with inactive ingredients. The term also includes a finished dosage form that does not contain an active ingredient but is intended to be used as a placebo. [21 CFR § 210]

> ***Drug product*** means a finished dosage form, for example, tablet, capsule, or solution, that contains a drug substance, generally, but not necessarily, in association with one or more other ingredients. [21 CFR § 314]

> ***Drug product*** means a finished dosage form, e.g., tablet, capsule, or solution, that contains the active drug ingredient, generally, but not necessarily, in association with inactive ingredients. [21 CFR § 320]

Drug substance means an active ingredient that is intended to furnish pharmacological activity or other direct effect in the diagnosis, cure, mitigation, treatment, or prevention of disease or to affect the structure or any function of the human body, but does not include intermediates use in the synthesis of such ingredient. [21 CFR § 314]

E, F

Efficacy supplement means a supplement to an approved application proposing to make one or more related changes from among the following changes to product labeling: [21 CFR § 314]

(1) Add or modify an indication or claim;

(2) Revise the dose or dose regimen;

(3) Provide for a new route of administration;

(4) Make a comparative efficacy claim naming another drug product;

(5) Significantly alter the intended patient population;

(6) Change the marketing status from prescription to over-the-counter use;

(7) Provide for, or provide evidence of effectiveness necessary for, the traditional approval of a product originally approved under subpart H of part 314; or

(8) Incorporate other information based on at least one adequate and well-controlled clinical study.

Electronic record means any combination of text, graphics, data, audio, pictorial, or other information representation in digital form that is created, modified, maintained, archived, retrieved, or distributed by a computer system. [21 CFR § 11]

Electronic signature means a computer data compilation of any symbol or series of symbols executed, adopted, or authorized by an individual to be the legally binding equivalent of the individual's handwritten signature. [21 CFR § 11]

Emergency use means the use of a test article on a human subject in a life-threatening situation in which no standard acceptable treatment is available, and in which there is not sufficient time to obtain IRB approval. [21 CFR § 56]

Family member means any one of the following legally competent persons: Spouse; parents; children (including adopted children); brothers, sisters, and spouses of brothers and sisters; and any individual related by blood or affinity whose close association with the subject is the equivalent of a family relationship. [21 CFR § 50]

FDA means the Food and Drug Administration. [21 CFR § 312, § 314, § 812, § 814]

Fiber means any particulate contaminant with a length at least three times greater than its width. [21 CFR § 210]

G, H

Gang-printed labeling means labeling derived from a sheet of material on which more than one item of labeling is printed. [21 CFR § 210]

Guardian means an individual who is authorized under applicable State or local law to consent on behalf of a child to general medical care when general medical care includes participation in research. For purposes of subpart D of this part, a guardian also means an individual who is authorized to consent on behalf of a child to participate in research. [21 CFR § 50]

Handwritten signature means the scripted name or legal mark of an individual handwritten by that individual and executed or adopted with the present intention to authenticate a writing in a permanent form. The act of signing with a writing or marking instrument such as a pen or stylus is preserved. The scripted name or legal mark, while conventionally applied to paper, may also be applied to other devices that capture the name or mark. [21 CFR § 11]

HDE means a premarket approval application submitted pursuant to this subpart seeking a humanitarian device exemption from the effectiveness requirements of sections 514 and 515 of the act as authorized by section 520(m)(2) of the act. [21 CFR § 814]

HUD (humanitarian use device) means a medical device intended to benefit patients in the treatment or diagnosis of a disease or condition that affects or is manifested in fewer than 4,000 individuals in the United States per year. [21 CFR § 814]

Human subject means an individual who is or becomes a participant in research, either as a recipient of the test article or as a control. A subject may be either a healthy human or a patient. [21 CFR § 50]

Human subject means an individual who is or becomes a participant in research, either as a recipient of the test article or as a control. A subject may be either a healthy individual or a patient. [21 CFR § 56]

I

IDE means an approved or considered approved investigational device exemption under section 520(g) of the act and parts 812 and 813. [21 CFR § 814]

Implant means a device that is placed into a surgically or naturally formed cavity of the human body if it is intended to remain there for a period of 30 days or more. FDA may, in order to protect public health, determine that devices placed in subjects for shorter periods are also "implants" for purposes of this part. [21 CFR § 812]

Inactive ingredient means any component other than anactive ingredient. [21 CFR § 210]

Increased frequency of adverse drug experience is an increased rate of occurrence of a particular serious adverse drug event, expected or unexpected, after appropriate adjustment for drug exposure. [21 CFR § 514]

IND means an investigational new drug application. For purposes of this part, "IND" is synonymous with "Notice of Claimed Investigational Exemption for a New Drug." [21 CFR § 312]

Independent ethics committee (IEC) means a review panel that is responsible for ensuring the protection of the rights, safety, and well-being of human subjects involved in a clinical investigation and is adequately constituted to provide assurance of that protection. An institutional review board (IRB), as defined in 56.102(g) of this chapter and subject to the requirements of part 56 of this chapter, is one type of IEC. [21 CFR § 312]

In-process material means any material fabricated, compounded, blended, or derived by chemical reaction that is produced for, and used in, the preparation of the drug product.

Institution means any public or private entity or agency (including Federal, State, and other agencies). The wordfacility as used in section 520(g) of the act is deemed to be synonymous with the terminstitution for purposes of this part. [21 CFR § 50, § 56]

Institution means a person, other than an individual, who engages in the conduct of research on subjects or in the delivery of medical services to individuals as a primary activity or as an adjunct to providing residential or custodial care to humans. The term includes, for example, a hospital, retirement home, confinement facility, academic establishment, and device manufacturer. The term has the same meaning as "facility" in section 520(g) of the act. [21 CFR § 812]

Institutional review board (IRB) means any board, committee, or other group formally designated by an institution to review biomedical research involving humans as subjects, to approve the initiation of and conduct periodic review of such research. The term has the same meaning as the phraseinstitutional review committee as used in section 520(g) of the act. [21 CFR § 50]

> ***Institutional Review Board (IRB)*** means any board, committee, or other group formally designated by an institution to review, to approve the initiation of, and to conduct periodic review of, biomedical research involving human subjects. The primary purpose of such review is to assure the protection of the rights and welfare of the human subjects. The term has the same meaning as the phraseinstitutional review committee as used in section 520(g) of the act. [21 CFR § 56]

> ***Institutional review board (IRB)*** means any board, committee, or other group formally designated by an institution to review biomedical research involving subjects and established, operated, and functioning in conformance with part 56. The term has the same meaning as "institutional review committee" in section 520(g) of the act. [21 CFR § 812]

Investigation means a clinical investigation or research involving one or more subjects to determine the safety or effectiveness of a device. [21 CFR § 812]

Investigational device means a device, including a transitional device, that is the object of an investigation. [21 CFR § 812]

Investigational new drug means a new drug or biological drug that is used in a clinical investigation. The term also includes a biological product that is used in vitro for diagnostic purposes. The terms "investigational drug" and "investigational new drug" are deemed to be synonymous for purposes of this part. [21 CFR § 312]

Investigator means an individual who actually conducts a clinical investigation, i.e., under whose immediate direction the test article is administered or dispensed to, or used involving, a subject, or, in the event of an investigation conducted by a team of individuals, is the responsible leader of that team. [21 CFR § 50, § 56]

> *Investigator* means an individual who actually conducts a clinical investigation (i.e. , under whose immediate direction the drug is administered or dispensed to a subject). In the event an investigation is conducted by a team of individuals, the investigator is the responsible leader of the team. "Subinvestigator" includes any other individual member of that team. [21 CFR § 312]

> *Investigator* means an individual who actually conducts a clinical investigation, i.e., under whose immediate direction the test article is administered or dispensed to, or used involving, a subject, or, in the event of an investigation conducted by a team of individuals, is the responsible leader of that team. [21 CFR § 812]

IRB approval means the determination of the IRB that the clinical investigation has been reviewed and may be conducted at an institution within the constraints set forth by the IRB and by other institutional and Federal requirements. [21 CFR § 56]

J, K, L

Legally authorized representative means an individual or judicial or other body authorized under applicable law to consent on behalf of a prospective subject to the subject's particpation in the procedure(s) involved in the research. [21 CFR § 50]

Listed drug means a new drug product that has an effective approval under section 505(c) of the act for safety and effectiveness or under section 505(j) of the act, which has not been withdrawn or suspended under section 505(e)(1) through (e)(5) or (j)(5) of the act, and which has not been withdrawn from sale for what FDA has determined are reasons of safety or effectiveness. Listed drug status is evidenced by the drug product's identification as a drug with an effective approval in the current edition of FDA's "Approved Drug Products with Therapeutic Equivalence Evaluations" (the list) or any current supplement thereto, as a drug with an effective approval. A drug product is deemed to be a listed drug on the date of effective approval of the application or abbreviated application for that drug product. [21 CFR § 314]

Lot means a batch, or a specific identified portion of a batch, having uniform character and quality within specified limits; or, in the case of a drug product produced by continuous process, it is a specific identified amount produced in a unit of time or quantity in a manner that assures its having uniform character and quality within specified limits. [21 CFR § 210]

Lot number, control number, or batch number means any distinctive combination of letters, numbers, or symbols, or any combination of them, from which the complete history of the manufacture, processing, packing, holding, and distribution of a batch or lot of drug product or other material can be determined. [21 CFR § 210]

M

Manufacture, processing, packing, or holding of a drug product includes packaging and labeling operations, testing, and quality control of drug products. [21 CFR § 210]

Marketing application means an application for a new drug submitted under section 505(b) of the act or a biologics license application for a biological product submitted under the Public Health Service Act. [21 CFR § 312]

Master file means a reference source that a person submits to FDA. A master file may contain detailed information on a specific manufacturing facility, process, methodology, or component used in the manufacture, processing, or packaging of a medical device. [21 CFR § 814]

Medicated feed means any Type B or Type C medicated feed as defined in 558.3 of this chapter. The feed contains one or more drugs as defined in section 201(g) of the act. The manufacture of medicated feeds is subject to the requirements of part 225 of this chapter. [21 CFR § 210]

Medicated premix means a Type A medicated article as defined in 558.3 of this chapter. The article contains one or more drugs as defined in section 201(g) of the act. The manufacture of medicated premixes is subject to the requirements of part 226 of this chapter. [21 CFR § 210]

Minimal risk means that the probability and magnitude of harm or discomfort anticipated in the research are not greater in and of themselves than those ordinarily encountered in daily life or during the performance of routine physical or psychological examinations or tests. [21 CFR § 50, § 56]

Monitor, when used as a noun, means an individual designated by a sponsor or contract research organization to oversee the progress of an investigation. The monitor may be an employee of a sponsor or a consultant to the sponsor, or an employee of or consultant to a contract research organization.Monitor, when used as a verb, means to oversee an investigation. [21 CFR § 812]

N

NADA is a new animal drug application including all amendments and supplements. [21 CFR § 514]

Newly acquired information means data, analyses, or other information not previously submitted to the agency, which may include (but are not limited to) data derived from new clinical studies, reports of adverse events, or new analyses of previously submitted data (e.g., meta-analyses) if the studies, events or analyses reveal risks of a different type or greater severity or frequency than previously included in submissions to FDA. [21 CFR § 314, § 814]

Nonapplicant is any person other than the applicant whose name appears on the label and who is engaged in manufacturing, packing, distribution, or labeling of the product. [21 CFR § 514]

Nonclinical laboratory study means in vivo or in vitro experiments in which test articles are studied prospectively in test systems under laboratory conditions to determine their safety. The term does not include studies utilizing human subjects or clinical studies or field trials in animals. The term does not include basic exploratory studies carried out to determine whether a test article has any potential utility or to determine physical or chemical characteristics of a test article. [21 CFR § 58]

Nonfiber releasing filter means any filter, which after appropriate pretreatment such as washing or flushing, will not release fibers into the component or drug product that is being filtered. [21 CFR § 210]

Noninvasive, when applied to a diagnostic device or procedure, means one that does not by design or intention: (1) Penetrate or pierce the skin or mucous membranes of the body, the ocular cavity, or the urethra, or (2) enter the ear beyond the external auditory canal, the nose beyond the nares, the mouth beyond the pharynx, the anal canal beyond the rectum, or the vagina beyond the cervical os. For purposes of this part, blood sampling that involves simple venipuncture is considered noninvasive, and the use of surplus samples of body fluids or tissues that are left over from samples taken for noninvestigational purposes is also considered noninvasive. [21 CFR § 812]

O, P

Open system means an environment in which system access is not controlled by persons who are responsible for the content of electronic records that are on the system. [21 CFR § 11]

Original application means a pending application for which FDA has never issued a complete response letter or approval letter, or an application that was submitted again after FDA had refused to file it or after it was withdrawn without being approved. [21 CFR § 314]

Parent means a child's biological or adoptive parent. [21 CFR § 50]

Percentage of theoretical yield means the ratio of the actual yield (at any appropriate phase of manufacture, processing, or packing of a particular drug product) to the theoretical yield (at the same phase), stated as a percentage. [21 CFR § 210]

Permission means the agreement of parent(s) or guardian to the participation of their child or ward in a clinical investigation. Permission must be obtained in compliance with subpart B of this part and must include the elements of informed consent described in 50.25. [21 CFR § 50]

Person includes an individual, partnership, corporation, association, scientific or academic establishment, government agency, or organizational unit thereof, and any other legal entity. [21 CFR § 58]

> *Person* includes any individual, partnership, corporation, association, scientific or academic establishment, Government agency or organizational unit of a Government agency, and any other legal entity. [21 CFR § 812]

> *Person* includes any individual, partnership, corporation, association, scientific or academic establishment, Government agency, or organizational unit thereof, or any other legal entity. [21 CFR § 814]

Pharmaceutical alternatives means drug products that contain the identical therapeutic moiety, or its precursor, but not necessarily in the same amount or dosage form or as the same salt or ester. Each such drug product individually meets either the identical or its own respective compendial or other applicable standard of identity, strength, quality, and purity, including potency and, where applicable, content uniformity, disintegration times and/or dissolution rates. [21 CFR § 320]

Pharmaceutical equivalents means drug products in identical dosage forms that contain identical amounts of the identical active drug ingredient,i.e. , the same salt or ester of the same therapeutic moiety, or, in the case of modified release dosage forms that require a reservoir or overage or such forms as prefilled syringes where residual volume may vary, that deliver identical amounts of the active drug ingredient over the identical dosing period; do not necessarily contain the same inactive ingredients; and meet the identical compendial or other applicable standard of identity, strength, quality, and purity, including potency and, where applicable, content uniformity, disintegration times, and/or dissolution rates. [21 CFR § 320]

PMA means any premarket approval application for a class III medical device, including all information submitted with or

---

incorporated by reference therein. "PMA" includes a new drug application for a device under section 520(1) of the act. [21 CFR § 814]

PMA amendment means information an applicant submits to FDA to modify a pending PMA or a pending PMA supplement. [21 CFR § 814]

PMA supplement means a supplemental application to an approved PMA for approval of a change or modification in a class III medical device, including all information submitted with or incorporated by reference therein. [21 CFR § 814]

> **30-day PMA supplement** means a supplemental application to an approved PMA in accordance with 814.39(e). [21 CFR § 814]

Potential applicant means any person: [21 CFR § 514]

(1) Intending to investigate a new animal drug under section 512(j) of the Federal Food, Drug, and Cosmetic Act (the act),

(2) Investigating a new animal drug under section 512(j) of the act,

(3) Intending to file a new animal drug application (NADA) or supplemental NADA under section 512(b)(1) of the act, or

(4) Intending to file an abbreviated new animal drug application (ANADA) under section 512(b)(2) of the act.

Presubmission conference means one or more conferences between a potential applicant and FDA to reach a binding agreement establishing a submission or investigational requirement. [21 CFR § 514]

Presubmission conference agreement means that section of the memorandum of conference headed "Presubmission Conference Agreement" that records any agreement on the submission or investigational requirement reached by a potential applicant and FDA during the presubmission conference. [21 CFR § 514]

Product defect/manufacturing defect is the deviation of a distributed product from the standards specified in the approved application, or any significant chemical, physical, or other change, or deterioration in the distributed drug product, including any microbial or chemical contamination. A manufacturing defect is a product defect caused or aggravated by a manufacturing or related process. A manufacturing defect may occur from a single event or from deficiencies inherent to the manufacturing process. These defects are generally associated with product contamination, product deterioration, manufacturing error, defective packaging, damage from disaster, or labeling error. For example, a labeling error may include any incident that causes a distributed product to be mistaken for, or its labeling applied to, another product. [21 CFR § 514]

Proprietary interest in the tested product means property or other financial interest in the product including, but not limited to, a patent, trademark, copyright or licensing agreement. [21 CFR § 54]

Q, R

Quality assurance unit means any person or organizational element, except the study director, designated by testing facility management to perform the duties relating to quality assurance of nonclinical laboratory studies. [21 CFR § 58]

Quality control unit means any person or organizational element designated by the firm to be responsible for the duties relating to quality control. [21 CFR § 210]

Raw data means any laboratory worksheets, records, memoranda, notes, or exact copies thereof, that are the result of original observations and activities of a nonclinical laboratory study and are necessary for the reconstruction and evaluation of the report of that study. In the event that exact transcripts of raw data have been prepared (e.g., tapes which have been transcribed verbatim, dated, and verified accurate by signature), the exact copy or exact transcript may be substituted for the original source as raw data.Raw data may include photographs, microfilm or microfiche copies, computer printouts, magnetic media, including dictated observations, and recorded data from automated instruments. [21 CFR § 58]

Reasonable probability means that it is more likely than not that an event will occur. [21 CFR § 814]

Reference listed drug means the listed drug identified by FDA as the drug product upon which an applicant relies in seeking approval of its abbreviated application. [21 CFR § 314]

Representative sample means a sample that consists of a number of units that are drawn based on rational criteria such as random sampling and intended to assure that the sample accurately portrays the material being sampled. [21 CFR § 210]

Resubmission means submission by the applicant of all materials needed to fully address all deficiencies identified in the complete response letter. An application or abbreviated application for which FDA issued a complete response letter, but which was withdrawn before approval and later submitted again, is not a resubmission. [21 CFR § 314]

Right of reference or use means the authority to rely upon, and otherwise use, an investigation for the purpose of obtaining approval of an application, including the ability to make available the underlying raw data from the investigation for FDA audit, if necessary. [21 CFR § 314]

S

Same drug product formulation means the formulation of the drug product submitted for approval and any formulations that have minor differences in composition or method of manufacture from the formulation submitted for approval, but are similar enough to be relevant to the agency's determination of bioequivalence. [21 CFR § 320]

Serious adverse drug experience is an adverse event that is fatal, or life-threatening, or requires professional intervention, or causes an abortion, or stillbirth, or infertility, or congenital anomaly, or prolonged or permanent disability, or disfigurement. [21 CFR § 514]

Serious, adverse health consequences means any significant adverse experience, including those which may be either life-threatening or involve permanent or long term injuries, but excluding injuries that are nonlife-threatening and that are temporary and reasonably reversible. [21 CFR § 814]

Significant equity interest in the sponsor of a covered study
means any ownership interest, stock options, or other financial
interest whose value cannot be readily determined through
reference to public prices (generally, interests in a nonpublicly
traded corporation), or any equity interest in a publicly traded
corporation that exceeds $50,000 during the time the clinical
investigator is carrying out the study and for 1 year following
completion of the study. [21 CFR § 54]

Significant payments of other sorts means payments made by the
sponsor of a covered study to the investigator or the institution to
support activities of the investigator that have a monetary value of
more than $25,000, exclusive of the costs of conducting the
clinical study or other clinical studies, (e.g., a grant to fund
ongoing research, compensation in the form of equipment or
retainers for ongoing consultation or honoraria) during the time
the clinical investigator is carrying out the study and for 1 year
following the completion of the study. [21 CFR § 54]

Significant risk device means an investigational device that: [21 CFR
§ 812]

(1) Is intended as an implant and presents a potential for serious
risk to the health, safety, or welfare of a subject;

(2) Is purported or represented to be for a use in supporting or
sustaining human life and presents a potential for serious risk
to the health, safety, or welfare of a subject;

(3) Is for a use of substantial importance in diagnosing, curing,
mitigating, or treating disease, or otherwise preventing
impairment of human health and presents a potential for
serious risk to the health, safety, or welfare of a subject; or

(4) Otherwise presents a potential for serious risk to the health,
safety, or welfare of a subject.

Specification means the quality standard (i.e. , tests, analytical
procedures, and acceptance criteria) provided in an approved
application to confirm the quality of drug substances, drug
products, intermediates, raw materials, reagents, components, in-
process materials, container closure systems, and other materials
used in the production of a drug substance or drug product. For
the purpose of this definition,acceptance criteria means numerical
limits, ranges, or other criteria for the tests described. [21 CFR §
314]

Specimen means any material derived from a test system for examination or analysis. [21 CFR § 58]

Sponsor means a person who initiates a clinical investigation, but who does not actually conduct the investigation, i.e., the test article is administered or dispensed to or used involving, a subject under the immediate direction of another individual. A person other than an individual (e.g., corporation or agency) that uses one or more of its own employees to conduct a clinical investigation it has initiated is considered to be a sponsor (not a sponsor-investigator), and the employees are considered to be investigators. [21 CFR § 50]

> ***Sponsor*** means a person or other entity that initiates a clinical investigation, but that does not actually conduct the investigation, i.e., the test article is administered or dispensed to, or used involving, a subject under the immediate direction of another individual. A person other than an individual (e.g., a corporation or agency) that uses one or more of its own employees to conduct an investigation that it has initiated is considered to be a sponsor (not a sponsor-investigator), and the employees are considered to be investigators. [21 CFR § 56]

> ***Sponsor*** means: [21 CFR § 58]
>
> > (1) A person who initiates and supports, by provision of financial or other resources, a nonclinical laboratory study;
> >
> > (2) A person who submits a nonclinical study to the Food and Drug Administration in support of an application for a research or marketing permit; or
> >
> > (3) A testing facility, if it both initiates and actually conducts the study.

> ***Sponsor*** means a person who takes responsibility for and initiates a clinical investigation. The sponsor may be an individual or pharmaceutical company, governmental agency, academic institution, private organization, or other organization. The sponsor does not actually conduct the investigation unless the sponsor is a sponsor-investigator. A person other than an individual that uses one or more of its own employees to conduct an investigation that it has initiated is a sponsor, not

a sponsor-investigator, and the employees are investigators. [21 CFR § 312]

Sponsor means a person who initiates, but who does not actually conduct, the investigation, that is, the investigational device is administered, dispensed, or used under the immediate direction of another individual. A person other than an individual that uses one or more of its own employees to conduct an investigation that it has initiated is a sponsor, not a sponsor-investigator, and the employees are investigators. [21 CFR § 812]

Sponsor of the covered clinical study means the party supporting a particular study at the time it was carried out. [21 CFR § 54]

Sponsor-investigator means an individual who both initiates and actually conducts, alone or with others, a clinical investigation, i.e., under whose immediate direction the test article is administered or dispensed to, or used involving, a subject. The term does not include any person other than an individual, e.g., corporation or agency. [21 CFR § 50]

Sponsor-investigator means an individual who both initiates and actually conducts, alone or with others, a clinical investigation, i.e., under whose immediate direction the test article is administered or dispensed to, or used involving, a subject. The term does not include any person other than an individual, e.g., it does not include a corporation or agency. The obligations of a sponsor-investigator under this part include both those of a sponsor and those of an investigator. [21 CFR § 56]

Sponsor-Investigator means an individual who both initiates and conducts an investigation, and under whose immediate direction the investigational drug is administered or dispensed. The term does not include any person other than an individual. The requirements applicable to a sponsor-investigator under this part include both those applicable to an investigator and a sponsor. [21 CFR § 312]

Sponsor-investigator means an individual who both initiates and actually conducts, alone or with others, an investigation, that is, under whose immediate direction the investigational device is administered, dispensed, or used. The term does not include any person other than an individual. The obligations of a sponsor-investigator under this part include those of an investigator and those of a sponsor. [21 CFR § 812]

Statement of material fact means a representation that tends to show that the safety or effectiveness of a device is more probable than it would be in the absence of such a representation. A false affirmation or silence or an omission that would lead a reasonable person to draw a particular conclusion as to the safety or effectiveness of a device also may be a false statement of material fact, even if the statement was not intended by the person making it to be misleading or to have any probative effect. [21 CFR § 814]

Strength means: [21 CFR § 210]

    (i) The concentration of the drug substance (for example, weight/weight, weight/volume, or unit dose/volume basis), and/or

    (ii) The potency, that is, the therapeutic activity of the drug product as indicated by appropriate laboratory tests or by adequately developed and controlled clinical data (expressed, for example, in terms of units by reference to a standard).

Study completion date means the date the final report is signed by the study director. [21 CFR § 58]

Study director means the individual responsible for the overall conduct of a nonclinical laboratory study. [21 CFR § 58]

Study initiation date means the date the protocol is signed by the study director. [21 CFR § 58]

Subject means a human who participates in an investigation, either as a recipient of the investigational new drug or as a control. A subject may be a healthy human or a patient with a disease. [21 CFR § 312]

    Subject means a human who participates in an investigation, either as an individual on whom or on whose specimen an investigational device is used or as a control. A subject may be in normal health or may have a medical condition or disease. [21 CFR § 812]

T

Termination means a discontinuance, by sponsor or by withdrawal of IRB or FDA approval, of an investigation before completion. [21 CFR § 812]

Test article means any drug (including a biological product for human use), medical device for human use, human food additive, color additive, electronic product, or any other article subject to regulation under the act or under sections 351 and 354-360F of the Public Health Service Act (42 U.S.C. 262 and 263b-263n). [21 CFR § 50]

> **Test article** means any drug for human use, biological product for human use, medical device for human use, human food additive, color additive, electronic product, or any other article subject to regulation under the act or under sections 351 or 354-360F of the Public Health Service Act. [21 CFR § 56]

> **Test article** means any food additive, color additive, drug, biological product, electronic product, medical device for human use, or any other article subject to regulation under the act or under sections 351 and 354-360F of the Public Health Service Act. [21 CFR § 58]

Test system means any animal, plant, microorganism, or subparts thereof to which the test or control article is administered or added for study. Test system also includes appropriate groups or components of the system not treated with the test or control articles. [21 CFR § 58]

Testing facility means a person who actually conducts a nonclinical laboratory study, i.e., actually uses the test article in a test system. Testing facility includes any establishment required to register under section 510 of the act that conducts nonclinical laboratory studies and any consulting laboratory described in section 704 of the act that conducts such studies. Testing facility encompasses only those operational units that are being or have been used to conduct nonclinical laboratory studies. [21 CFR § 58]

The list means the list of drug products with effective approvals published in the current edition of FDA's publication "Approved

Drug Products with Therapeutic Equivalence Evaluations" and any current supplement to the publication. [21 CFR § 314]

Theoretical yield means the quantity that would be produced at any appropriate phase of manufacture, processing, or packing of a particular drug product, based upon the quantity of components to be used, in the absence of any loss or error in actual production. [21 CFR § 210]

Transitional device means a device subject to section 520(l) of the act, that is, a device that FDA considered to be a new drug or an antibiotic drug before May 28, 1976. [21 CFR § 812]

U, V

Unanticipated adverse device effect means any serious adverse effect on health or safety or any life-threatening problem or death caused by, or associated with, a device, if that effect, problem, or death was not previously identified in nature, severity, or degree of incidence in the investigational plan or application (including a supplementary plan or application), or any other unanticipated serious problem associated with a device that relates to the rights, safety, or welfare of subjects. [21 CFR § 812]

Unexpected adverse drug experience is an adverse event that is not listed in the current labeling for the new animal drug and includes any event that may be symptomatically and pathophysiologically related to an event listed on the labeling, but differs from the event because of greater severity or specificity. For example, under this definition hepatic necrosis would be unexpected if the labeling referred only to elevated hepatic enzymes or hepatitis. [21 CFR § 514]

W, X, Y, Z

Ward means a child who is placed in the legal custody of the State or other agency, institution, or entity, consistent with applicable Federal, State, or local law. [21 CFR § 50]

Index

---

labeling, 3, 5, 11, 15, 17, 105, 120,
124, 126, 129, 131, 135, 142, 166,
209, 210, 212, 214, 219 — 223,
227, 231, 236, 239, 242, 247, 250,
254 — 257, 259, 261 — 264, 267,
270, 272, 273, 276, 283 — 290,
293, 294, 297, 310, 311, 318, 321,
325, 326, 332, 333, 335, 337 —
339, 352, 353, 358, 369, 370, 372,
374, 378, 380, 381, 385, 389 —
391, 394 — 396, 398, 404, 409,
419 — 424, 427, 429, 431 — 435,
437 — 441, 450 — 452, 459, 460,
463, 465, 466, 469 — 472, 474 —
476, 478 — 480, 492, 496, 497,
502 — 505, 508, 509, 512, 514,
515, 517, 519, 523, 524, 531, 539,
541, 542, 545, 547, 550, 554, 555,
560, 563, 593, 594, 598, 603 —
607, 610, 616, 619 — 621, 624,
630, 637 — 639, 642 — 644, 649,
653, 660
Labeling, 13, 17, 19, 129, 142, 231,
272, 277, 289, 290, 297, 347, 353,
419, 450 — 452, 457, 459, 463,
502, 503, 505, 513, 520, 550, 555,
597, 599
labeling materials, 459
labels, 142, 272, 325, 459, 490, 505,
509
Labels, 504, 544
laboratories, 222, 223, 298
Laboratories, 24
laboratory animals, 143, 151, 428,
434, 546, 550
laboratory test, 17, 123, 141, 172,
198, 425, 426, 556, 563, 658
language, 45, 145, 417, 429, 451, 469,
473
law, 4 — 7, 9, 21, 25, 44, 48, 51, 56,
59, 61, 63, 79, 116, 129, 469, 473,
504, 550, 616, 639, 644, 647, 660
Law, 5, 6, 486
legally authorized, 45, 50 — 53, 56,
57, 81, 84, 189
Legally authorized, 44, 647

license, 16, 41, 73, 93, 120, 129, 227,
294, 489, 491 — 496, 501, 505 —
508, 514 — 516, 519, 523, 532,
533, 535, 632, 634, 636, 648
License, 25
listed drug, 209, 211, 246, 247, 282
— 287, 289 — 294, 296 — 299,
306, 312, 314, 315, 323, 324, 331,
332, 334, 335, 339 — 346, 384,
637, 648, 654
Listed drug, 210, 289, 647
location, 148, 411, 425, 430, 490,
493, 494, 496, 506, 507, 567, 575,
593
lot, 95, 123, 124, 216, 246, 247, 291,
422 — 424, 490, 505, 534, 629,
638, 648
Lot, 122, 123, 648
Lot number, control number, or
batch number, 123, 648
lot or batch, 124, 629
lubricants, 401
maintenance, 35, 69, 102, 112, 403,
491
Maintenance, 102, 103, 610, 611
management, 38, 95, 97, 99, 100,
103, 168, 309, 525, 526, 653
Management, 172, 192, 341, 343,
344, 348, 361, 509, 516, 533, 566,
569, 585, 603, 694, 698
Mandatory, 20
manufacture, 119, 120, 122, 123,
132, 133, 141, 142, 215, 216, 226,
235 — 237, 239, 242, 243, 246,
247, 255, 277, 280, 282, 291, 293,
314, 325, 326, 331, 336, 337, 346,
358, 379, 419 — 421, 424, 430 —
432, 444, 457, 468, 471, 472, 474,
478, 480, 490, 491, 493, 506, 507,
551, 553, 583, 591, 597, 599, 630,
638, 641, 648, 649, 654
Manufacture, 123, 648
manufacture, processing, 119, 120,
123, 216, 325, 326, 331, 337, 358,
421, 457, 468, 472, 474, 478, 480,
553, 583, 591, 648

status, 50, 61, 99, 104, 136, 153, 161,
162, 164, 165, 167, 204, 210, 219,
274 — 276, 308, 349, 351, 354,
472, 524, 526, 535 — 537, 613,
618, 643, 648
Status, 119, 274, 276, 524
sterile, 423
sterility, 215, 216, 255, 424, 444, 498,
597
sterility testing, 597
stock, 64, 655
storage, 101 — 104, 106, 108, 110,
112, 120, 175, 178, 366, 405, 422,
423, 471, 553, 557, 591
Storage, 101, 106, 110
storage conditions, 106
storage of reserve samples, 405
strength, 4, 46, 97, 101, 105, 106,
109, 119, 141, 142, 162, 198, 209,
212, 215, 216, 234, 236, 237, 244,
246, 255, 257, 259 — 261, 271,
282 — 284, 286, 288, 300, 316,
325, 330 — 332, 337, 378, 380,
383, 392, 421, 422, 425, 426, 441,
442, 444, 446, 448, 449, 457, 463,
472, 473, 475, 478, 480, 497, 498,
500, 501, 503, 599, 637, 651
Strength, 4, 123, 237, 240, 658
Study completion date, 95, 658
study director, 95, 97 — 100, 103,
108, 110, 653, 658
Study director, 95, 98, 658
study initiation, 106, 107
Study initiation, 95, 658
subject, 7, 8, 11, 32, 35, 36, 42 — 48,
50 — 53, 55 — 58, 65, 66, 74 —
77, 81, 84, 85, 87, 92, 120, 121,
123, 126 — 129, 134, 136, 137,
144 — 146, 150, 154, 155, 162 —
164, 169, 171, 174, 178, 180, 183
— 185, 189, 200, 207, 217, 218,
221, 229, 233, 235, 249, 256, 264,
265, 269, 272, 276, 279, 283, 284,
287 — 289, 296, 297, 299, 305,
306, 311, 326, 338 — 340, 343 —
349, 351, 355, 357, 358, 367, 369,

371, 374, 379 — 382, 384, 389 —
391, 394, 398, 399, 401, 402, 415,
428, 429, 444, 452, 457, 462, 466,
473, 474, 476, 479, 481, 490, 491,
495, 506, 507, 519 — 521, 528,
531, 538, 541, 544 — 546, 548,
549, 551, 553, 558, 565, 568, 571,
574, 575, 577, 585, 590, 592, 594,
595, 600, 606, 607, 609, 616, 622
— 624, 639, 641, 643 — 645,
647, 649, 655 — 660
Subject, 22, 129, 549, 658
sufficient time, 74, 643
supervision, 6, 96, 140, 176, 571
supervisory personnel, 110
supplement, 104, 120, 141, 191, 208,
210, 212, 213, 230, 235, 238 —
240, 242, 244, 245, 251, 252, 254
— 259, 261, 262, 267, 271, 274,
279, 286, 322, 359, 385, 443, 445
— 447, 450 — 452, 457, 470,
491, 492, 497 — 504, 535, 558,
559, 596 — 600, 617, 622, 623,
631, 643, 648, 660
Supplement, 28, 257, 258, 445, 446,
447, 448, 452, 498, 499, 503, 598
supply, 101, 107, 110, 133, 176, 281,
507, 568, 571
supporting data, 177, 223, 359, 503,
574
system, 18, 33 — 38, 47, 95, 106,
112, 154, 208, 216, 256, 260, 337,
395, 396, 431, 444, 449, 478, 500,
639, 650, 659
open, 18, 33, 34, 35, 36, 37, 38,
639, 643, 650
System, 28, 695
tapes, 95, 224, 653
temperature, 422
termination, 56, 81, 85, 115, 116,
161, 163, 411, 412, 414, 567, 571,
577, 578
Termination, 116, 161, 195, 370,
374, 414, 531, 541, 549, 568, 659
test, 21, 39, 42, 43, 45, 46, 49, 51, 74,
75, 77, 92, 94, 95, 97 — 101, 103,

ward, 44, 61, 651
Ward, 44, 660
washing, 122, 650
water, 12, 16, 92, 105, 334, 401, 423,
427, 435, 436, 437, 641
who, 4, 6, 21, 3 — 35, 37, 39, 42 —
47, 49 — 51, 53 — 55, 61, 64 —
66, 68, 74, 75, 78, 80, 94, 117,
120, 128, 129, 131, 132, 136 —
138, 143, 145, 153, 154, 157, 158,
164, 171, 173 — 175, 177, 179,
180, 185 — 188, 190, 195, 199,
208, 213, 220, 224, 225, 227 —
229, 235, 238, 241, 277, 28 —
283, 294 — 296, 317, 324, 336,
337, 346 — 349, 352, 354, 355,

359, 368, 373, 403, 408, 409, 411,
413, 414, 418, 421, 422, 428, 430,
432, 438, 530, 540, 547 — 549,
551, 554, 563, 568, 569, 572, 573,
576, 577, 586, 592, 594, 630, 631,
639, 640, 644, 646, 647, 649, 650,
656 — 660
withdrawal period, 411, 426, 470,
472, 475
written procedure, 80, 81, 100, 265,
555
written procedures, 80, 81, 100, 265,
555
written record, 176
written records, 176

About the author

Mindy J. Allport-Settle was born in Beckley and raised in Oak Hill, West Virginia. She moved to North Carolina to attend the N.C. School of the Arts for high school and now lives near Raleigh. Following in the footsteps of Gordon Allport, all of her books are built on a foundation of psychology and sociology with a focus on improving some aspect of industry through research and education.

Her career in healthcare began when she was a teenager working as an emergency medical technician. Since then, she has joined the U.S. Navy's advanced hospital corps, worked in organ and human tissue procurement, specialized in ophthalmology, and moved on to serve as a key executive, board member, and consultant for some of the best companies in the pharmaceutical, medical device, and biotechnology industry. She has provided guidance in regulatory compliance, corporate structuring, restructuring and turnarounds, new drug submissions, research and development and product commercialization strategies, and new business development. Her experience and dedication have resulted in international recognition as the developer of the only FDA-recognized and benchmarked quality systems training and development business methodology.

Her education includes a Bachelor's degree from the University of North Carolina, an MBA in Global Management from the University of Phoenix, and completion of the corporate governance course series in audit committees, compensation committees, and board effectiveness at Harvard Business School.

About PharmaLogika

Since 2002, PharmaLogika, Inc has established itself as one of the world's premier consulting firms for Pharmaceutical, Biotech, and Medical Device companies across the globe. In so doing, it has earned the trust of executives in Life Sciences for its integrity, accuracy, and unwavering commitment to independent thought with regard to its products and services as well as those of its customers. Through www.PharmaLogika.com, its involvement in sponsored events, and personal references it has reached millions in print and online. Its mission, to provide flawlessly designed and executed products and services to startups as well as established industry leaders to facilitate their growth from discovery and clinical trial navigation to the commercialization and marketing of their products.

PharmaLogika consults with pharmaceutical, biotech, and medical device quality units to provide third party audits, training, pre approval inspections (PAIs), compliance remediation, and a portfolio of related quality and regulatory affairs products and services. Those products include but are not limited to Quality Assurance Forms, SOP and clinical templates, and the highly successful Integrated Development Training System.

Regulatory action guidance as well as quality systems guidance are delivered as part of its standard products and services. Through the use of highly skilled resources throughout the process, each offering is designed to enact a comprehensive quality systems approach in addressing Quality Assurance (QA) issues. The results insure a close adherence to current Good Manufacturing Practice (cGMP) standards.

PharmaLogika also has a Research and Development OTC line for human consumption that targets alpha 1-antitrypsin deficiency, Fibromyalgia, Restless Legs Syndrome, and Attention Deficit Disorder. A veterinary OTC is currently available that provides canine and feline oral debriding and cleansing agents as well as a stain remover and topical antiseptic. These products combine to provide a strong pipeline of both current and future deliverables.

Other books available

Current Good Manufacturing Practices: Pharmaceutical, Biologics, and Medical Device Regulations and Guidance Documents Concise Reference

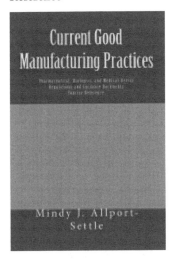

Good Manufacturing Practice (GMP) Guidelines: The Rules Governing Medicinal Products in the Eurpean Union, EudraLex Volume 4 Concise Reference

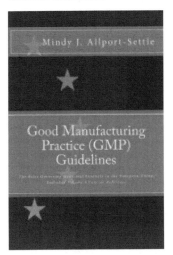

International Conference on Harmonisation (ICH) Quality Guidelines:
Pharmaceutical, Biologics, and Medical Device Guidance Documents
Concise Reference

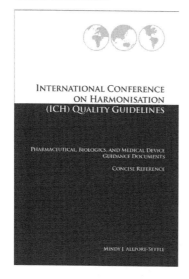

FDA Acronyms, Abbreviations and Terminology: Human and Veterinary
Regualtory Reference

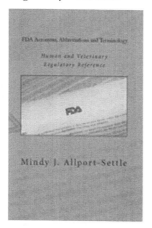

Course Development 101: Developing Training Programs for Regulated Industries

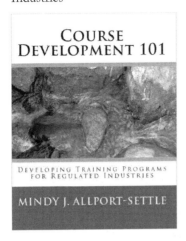

Compliance Remediation for Pharmaceutical Manufacturing: A Project Management Guide for Re-establishing FDA Compliance

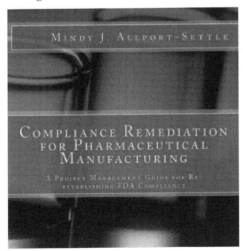

Investigations Operations Manual: FDA Field Inspection and
Investigation Policy and Procedure Concise Reference

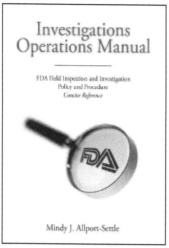

FDA Establishment Inspections: Pharmaceutical, Biotechnology, Medical
Device and Food Manufacturing Concise Reference

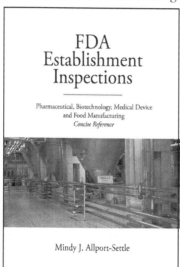

Canadian Good Manufacturing Practices: Pharmaceutical, Biotechnology, and Medical Device Regulations and Guidance Concise Reference

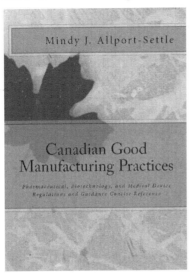

Please visit www.PharmaLogika.com for additional titles and for a list of resellers

or visit your favorite local or internet book seller.

* Companion products and bulk discounts are only available at

www.PharmaLogika.com

Made in the USA
Charleston, SC
22 October 2011